NATIONAL
HEALTH SYSTEMS
OF THE WORLD

NATIONAL HEALTH SYSTEMS OF THE WORLD

Volume Two

The Issues

Milton I. Roemer

New York   Oxford   OXFORD UNIVERSITY PRESS   1993

Oxford University Press

Oxford   New York   Toronto
Delhi   Bombay   Calcutta   Madras   Karachi
Kuala Lumpur   Singapore   Hong Kong   Tokyo
Nairobi   Dar es Salaam   Cape Town
Melbourne   Auckland

and associated companies in
Berlin   Ibadan

Published by Oxford University Press, Inc.,
198 Madison Avenue, New York, New York 10016-4314

Oxford is a registered trademark of Oxford University Press

Library of Congress Cataloging-in-Publication Data
(revised for vol. 2)
Roemer, Milton Irwin, 1916–
National health systems of the world.
Includes bibliographical references and index.
Contents: v. 1. The countries—v. 2. The issues.
1. Medical policy.
2. Medical care.
3. Public health.
4. Insurance, Health.   I. Title.
RA393.R593   1991   362.1
ISBN 0-19-505320-6 (v. 1)
ISBN 0-19-507845-4 (v. 2)
90-7336

Printing (last digit): 9 8 7 6 5 4 3 2

Printed in the United States of America
on acid-free paper

Preface

Volume II of this work is the complement to Volume I. The first volume analyzes the national health systems of countries of three economic levels: (1) with gross national product (GNP) per capita of $5,000 or more around 1985—designated as *industrialized* countries; (2) with GNP per capita of $500 to $5,000—designated as *transitional*; and (3) with GNP per capita of less than $500—designated as *very poor.*

At each economic level, the health systems of countries are scaled according to the degree of free market intervention by government. This degree ranges from minimal to maximal in four steps as follows: (1) *entrepreneurial,* (2) *welfare oriented,* (3) *comprehensive,* and (4) *socialist.* It may be noted that these four attributes apply to the health system, whereas the economic level applies to the country. Both the types of health system and the country's economic level are constantly changing, and in Volume I the situation is described as it was around the mid-1980s.

Volume II examines issues or components of health systems *across* countries. Selection of these issues has been based on the general model of a health system employed in Volume I. This consists of an interlocking framework of five major components: (1) production of *resources,* (2) organization of *programs,* (3) *economic support,* (4) system *management,* and (5) *delivery of services.* Subdivisions of these major components define the issues that are explored in Volume II.

Issues within these five components are presented in Parts I to IV, by combining economic support and management in Part III. Then Part V is devoted to a "world perspective" on international health activities and world trends in health systems.

Within each of the chapters under Parts I to IV, the cross-national comparisons are necessarily selective. In Chapter 3, for example, health centers are discussed in countries of the three economic levels; at each level, however, it is possible to discuss only *examples* of health systems in which health centers are used. In Chapter 5, in which Ministries of Health are discussed, their structure and functions are elaborated only in illustrative types of health systems. The comparisons, in other words, are not encyclopedic, but based on examples intended to reflect whole classes of health systems and countries.

With respect to nearly every issue, the historic background is explored. In the biomedical sciences, history may not be essential to an understanding of modern physiology or pathology. But for an understanding of modern issues in health care, knowledge of the sociomedical background is essential. The structure and function of the British National Health Service can be understood only in light of its evolution, and the same applies to health centers in Finland, "barefoot doctors" in China, worker hospitals in Peru, or Blue Cross insurance in the United States.

Aside from its value in clarifying any contemporary issue in a health system, historic background may have special meaning for other countries. Evolution of health programs proceeds at different rates among countries, and past developments in one country may suggest an effective strategy in another country today.

A volume of this scope necessarily suffers from certain deficiencies. For many issues there are inadequate data. Much of the information, of course, is drawn from the country accounts in Volume I. Despite use of automated library searches (Medlines, Medlars, etc.) on numerous subjects, little further information was turned up. The greatest gaps were in the "developing" countries—both transitional and very poor in our terminology. Even in the industrialized countries, available information often applied to only a few, especially the United States, which has been the subject of exceptionally rich reporting. In the absence of more specific information, it is sometimes necessary to offer broad comments on two categories of the world—developing and industrialized countries.

Another problem is the duplication of the same material in different chapters. The five major components of a health system are inevitably interconnected and overlapping. The training and functions of community health workers (CHW), for example, are explored in Chapter 2 under "Resources." In Chapter 5, the work of CHWs in Ministries of Health is explored under "Programs." In Chapter 11 under "Management," there are the laws governing CHWs. In Chapter 12 under "Health Service Delivery," CHWs figure prominently in the experience with primary health care. Even in the closing chapter on "World Trends," CHWs are treated as a significant feature of health manpower development. Each reference to CHWs, however, is in a different context.

Another issue is illustrated by the world review of health insurance in Chapter 6. Then in Chapter 9, health insurance is treated as one of the main sources of health expenditures. In Chapter 11, it is a subject of legislation. In Chapter 18, health insurance is one of the strongest trends for strengthening national health systems. Each of these contexts is important and different.

Each chapter, in other words, is intended to stand as an account of its own. The objective is to present each health system subject as a self-contained story, despite the duplication of points appearing also in other chapters. Thus the story of voluntary health agencies, as a worldwide activity, is intended to be complete in Chapter 7. An overview of health planning is given in Chapter 10. Likewise, even a subdivision such as health programs for rural people in Chapter 14 is intended to be a comprehensive though brief account.

Finally, everyone who writes about cross-national comparisons in health activities or any other field must face the question: Why? What is the value of these comparative studies? I would suggest that five major purposes are served:

1. The acquisition of knowledge is in itself a valid purpose. Facts and ideas clarified today may have unexpected value at a future time.
2. Generalizations may be formulated on the social, economic, and political conditions in a country that gave rise to various types of health system policy. Such information can provide guidance in the health planning of other countries.
3. Lessons on health system policies can be learned by one country from another. Examples of such lessons are countless in every component of health systems—in the training of personnel, the organization of preventive services, economic support through social security, teamwork in the organized delivery of ambulatory services, and so on. The United States has special lessons to learn on the use of trained midwives and the development of health service financial protection for the entire national population.
4. As long as most of the world population is in developing countries, and most of the world's wealth is in the industrialized countries, socioeconomic assistance from the rich to the poor countries must be expected. Comparative studies of the health systems in both types of country can facilitate programs of cross-national support and cooperation.
5. Cross-national studies of health systems can reveal world trends in each of the major system components. They can show the trends and undulations in the concept of health care as a market commodity, as against the concept of health care as a basic human right. The more closely this issue is examined, the more complex it is found to be. The health leadership of most countries, however, supports the doctrine of the World Health Organization that "Health for All" must be the goal of all national health policies.

Los Angeles   M.I.R.
June 1992

Contents

PART ONE:
RESOURCES

CHAPTER ONE

Physicians and Healers

In primitive societies, the totality of health service consisted of the ministrations of the healer or "medicine man." Since disease was believed to arise from supernatural forces, various magical measures were used to counteract those forces. Certain physical or medicinal interventions were also found helpful, from experience, to cope with disease. The relationship between patient and doctor was on a one-to-one basis, uncomplicated by laws or regulations, except for the influence of custom.

The healing arts of preliterate societies that have survived to modern times are generally described as "traditional medicine" or "traditional healing." They constitute a wide variety of practices that are seen, with different degrees of prominence, throughout the world. Before tracing the evolution of the traditional healer into the modern physician, we will review the current place of such healers in various national health systems. A closely related practitioner, the traditional birth attendant, will be discussed later in a section on midwives.

TRADITIONAL HEALERS

In many countries where modern scientific health service has been developed relatively recently, traditional healing still plays an important role. Although based on concepts originating centuries before, it is often the most readily available form of help that sick people can get—especially in the rural areas of developing countries. In Africa and Latin America, the doctrines and principles of traditional healing have been transmitted from generation to generation in diverse informal ways. In Asia, equivalent practices have been highly systematized and transmitted through literature and schools. Everywhere, however, the procedures

and performance of traditional healers have been changing with the social circumstances and the policies in health systems.

Traditional Healing in Africa

In subSahara Africa it is often claimed that the initial response to illness of the great majority of people is to consult a traditional healer. Such healers are likely to live nearby, to be known by the family, to be regarded as sympathetic, and to charge very little (perhaps only some barter) for their services. They are part of the local culture and people trust them.

Among the thousands of different tribes of Africa, the precepts underlying traditional healing differ in countless ways. Most doctrines, however, embody some notion of balances and imbalances. These involve relationships between different parts of the human body and also between the human body and various elements in the environment. Various imbalances are believed to be correctable through medical interventions or through certain physical measures.

Attempts have been made to classify the main types of African healer. Broadly speaking, there are (1) those relying mainly on magic and magical procedures, (2) those using various medicinal products from herbs or animals, and (3) those combining both of these approaches. The third category is probably most numerous.

Anthropological studies have indicated that magical procedures—usually rituals and incantations—are most effective in treating ailments with strong psychosomatic content, such as hypertension or rheumatism. Medicinal therapy is believed more effective for febrile disorders. If one method is not successful, the other is tried. Both methods may be regarded as effective, insofar as they withdraw from the body harmful influences responsible for imbalances.

The numbers of traditional healers in countries are not clear, although whenever they can be enumerated, through registration, they exceed greatly the supply of modern physicians. Liberia, for example, had 300 physicians in 1985 and an estimated 1,800 traditional healers. Estimates of healers are often based on an assumed ratio of between 1:500 and 1:1,000 population. Many traditional practitioners, however, are mainly farmers or shopkeepers, engaged in healing only part time.

Attitudes of African governments toward healers have changed substantially in recent decades. Under colonial authorities they were, at best, tolerated and sometimes regarded as illegal. In the newly self-governed nations of Africa, they have generally been regarded as proper manpower resources of the health system in its private sector. Many African ministries of health have established research institutes to examine and test, according to conventional scientific methods, the value of various traditional medicinal products. Such investigations have been encouraged by the World Health Organization.

Traditional Healing in Latin America

Although tribal groups in Latin America are not as diverse as in Africa, several large cultures have their own forms of traditional healer or *curandero*. In the various traditional theories of disease and its treatment, the concept of hot and cold has a prominent place, both for the achievement of balance within the body and in relations of people to the environment, as in the consumption of food. Therapy calls for certain foods or environmental changes to counteract the excess of hot or cold. Medicinal plants may also be used.

Beyond the hot–cold concept, Latin American Indian theories of healing recognize various spiritual forces. An individual may experience fright, which then affects the entire central nervous system and all bodily functions. Illness may be caused by spirits, which may come from the dead, and are carried through the air. A common source of harmful

spirits is the "evil eye," projected deliberately or inadvertently. Various ceremonies may be necessary to remove these harmful influences.

One categorization of healers in Mexico probably applies to Latin American countries more generally: (1) witches, who can cause disease as well as cure it, through some strange intrinsic power; (2) spiritualistic mediums, who can invoke supernatural powers to counteract harmful processes in the body; (3) herbalists, who prescribe plant or animal medications; and (4) empirical health workers such as midwives or masseurs.

Various kinds of *curandero* are found in the rural areas of every Latin American country, and to some extent even in the cities. Estimates of their numbers, however, are hard to find; unlike the pattern in Africa, they are never registered with a government agency. In most of these countries, they are explicitly illegal. Household surveys of health care utilization, made over recent decades, show a clear decline in their use. A study in Colombia in 1967 found that 11 percent of households had contacts with a traditional healer in the previous month; in Bolivia (with lower standards of living) a 1977 study found the equivalent contacts to be only 6 percent. The increasing literacy of the population in Latin America, the greater availability of modern health resources, and the negative posture of government have all contributed to this decline in the use of healers. In socialist Cuba, the *curanderos* are aggressively prohibited as being unscientific, fraudulent, and harmful.

Ayurvedic Practitioners in Asia

Traditional healers in Asia represent something very different. In India, Ayurvedic medicine can be traced to religious origins more than a thousand years before Christ. Disease was thought to be caused by sin and the invasion of demons. Treatment was through confessions and rituals to drive out the evil spirits. In a later period, when Hindu culture was influenced by Islamic Arabs, medical practice became dominated by priests from the high Brahman caste.

India also had doctors of lower caste, trained in schools, who regarded disease as due to an imbalance among various physical elements. The environment was composed of five basic substances: earth, water, fire, air, and sky; it had two qualities: hot and cold. The human body was composed of six elements: chyle, blood, flesh, bone, marrow, and semen, plus the so-called vital force. In addition, there were three body humors: air, bile, and phlegm. Ayurvedic theory attributed disease to disturbances in the amounts or characters of these body elements and humors. Treatment was by drugs derived from minerals, animals, or plants. Special diets were prescribed. Surgery was also performed, especially for the removal of foreign bodies. All types of treatment were usually accompanied by prayers or spells.

Over the centuries, the doctrines and practices of Ayurvedic medicine have changed. Although religious concepts have not completely disappeared, various forms of empirical therapy with diet and drugs have become more systematically developed. By the time Western medicine was brought into India with European imperialism, Ayurvedic medicine had become fully recognized by the government of India as part of the health system, although mainly in the private sector. The same applied to the much smaller but also ancient traditional field of Unani medicine. Many schools training these practitioners are partially supported by the state governments of India, and a certain number of graduates of these schools are appointed to positions in the government health services.

In 1975 there were 102 colleges of traditional medicine in India—91 Ayurvedic and 11 based on other doctrines. The duration of training varies, and may be as long as 5 years after secondary school. Most of these schools include some basic principles of modern medicine in their instruction, so that practitioners may be capable of referring patients to Western or "allopathic" doctors.

Some 200,000 traditional practitioners were officially registered with state governments of India in the mid-1970s. Registration requires certain educational qualifications. Another 200,000 practitioners were estimated to be providing services mainly in rural areas, without being registered; they learned their skills simply by apprenticeship with an older traditional doctor. In addition to this group of 400,000 traditional practitioners, India had 330,000 scientifically prepared physicians in 1987. Ayurvedic hospitals also function in India. In 1978 there were 195 of them under either private or public sponsorship; their average capacity was small, with an aggregate total of 9,000 beds.

The Ayurvedic doctor typically is close by, charges low fees, and usually combines dispensing of drugs with advice about diet and other aspects of daily life. His charges theoretically are for the medication; the consultative service is free. Variants of Ayurvedic medicine are practiced in Burma, Sri Lanka, Malaysia, and other Asian countries, where Hindu culture has spread. It has also had an influence on traditional Chinese medicine.

Traditional Chinese Medicine

The major doctrines of ancient Chinese medicine can be traced to more than 1,000 years before Christ, although the great written classics are dated to about 200 B.C. Disease was attributed to imbalances between basic forces of nature, expressed in the human body. Best known is the doctrine of *yang,* meaning male or sunny principle, and *yin,* meaning female or shadowy principle. Another theory related disease to changed relationships among five elements: wood, fire, earth, metal, and water. In the famous *Yellow Emperor's Classic of Internal Medicine* (around 200 B.C., but appearing in many subsequent editions), there are many references to physical treatments, such as acupuncture and massage, but little about drugs. It is likely that these doctrines were applied mainly to the upper social classes.

Quite separate was another type of healing used mainly by the masses of common people. Based largely on magic and religious doctrines (both Taoism and Buddhism), this approach applied magico-religious ceremonies, combined with drugs made from herbs and animal parts.

Over the years, these two schools of traditional healing intermingled. Herbal therapy grew stronger. A *Great Pharmacopoeia* of traditional herbal drugs was issued in 1596. Educational programs for training in traditional

Chinese medicine, including both herbal and physical therapy (acupuncture and massage), became increasingly standardized. By the Communist Revolution in 1949, there were an estimated 400,000 traditional practitioners in China, compared with only 12,000 Western-trained physicians. Traditional doctors were doubtless the major source of health service for the vast rural population of China. Their services, mainly drugs, commanded private fees, but they were relatively low.

The Great Proletarian Cultural Revolution in China (1965–1975) led to strong support for traditional Chinese medicine. A few colleges of traditional medicine were increased to 24 around 1970, and their enrollments were enlarged. The course of study was standardized at 5 years after middle school, and various principles of Western medicine were incorporated in the curricula. Government policy was to integrate traditional and Western medicine at every level of the health system.

After the Cultural Revolution and the onset of the period of the Four Modernizations, China concentrated its health manpower efforts on training Western-style doctors, and the number of traditional practitioners declined. The Ministry of Public Health registered 336,000 traditional Chinese doctors in 1986, which amounted to 32 per 100,000 population. The great majority of these were in private practice, both in cities and rural villages, but thousands were employed in governmental hospitals and health centers. In addition, there were 151,000 dispensers of traditional herbal drugs, trained in *secondary medical schools.* For surgical intervention, the traditional doctor is expected to refer patients to a Western-trained doctor. Acupuncture has shown remarkable value as a form of surgical anaesthesia—a special instance of the integration of traditional and Western medicine. As a form of pain control, acupuncture has become popular in many countries outside of China.

European Cultist Practitioners

In the European and other industrialized countries, traditional medical practice of ancient origin is no longer found, but several nonscientific cults, starting in recent centuries, exist to some extent. Most of these practices developed as a reaction to certain aspects of mainstream scientific medicine, and typically they were based on some unitary theory of disease, which would theoretically respond to a relatively simple form of therapy.

These cults are well illustrated by homeopathy, which originated in early nineteenth-century Germany as a reaction against strong medications. Drugs that cause symptoms similar to those of the disease are given in very low dosages. Homeopathy grew in Europe and America throughout the nineteenth century, but then declined in the twentieth century as scientific medicine flourished. In many industrialized countries, however, including Germany and the Soviet Union, it still persists in certain communities. There are also thousands of homeopaths in India and some other Asian countries. Pharmacies may sell "homeopathic" drugs, dispensed without a medical prescription.

Chiropractic was introduced in the United States in the late nineteenth century as a form of "drugless healing." It is based on the notion that all diseases come from pressures on the spinal nerves, caused by dislocation of the vertebrae; treatment therefore consists of manipulation of the vertebral column. Chiropractors have achieved licensed status in most states of the United States, where there were 14 schools turning out 2,000 graduates in 1980. For treatment of disorders of the lower back, chiropractors are even recognized under the U.S. Medicare insurance program for the elderly. To a lesser extent they practice in some European countries.

Somewhat similar to chiropractic is osteopathy, starting in America about the same time, but developing quite differently. It soon deviated from the principle of tracing all diseases to skeletal dislocations, and increasingly adopted the principles and practices of scientific medicine. By the 1980s, osteopaths were regarded essentially as regular physicians, contributing 4 percent of the total number in the United States. Since their training generally was less elaborate than that of conventional physicians, they concentrated their efforts on gaining recognition as broadly oriented *family practitioners.*

Faith healing is another form of medical cultism that assumes many forms in both developing and industrialized countries. The origins of all medicine from religion were bound to yield sacred places in the modern world, where miracles of healing could occur. Such is Lourdes Shrine in France or the Buddhist Temple of the Tooth in Sri Lanka. Buddhist temple ceremonies are considered an effective treatment for many cases of drug addiction in Thailand. Christian Science healing has been promoted by a well-organized church in North America, since its development in the 1860s; this form of divine healing is practiced to some extent in most countries with large Protestant populations.

Less structured are various forms of healing cult based on "natural" methods, especially diets. At several periods in the history of medical science, individuals have opposed the use of elaborate technology by emphasizing the benefits of the natural environment, food grown without chemical fertilizers, fresh air, and exercise. As a healing doctrine, *naturopathy* may even be taught in schools and subject to government licensure, although in the 1980s it was virtually eclipsed by the emphasis on prudent diet and health promotion in the mainstream of scientific medicine.

Comment

The place of traditional healing in the national health systems of different countries is obviously varied. In large countries of Asia, its role is substantial, and in many ways supported or even promoted by government. In Africa, it would seem that political leaders usually accept it and even acclaim its virtues—though without a firm rational basis. Research is pursued to explore its value. Among developing countries only in Latin America are official attitudes predominantly negative.

The posture of the World Health Organization toward traditional healing is noteworthy. As an assemblage of sovereign states, WHO must reflect the views of its members; many of these are former colonies, in which traditional medicine symbolized an aspect of the indigenous culture. Moreover, modern medical resources are still typically scarce, especially in

large rural regions, so that traditional healers are regarded as a source of primary health care. One can appreciate why newly independent governments usually seek to find value in traditional healing, and why they enhance its status through some linkage with the official services and sometimes special training. WHO encourages this policy and promotes evaluative research on traditional drugs.

BACKGROUND OF THE MODERN PHYSICIAN

The origin of the modern physician from the priestly representatives of religion was evident in several societies. In preliterate cultures, the priest and the healer were one person; there was usually no clear line between religious ritual and magic as a method of removing the evil spirits believed to cause disease.

Ancient Physicians

In ancient Babylonia physicians were priests. All Babylonian civilization was permeated by theology, and the task of priests was to placate the gods if various omens showed they were offended. The priest–physician was regarded as an important figure.

In ancient Egypt physicians were also sometimes priests, especially if they served the upper classes. For the common people, however, physicians belonged to the class of scribes, and sometimes were trained in special schools. Imhotep was an ancient physician who served a pharaoh about 2900 B.C. and was later made into a god of healing. According to records on ancient papyri, there were hundreds of prescriptions—compounded from minerals, plants, and animals—for the treatment of different ailments.

Physicians of early Greek civilization were likewise mainly priests. Asclepius was the god of medicine; his staff and holy snake are still the worldwide symbol of the medical profession. Aesculapian temples were established widely throughout Greece and Asia Minor; here patients would come to sleep, and during the night the god would come and prescribe for them. The practice was a combination of religion and empirical therapy. In later Greece, about 400 B.C., there emerged the purely empirical craft of medical practice, identified with the school of Hippocrates. His was the first school of thought that separated medicine clearly from religion, and rejected magic in favor of observation and careful description as the keys to understanding disease. In his *Airs, Waters, and Places,* Hippocrates even wrote of the influence of environment on health. Hippocratic and similar artisan–physicians traveled from town to town, setting up shops in the marketplace.

In ancient Rome, the first physicians were slaves brought from Greece and attached to the large agricultural latifundia. Later, free Greek physicians were attracted to Rome with offers of citizenship and exemption from taxes if they would settle in the towns. Some were also attached to the Roman armies as military surgeons.

With the advent of Christianity, Greek and Roman doctors came to be regarded as practitioners of a pagan art, and most new physicians were monks. This meant that their activities became governed by an increasingly organized church. Monasteries sometimes had special quarters for the care of the sick and destitute (later evolving into hospitals). By the twelfth century, however, the Church hierarchy reacted against the preoccupation of monks, or sometimes priests, with so worldly a matter as treatment of the human body. Surgery was particularly unsuitable. Therefore lay artisans became engaged in medicine—using drugs and physical procedures—and barbers (sometimes called barber—surgeons) performed surgery.

Medical Education

The first formal medical school for training physicians of a modern mold was founded at Salerno, Italy in the ninth century. It gradually acquired wide influence in Europe, reaching its height in the twelfth century—after which it gradually declined and closed in the early nineteenth century.

After Salerno, the next medical school arose in the Arab world. Although most of Europe was still in its Dark Ages, a medical school was founded in 972 A.D. in Cairo, where ancient classical culture was being kept alive by Arabian scholars. Up to the sixteenth century, university training for medicine was developed in the major cities of Europe, including Oxford and Cambridge in England, Krakow and Rostow in the eastern Slavic regions, and Copenhagen in the north. Medical education, however, was most highly developed in southern and central Europe—Italy, France, and Germany. It was not until 1551 that the first medical school was established in the Western Hemisphere—at Mexico City under the influence of Spain.

In the British colonies of North America, the first medical school was established in 1765 in Philadelphia, sponsored by the University of Pennsylvania. The Harvard theological seminary was started in Boston 1636, and the Harvard Medical School began in 1782, soon after the American Revolution. Other medical faculties were organized in Latin America at Caracas, Venezuela in 1725, Santiago, Chile in 1743, Rio de Janeiro, Brazil in 1808, Buenos Aires, Argentina in 1821, and Montevideo, Uruguay in 1840. The first medical school in English Canada (Dalhousie University) was founded at Halifax in 1818 and in French Canada at Quebec City in 1852. Not until 1868 was a medical school started on any other continent—in Tokyo, Japan. Another was founded by the British in Hong Kong in 1887. In Thailand the first school was founded in 1889. The University of the Philippines, under American influence, established a medical school in 1908. American foundations financed the development of several of these schools, but their "high-tech" policies have been severely criticized as inappropriate.

The vast majority of medical schools in the world today, however, are of relatively recent origin. A compilation of all known medical schools in 1922 identified 229. In 1955, a World Health Organization survey found 631 medical schools in the world. In 1974, when another WHO survey was done, the number had risen to 1,124. By 1985, WHO could report that 1,351 medical schools had been established in 127 countries. It is evident that in the last few decades, more schools for training doctors have been established than in all previous centuries. Medical schools have become not only places for training physicians, but centers for research and consultation in the national health systems of their countries.

The most schools—142, counting those for training osteopathic physicians—were in the United States, and more than 50 schools were operating in China (114), India (106), the Soviet Union (87), Japan (80), Brazil (76), and Mexico (57). The medical school curriculum typically requires 5 or 6 years of full-time study, with much laboratory and clinical training, after completion of secondary school (usually 12 years). An additional year of hospital internship is usually required at the end, although sometimes this is equivalent to the sixth academic year. The U.S. policy of requiring a "premedical" baccalaureate, preceding 4 years of medical school, is unusual in the world scene.

The content and viewpoint of medical education have evolved over the years. With the vast scientific discoveries of the nineteenth century, much greater attention has been given to the basic sciences as a foundation for the study of clinical diagnosis and treatment. The first years of training were based mainly in laboratories and the later years mainly in hospitals. Unfortunately, many developing countries, that had been colonies, emulated the medical education patterns of the former mother country, instead of being well adapted to the main health realities at home. Even in industrialized countries rare diseases may receive great attention, whereas the common disorders of the population receive only limited attention.

Critical to this evolution was the Flexner Report of 1910 in the United States and Canada, also influencing Europe. It led to enormous improvement in the quality of teaching of the basic sciences and established the pattern of medical schools within universities. Clinical experience was to be provided in university-affiliated hospitals. On the other hand, it contributed to the aggrandizement of tertiary medicine and made medical education very costly.

After around 1965, the low-income developing countries became more sensitive to the major health problems of their own people,

modifying medical curricula accordingly. Periods of work in small villages became a frequent educational requirement. Also in medical schools in all countries, a new appreciation arose for understanding the daily problems of the patient as a whole, along mental and social, as well as physicochemical dimensions. Medical education became reoriented to emphasize family and community circumstances contributing to health and disease.

NUMBERS AND DISTRIBUTION OF PHYSICIANS

With appreciation of the important place of medical science in national health systems, almost every country has taken steps to increase its output of physicians. Medical education is expensive, so that a country's capability of preparing doctors depends largely on its national wealth; but, as we shall see, many other factors, political and cultural, are also influential.

In 1987 there were about 5,000,000 physicians in the world or roughly one per 1,000 population. This applies to the doctors that each country regards as fully qualified, and does not include traditional practitioners or any of the variety of medical assistants, with limited training, who work in so many countries. Physician distribution, of course, is very uneven among districts in a country, as well as among countries. The economic level of the local population is usually the most prominent determinant of these variations.

Economic Influences

Using the most elementary approach, we may compare the supply of physicians in the industrialized countries (with GNPs per capita of $5,000 per year or more) with that in the developing countries, (nearly all with GNPs per capita of under $3,000 per year). In 1986, physicians in industrialized countries numbered 265 per 100,000, compared with 51 per 100,000 in all developing countries. Such a crude comparison, however, is a great oversimplification. Among industrialized countries, for example, the United States had three times the GNP per capita of Spain in 1986; yet U.S.

physicians numbered 216 per 100,000 people compared with 314 per 100,000 in Spain.

Among developing countries, the disparities in physician supply are equally or more striking. The transitional or middle-income country, South Korea (GNP per capita $2418 in 1986), had 75 doctors per 100,000, whereas Argentina with slightly lower wealth had 264 doctors per 100,000. Among the very poor developing countries, Indonesia (GNP per capita $491 in 1986) had 11 physicians per 100,000, whereas India with even lesser per capita wealth had 41 physicians per 100,000.

Explanations of these differences in physician supply must be sought in the political, social, and historical developments of each country. The supply of physicians in countries of three economic levels and various health system types are listed in Table 1.1. The economic levels are based on the country's GNP per capita in a recent year, and the classification of systems is from Volume I. These system types are based mainly on the degree of market intervention by government, ranging from minimum to maximum. The countries selected are those with the largest populations for each system category. Within almost every country in the world, the concentration of wealth in cities has led to a corresponding concentration of doctors, leaving relatively few

Table 1.1. Supply of Physicians in Countries of Three Economic Levels, according to Health Systems of Different Types, 1986

Country and Health System Type	Physicians per 100,000
Affluent industrialized	
Entrepreneurial (United States)	216.5
Welfare oriented (West Germany)	271.0
Comprehensive (Great Britain)	144.7
Socialist (Soviet Union)	423.7
Transitional	
Entrepreneurial (Philippines)	15.2
Welfare oriented (Brazil)	89.1
Comprehensive (Nicaragua)	70.9
Socialist (Cuba)	219.8
Very poor	
Entrepreneurial (Indonesia)	10.9
Welfare oriented (India)	40.7
Comprehensive (Sri Lanka)	13.5
Socialist (China)	59.8

Source: Derived from Sivard, Ruth, *World Military and Social Expenditures, 13th Edition,* Washington, DC: World Priorities, 1989.

doctors for rural populations. In Thailand, for example, around 1980 the national capital Bangkok, with 9.2 percent of the population, had 75 percent of the doctors. In Peru (1985) Lima had 16.1 percent of the national population but more than 60 percent of all doctors. Similar maldistributions are found in most industrialized countries, although the disparities may not be so extreme.

Some urban concentration of physicians and other health manpower, of course, is reasonable for staffing tertiary-level medical centers, medical schools, research institutes, and so on. People from outside the cities and small towns, moreover, come to the cities for medical care. Much primary health care, nevertheless, requires services nearby and conveniently available, so that most developing countries have trained paramedical and auxiliary health personnel to provide such services in rural areas.

Aside from the urban–rural maldistribution problem, the economic level of whole provinces or states obviously influences the supply of doctors. India has about 41 physicians per 100,000 population, but among its 31 states and union territories, the ratios vary from 130 to 6.0 per 100,000, and a broad range in between (1987). Among the 50 states of the United States, the doctor supply in 1986 ranged from 122 per 100,000 in Mississippi to 306 per 100,000 in Massachusetts. These differences among regions, of course, affect living standards, schools, cultural opportunities, and more; at their roots, however, are economic factors.

Even within large cities, different sections or neighborhoods reflect the income levels of their residents. In most, though not all, industrialized countries there are very low-income areas, even miserable slums, in the older "inner cities"; slums and shanty towns tend to develop around the periphery of large cities of the developing countries, both transitional and very poor. In all these depressed areas, the supply of physicians is meager, much lower than in the attractive neighborhoods of the same cities. In more welfare-oriented health systems, this discrepancy may be compensated by the organization of special health programs for slum-dwellers.

One other clearly economic determinant of a country's output of physicians has been evident in recent years. As medical practice has become a lucrative occupation, entrepreneurial interests in certain countries have established medical schools as profit-making businesses. Other factors may play a part, but the presence of a demand for medical training and the availability of investment funds have led to the funding of several small proprietary schools. Many of these are close to the United States, where young people, denied admission to U.S. schools, are able to pay the cost of schooling. In the Dominican Republic, for example, with a 1986 population of 6.6 million, there were 5 medical schools in 1975; by 1985 there were 12 medical schools, the majority of whose students were U.S. residents. Similar "off-shore" medical schools, catering to the U.S. applicants, have been established in other Caribbean islands states, such as Grenada and Saint Lucia, and also in Mexico. Many of the 18 medical schools established in the Philippines between 1975 and 1985 have also trained their graduates largely for "export."

The economic roots of a country's doctor supply have been perversely reflected by the growth in some countries of numbers beyond what the economy can sustain. There results, it is claimed, an excess of physicians—in spite of vast unmet needs in the rural areas. The policy question comes down to whether we should judge doctor supply by market criteria or health needs. If health needs are the criteria, strategies can be designed to assign physicians to areas where they are lacking.

Economic determinants of a country's supply and distribution of doctors are obviously intermingled with political and other social influences. Examining countries of similar economic level, with very different supplies of physicians, we may draw inferences about these noneconomic influences (see Table 1.1).

Political and Social Influences

The multiplicity of influences on a country's stock of physicians is so great and complex that a simple direct relationship to the national political ideology or to its health system policies can hardly be drawn. The impact of spe-

cial policies in the universities, the business interests of medical associations, the freedom of religious groups, and the variability of national technical standards all play a role—aside from any political will in the health system to increase the availability of physicians.

The United States in 1986 had 216.5 physicians per 100,000 population—a substantial increase over previous decades and yet a ratio reflecting constraints from many sources. To limit competition, the medical profession has managed to retard the rate of admission to medical schools. Government support for medical education was relatively weak until the 1960s. For several decades after 1910, standards were raised to advance the quality of medical education, without regard to meeting societal needs.

In a welfare-oriented health system such as that of West Germany, physicians numbered 271 per 100,000 in 1986. Although the medical profession is strong in defending its business interests, the labor movement and the welfare orientation of government have prevailed. Most of the German medical schools have a very permissive admission policy, and large classes are accepted. Despite wartime destruction, the old schools were rebuilt and several new ones established. The social insurance program ensures comfortable incomes to doctors in community practice, as well as in the hospitals. On the other hand, in Japan, also with a welfare-oriented health system, a powerful medical profession has successfully limited the intake of new medical students rather rigidly. In spite of a high demand for medical care and a robust economy, the supply of physicians in 1986 was only 153 per 100,000.

In Sweden, with a comprehensive health system, there were 263 physicians per 100,000 in 1986, even though the demand for services was relatively modest. The hospital bed supply is large, and hospitals are very well staffed medically. Great Britain, however, with a much larger population and a system of equally comprehensive character, has kept its stock of physicians down to 144.7 per 100,000. This has resulted from a deliberate policy limiting national health expenditures by supply-side restrictions. It has led to very long capitation lists in general practitioner practices, long waiting periods for elective surgery, and hospital out-patient services that are often considered per-functory.

The Soviet Union's 423.7 physicians per 100,000 is a greater supply than that in any of the other industrialized countries. In this so-cialist health system, the salaries paid physi-cians have been low, and policy calls for abun-dant medical staffing of all health facilities. The medical school or "institute" classes are very large, the great majority of students and doctors are women, the working day is rela-tively short (6 or 7 hours), and physicians do work—such as emergency service on ambu-lances—that paramedical personnel would do elsewhere. Other industrialized socialist coun-tries, such as Poland with 201 or Yugoslavia with 182 doctors per 100,000, have less lavish doctor supplies, but, in light of their modest GNPs per capita, these ratios are large.

In transitional-level countries with varying health system policies, one may also find sharp contrasts in physician supply. Thailand and the Philippines had GNPs per capita of $590 and $783 in 1986; Thailand's entrepreneurial type system had 17 physicians per 100,000 whereas the similar health system in the Phil-ippines had 15.2.

Brazil's welfare-oriented health system had 89.1 doctors per 100,000 in 1986, and Chile's similar system had 80.3 doctors. Both these countries had GNPs per capita between $500 and $2,000 per year. Another welfare-oriented health system is in Egypt, with 143.2 doctors per 100,000. Egypt, after the monarch was overthrown in 1952, had established a consti-tution that guarantees that every secondary school graduate, wishing to study medicine, has the right to do so.

The comprehensive health system in Nica-ragua was greatly handicapped by hostilities of the *contras* in the 1980s. Yet in 1986, it had 70.9 physicians per 100,000. The socialist health system of Cuba, with a GNP of nearly $2,000 per capita in 1986, had 219.8 doctors per 100,000. Cuba's health policies give very high priority to training physicians, even for managing childbirth, which had previously been handled by midwives or traditional birth attendants.

Among very poor countries, Indonesia with

its entrepreneurial type of health system had 10.9 doctors per 100,000 in 1986; Kenya, a smaller African country with the same type of health system, had 9.9 doctors per 100,000 in 1986; India, much the largest very poor coun-try with a welfare-oriented system, had 40.7 physicians per 100,000 people in 1986; and Zimbabwe, a very poor African country with a welfare-oriented health system, had a supply of 15.2 doctors per 100,000 in 1986.

Sri Lanka, a very poor country with a com-prehensive health system, had only 13.5 phy-sicians per 100,000 in 1986. This relatively low supply reflects a deliberate government policy of using mid-level health personnel exten-sively, the unrestricted freedom of emigration of doctors, and a large stock of Ayurvedic prac-titioners. The socialist health system of China had 59.8 Western-type physicians per 100,000 in 1986—without counting the large numbers of traditional Chinese practitioners.

The supply of physicians in countries is ob-viously influenced by their basic economic lev-els. But it is clear that the political orientation of the health system also plays a large part. Even after political ideologies change, previ-ously established health policies often linger on. Long-term trends in science and in society have had major impacts on the characteristics of the medical profession.

MAJOR DEVELOPMENTS IN THE MEDICAL PROFESSION

Since the scientifically trained physician has become the generally recognized leader in healing the sick throughout the world, several developments have shaped the medical profes-sion and its role in health systems. Because functions and relationships to patients of doc-tors have changed in countless ways, their characteristics now differ enormously from those of the ancient healer.

Specialization

As universities developed during the Renais-sance in Europe, physicians were trained with a broad knowledge of "natural philosophy." University graduates were the elite, and a coveted goal was to become attached to a feudal estate or a royal court as a salaried *body physician*. In this position, the doctor would serve the extended lordly family, as well as giving some care to the lowly serfs.

At the same time, some physicians and also a lower class of medical artisans settled in towns, selling their services to townspeople for small fees. Some developed special skills for setting bones, extracting teeth, or even removing from the eyes cataracts that caused blindness. The barbers often did blood-letting as well as minor surgery. Not until the nineteenth century was surgery regarded as a proper task for physicians. When hospitals were more extensively developed in the sixteenth century, physicians appointed to look after their patients were university graduates.

Specialization was not undertaken by the university medical graduate until later. With the flowering of medical science, particularly organ pathology and bacteriology, in the latter part of the nineteenth century, the whole character of the medical profession changed. Largely related to the rapid growth of hospitals after around 1880, specialization grew rapidly in medicine.

By the twentieth century, with anesthesia and antisepsis (later asepsis), surgery was absorbed fully into medicine as a specialty. Diseases of women became the province of gynecology and obstetrics. Problems of children gave rise to pediatrics. Special skills for dealing with visual problems had been acquired in the eighteenth century, with the development of optics, but ophthalmology as a medical specialty took shape later. In 1916, ophthalmology became the first specialty for which a definite schedule of training was required to attain "specialty qualifications." This was in the United States, where competition from nonmedical opticians or optometrists was keen. Numerous other subspecialties—with defined periods of training and examination—were soon established under surgery and internal medicine. With the further growth of technology, specialties arose in clinical pathology, radiology, hematology, and anesthesiology. Mental disorders became the special domain of psychiatry.

In most countries in the nineteenth century specialization became closely linked with hospitals. Large facilities could arrange their wards to keep patients with similar types of medical problems together. Then specialists in these fields would be appointed to supervise the medical care on a full-time or part-time basis. As hospitals grew larger and more complex, medical staffs of full-time specialists on salaries became the norm in Europe and the many colonies dominated by European powers. North America was the exception, in that hospitals were open to almost any physician, specialist, or generalist. Only for the care of indigent patients in charitable or public wards were salaried doctors sometimes appointed.

As medical science developed throughout the twentieth century, specialization expanded correspondingly. In the more affluent industrialized countries, new technology has been most extensive and with it greater degrees of specialization. Training specialists takes time and money, so that their services, whether paid by salaries or fees, are costly. The exceptionally large proportion of specialists in the U.S. medical profession, about 85 percent, is the result not only of the *open staff* general hospital policy but also of the high incomes and the financial support of medical care by voluntary insurance. Furthermore, a large percentage of physicians, known as specialists in some countries, are self-designated, rather than being certified by any recognized body.

Most national health systems have formalized some procedure for certifying specialty qualifications. Sometimes this may be through the same governmental channels as medical licensure or registration, but more often the responsibility is assigned to a nongovernmental professional society. Training for specialty status usually requires several years of supervised work in an approved hospital, and passing various examinations. Young doctors from developing countries must often go abroad for such hospital specialty training, as it is not available at home.

By the 1980s the majority of physicians in industrialized countries with health systems of any orientation had become specialists. In the welfare-oriented systems of European countries, 55 to 65 percent of physicians were specialists, mainly attached to hospitals. In the

United States, around 1970 even general practitioners "specialized" in family practice. In the industrialized former socialist countries, there were typically two grades of specialists; the lower grade served in polyclinics and the higher grade staffed the hospitals. Most pediatricians in socialist systems were regarded as general practitioners for children, and relatively few were qualified as genuine specialists.

The greater prestige and usually higher earnings of specialists and the needs for primary health care have generated a movement for strengthening general practice in many countries. This has brought about many programs of continuing education, encouragement of the grouping of generalists with ancillary personnel, and, in a growing number of countries, the development of specialty training programs in *general medicine* or *family practice.* The specialist in family practice has training as long and rigorous as the conventional specialists, but usually it includes supervised work in several older specialties, except for major surgery. Family practice has acquired great strength in many industrialized countries, and has grown more rapidly than other specialties. In Cuba, the entire polyclinic program has been modified, so that everyone has access, first, to a *family doctor* before visiting a polyclinic.

In the developing countries of both transitional and very poor economic levels, specialization is much less developed. In Latin American countries with large population coverage under social security programs, such as Mexico or Brazil, specialization is somewhat greater, but typically it involves only a small minority of physicians. In the very poorest countries only a handful of medical graduates are able to seek the necessary training for a specialty at home or abroad.

The linkage of specialization to hospitals, in which general practitioners customarily may not work, has caused an awkward dichotomy in the medical profession of many countries. Hospital doctors often became an elite group in relation to general practitioners. To counteract this attitude, hospitals in some countries invite generalists to clinical sessions within the hospital, and sometimes to serve in the outpatient department.

Broadening Medical Functions

The role of modern physicians is far broader than that of their historical antecedents. Aside from specialization, and within the scope of any physician, specialist or generalist, developments in society and in health systems have resulted in the doctor's assumption of an ever widening range of responsibilities. Diagnosis and treatment of the sick may still be the central functions of physicians, but they have increasingly come to be expected to provide personal preventive services. They are called on to educate allied and technical health personnel in hospitals and elsewhere, and often to engage in research. Where teams of health workers provide service, doctors are usually captains of the team and must perform certain administrative tasks. In factories and schools they may be expected to advise on the safety and hygiene of environmental conditions. In the courts of law they are the expert witnesses on many questions. In time of war they may serve in the military establishment. In rural communities everywhere, physicians are generally regarded as civic leaders and advisors on almost all social matters.

In hospitals, the physician is usually associated with nurses and other personnel, who do many tasks formerly regarded as requiring a doctor—injections, venupunctures, catheterizations, all sorts of diagnostic procedures, and surgical dressings. Large hospitals typically have a hierarchy of physicians, so that younger doctors in training perform medical examinations, make initial diagnoses, and prescribe treatment, and the senior physician simply reviews and approves the case management. The hospital specialist is the main teacher of the clinical sciences in medical schools.

In health centers and polyclinics for ambulatory care, more and more physicians function with a team of personnel. Most of the examination of infants is done by nurses, and in regions with insufficient doctors auxiliary personnel may be delegated to serve all patients who seem to have simple ailments. A dispenser maintains and dispenses drugs. The physician is expected to supervise the other personnel as well as to work with them.

The time available for the patient–doctor encounter is often very limited, so that medical service may be perfunctory. This is especially serious in health systems supported by public funds, where demands may be high and resources are inadequate. Physicians are then widely criticized for insensitivity to the patient's feelings. Innovations have been introduced in medical education to "humanize" services, but an adequate supply of health manpower remains basic. Complaints about the impersonality of physicians are articulated mostly in the affluent countries, where educational programs are strong, but they apply with greater force in the developing countries (both transitional and very poor), where class lines are very sharp. It is these attitudes, most evident in public programs, that may drive even the poorest people to seek care from a private doctor who makes time to be sympathetic.

Since the physician is usually captain of various health care teams, "professional dominance" has been a feature of most organized health programs. Sociologists have criticized the nondemocratic results of this situation. "Medical chauvinism" is another characterization of professional dominance. Yet, if we examine trends over recent decades, the degree of professional dominance in organized health programs is surely declining. The dynamics of group activity and the professionalization of allied health personnel are generating more democratic patterns of work.

Medical Associations

In the nineteenth century, before medical licensure was well established and when various medical cults (homeopathy, chiropractic, etc.) were competing for popular attention, extravagant claims were made by some practitioners. In several European countries advertising was common. To combat this, the British Medical Association was founded in 1832 to set standards of professional conduct. In 1845 the French Society of Medicine was founded and in 1847 the American Medical Association. Later equivalent associations were formed in other countries. The colonies of European powers often formed peripheral branches of the association in the ruling country.

By selectivity in granting membership, the medical associations attempted to denigrate practitioners they regarded as cultists or quacks. They also conducted educational programs for their members. A special strategy was to promulgate codes of ethics on the behavior of doctors toward their patients and toward each other. These codes were much more specific than the time-honored Hippocratic Oath; they banned advertising, they asserted the confidentiality of information about patients, and they sometimes even listed schedules of fees recommended for various procedures.

As organized health care programs were increasingly developed, the medical association gradually became the official representative of physicians. Negotiations with governments or sickness funds were often necessary to settle on rates of remuneration, whether by fees or salaries. Fee schedules were sometimes published by medical associations, to encourage fair prices and reduce competition. Often a medical association was outspokenly hostile to government programs, and sometimes might even call a physician's strike.

To provide for the registration or licensure of physicians, many countries set up *medical colleges* as semiautonomous bodies vested with legal authority. The ethical code is usually adopted by the college, and all new physicians are obligated to abide by its rules or risk their license to practice. In 1771 an English physician, Thomas Percival, began publishing a series of essays on proper "professional conduct." These covered subjects such as

- Professional conduct relative to hospital or other medical charities
- Professional conduct in private or general medical practice
- Conduct of physicians to apothecaries
- Professional duties in certain cases, which require a knowledge of law

These principles of the physician's conduct were translated into the language of ethical codes in Europe and North America—especially in the nineteenth century, when the private physician functioned in a highly competitive market. Unfortunately, some ethical codes were formulated to obstruct certain patterns of medical practice, rather than to promote truly ethical objectives.

In 1912, for example, the Code of Ethics of the American Medical Association stated:

> The poverty of a patient and the mutual professional obligation of physicians should command the gratuitous services of a physician. It is unprofessional for a physician to dispose of his services under conditions that make it impossible to render adequate service to his patient or which interfere with reasonable competition among physicians of a community. To do this is detrimental to the public and the individual physician and lowers the dignity of the profession.

This language was intended, of course, to retard the payment of physicians by salary, which is a matter of competitive business economics, and not ethics. Yet with all the complex relationships of physicians to organized health programs—whether solely financial or mainly supervisory—the traditional autonomy of the physician is becoming increasingly compromised. Physicians have naturally reacted strongly against this loss of autonomy, especially in countries where a large market of private patients enables them to work independently most of the time. Yet all the developments in health system structures have put physicians in a context of organized relationships, on which their daily work depends.

The method of paying physicians has been a matter of controversy in many industrialized countries. Payment by a fee for each identifiable service (or by fee-for-service) has usually been preferred by private practitioners. Sometimes fees may be replaced by barter. A second method, by capitation for each person on the doctor's list, has been instituted for paying general practitioners in Great Britain and for certain doctors in Denmark and the Netherlands. A third method, by full-time or part-time salary, is used for hospital specialists in most countries, and for publicly employed physicians in almost all countries. Indeed, in lower income developing countries, where private

medical markets are weak, salaried payment is usually preferred by most physicians. Each method of paying doctors has both advantages and hazards for both doctor and patient in various settings, as will be explored later.

To protect the doctor's economic and social position, medical associations often become protagonists against government or citizen groups. Doctors may claim that their viewpoints are meant to protect the consumer when they are really designed to advance their personal income and prestige. In the United States, Australia, and other affluent countries, the attitude of medical associations toward social insurance for medical care has typically been hostile, whereas that of their patients has been favorable. Codes of ethics of medical associations may not have the force of law, but they certainly influence the behavior of most physicians.

International Medical Migration

A few years after national independence, in the post-World War II period, physicians from India, the Philippines, and some other countries left their homes for North America and Europe. By 1972, approximately 6 percent of the world's total physicians or 140,000 had relocated in a country other than their own. About 119,000 of the emigrating physicians were settled in five countries—the United States (77,000 doctors), Great Britain, Canada, West Germany, and Australia.

Before World War II (1939–1945), most of the movement of physicians had been between industrialized countries or from the latter to developing countries. After World War II physician migration was principally from the low-income developing countries to the high-income industrialized countries. This *brain drain,* as it was called, caused concern in both the donor and recipient countries. In the recipient industrialized countries, "foreign medical graduates" (FMGs)—even though they might pass special examinations—were deemed to lower the professional standards. Yet in the United States, in 1970 FMGs constituted 20 percent of all physicians, in Canada they constituted 33 percent of the physicians, and in

Great Britain they constituted 25 percent of the physician stock.

For the donor developing countries, the problem was more serious. Emigration of physicians, trained usually at government expense, represented a serious loss of social investment in the face of vast unmet medical care needs. In India, for example, the estimated 15,000 physicians abroad in 1971 constituted a loss of 13 percent of the country's national stock of physicians. Iran's loss of 3,700 physicians abroad was equivalent to 39 percent of its national stock. The 9,500 Philippine physicians abroad in 1971 constituted 67 percent of the national supply. In Thailand, 30 percent of the national stock of physicians in 1971 left for greener pastures.

In the 1970s, the World Health Organization did an international study of the migration of physicians and nurses, and concluded that out-migration was due to the country's having a greater supply of physicians than it could absorb economically. Countries receiving migrant physicians were, in effect, those with a smaller supply of physicians than they could support economically. This was under conditions of very permissive immigration and emigration.

Around 1978, legislation in the United States, Canada, and Great Britain raised the barriers to in-migration, on the assumption that their national stocks of physicians were adequate. This greatly reduced the annual entry of noncitizens. The entry of FMGs, to the United States at least, became principally U.S. graduates of non-U.S. medical schools, especially those in the Caribbean region.

According to the WHO study, many developing countries faced an apparent "surplus" of physicians. The *brain drain* could no longer be considered a solution. Yet everyone knew that in these countries there were enormous unmet medical needs. Political pressure mounted, therefore, for some corrective policy within the country. Reducing the output of medical schools was undertaken in several countries. Mandating longer periods of rural service for new medical graduates was a more wholesome solution, but this naturally met opposition from the doctors. The best solution would be found only by political commitment to Health for All.

REFERENCES

Ackerknecht, Erwin H., *A Short History of Medicine: Revised Edition.* Baltimore: John Hopkins University Press, 1982.

Badgley, Robin F., "Health Worker Strikes: Social and Economic Bases of Conflict." *International Journal of Health Services,* 5(1):9–17, 1975.

Banerji, Debabar, "Place of the Indigenous and the Western Systems of Medicine in the Health Services of India." *International Journal of Health Services,* 9(2):511–519, 1979.

Bannerman, Robert H., et al. (Editors), *Traditional Medicine and Health Care Coverage.* Geneva: World Health Organization, 1983.

Berliner, Howard S., "A Larger Perspective on the Flexner Report." *International Journal of Health Services,* 5(4):573–592, 1975.

Bowers, John A., and Elizabeth F. Purcell, *The Impact of Health Services on Medical Education.* New York: Josiah Macy Jr. Foundation, 1978.

Brown, E. Richard, *Rockefeller Medicine Men: Medicine and Capitalism in America.* Berkeley, CA: University of California Press, 1979.

Bryant, John, *Health and the Developing World.* Ithaca, NY: Cornell University Press, 1969.

Bui Dang Ha Doan, "Specialization of Physicians: Levels and Trends in Some Industrialized Countries. *"World Health Statistics Quarterly,* 30(3):207–226, 1977.

Butter, Irene, and Alfonso Mejia, "Too Many Doctors!" *World Health Forum,* 8:494–500, 1987.

Commission for Alternative Systems of Medicine, "Alternative Medicine in the Netherlands." *World Health Forum,* 3(2):204–208, 1982.

Freidson, Eliot, *Professional Dominance: The Social Structure of Medical Care.* New York: Aldine Atherton Press, 1970.

Frenk, Julio, "Career Preferences under Conditions of Unemployment." *Medical Care,* 23(4):320–332, 1985.

Fulop, Tamas, and M. I. Roemer, *International Development of Health Manpower Policy.* Geneva: World Health Organization (Offset Pub. No. 61), 1982.

Gilpin, Margaret, "Update-Cuba: On the Road to a Family Medicine Nation." *Journal of Public Health Policy,* 12:83–102, Spring 1991.

Gish, O., and B. Godfrey, "A Reappraisal of the Brain Drain—With Special Reference to the Medical Profession." *Social Science and Medicine,* 13C, 1979.

Glaser, William A., *Paying the Doctor: Systems of Remuneration and Their Effects.* Baltimore, MD: Johns Hopkins Press, 1970.

Landy, David (Editor), *Culture, Disease, and Heal-*

ing: Studies in Medical Anthropology. New York: Macmillan, 1977.

Lashari, Mohammad Saleh, "Traditional and Modern Medicine—Is a Marriage Possible?" *World Health Forum,* 5:175–177, 1984.

Leake, Chauncey D. (Editor), *Percival's Medical Ethics.* Baltimore: Johns Hopkins Press, 1969.

Lee, Rance P.L., "Chinese and Western Medical Care in China's Rural Communes." *World Health Forum,* 3(3):301–306, 1982.

Mejia, Alfonso, "Health Manpower Out of Balance." *World Health Statistics Quarterly,* 40(4):335–348, 1987.

Mejia, A., H. Pizurki, and E. Royston, *Physician and Nurse Migration.* Geneva: World Health Organization, 1979.

Odegaard, C. E., *Dear Doctor—A Personal Letter to a Physician.* Menlo Park, CA: Henry J. Kaiser Family Foundation, 1986.

Page, Leigh, "Should There be Regulations on Use of MD Specialties?" *American Medical News,* 8 September 1989.

Purcell, Elizabeth (Editor), *World Trends in Medical Education, Faculty, Students, and Curriculum.* Baltimore, MD: Johns Hopkins Press, 1971.

Ransome-Kuti, Olikoye, "A New Breed of Doctors." *World Health Forum,* 11:265–268, 1990.

Reed, Louis S., *The Healing Cults: A Study of Sectarian Medical Practice* (Committee on the Costs of Medical Care Pub. 16). Chicago: University of Chicago Press, 1934.

Roemer, M. I., "Medical Ethics and Education for Social Responsibility." *Yale Journal of Biology and Medicine,* 53:251–266, 1980.

Roemer, Milton I., "Canadian Health Services and Manpower Policy." In M. I. Roemer, *National Strategies for Health Care Organization,* Ann Arbor, MI: Health Administration Press, 1985, pp. 193–222.

Roemer, M. I., "Judging Doctor Supply—Market or Health Criteria?" *World Health Forum,* 9:547–554, 1988.

Sigerist, Henry E., "The Physician's Profession Through the Ages." *Bulletin of New York Academy of Medicine,* 2nd series, 9:661–676, December 1933.

Sigerist, Henry E., "Medical Societies, Past and Present." *Yale Journal of Biology and Medicine,* 6:351–362, January 1934.

Veatch, Robert M. (Editor), *Cross-Cultural Perspectives in Medical Ethics: Readings,* Boston: Jones and Bartlett, 1989.

Vithoulkas, George, et al., "Homeopathy Today." *World Health Forum,* 4:99–113, 1983.

World Health Organization, "Report on Consultation on Health Services and Manpower Development." Geneva: WHO, September 1976 (processed document).

World Health Organization, *The Promotion and Development of Traditional Medicine.* Geneva: WHO (Technical Report Series 622), 1978.

World Health Organization, *Competency-Based Curriculum Development in Medical Education: An Introduction* (Public Health Papers 68). Geneva: WHO, 1978.

World Health Organization, *World Directory of Medical Schools,* 6th ed. Geneva: WHO, 1988.

CHAPTER TWO

Nurses, Pharmacists, and Other Health Personnel

The reach of the physician has been greatly extended over the years by the training of a wide variety of other health personnel. Strictly speaking, most of these personnel perform their functions under the general supervision of or according to orders issued by the physician. In practice, however, these associated health personnel have developed a proper scope of functions of their own, and a great deal of their work is carried out quite independently of the physician. The most abundant category of health personnel is the nurse, who plays a major role in the health system of nearly all countries. Often closely associated with the nurse, and oriented especially to pregnancy and childbirth, is the midwife.

In addition to nurses and midwives, who may have several levels of training, virtually all health systems have pharmacists (sometimes called chemists) with specialized knowledge of drugs. For analysis of blood, urine, and many other products of human life, there are diverse types of laboratory technicians or technologists. Many modalities of rehabilitation are the special skill of physical therapists and related personnel. A general health worker, who under certain circumstances may replace the physician, and who receives a relatively short period of training, exists in many countries. These workers, designated by different terms in various countries, are perhaps most commonly known as *medical assistants*. In recent times the term "community health worker" has come to be widely used for even more briefly trained personnel. Regarding dietary matters, there is the dietician and, on a more advanced level, the nutritionist. The written record of a patient's status may be handled by the medical record librarian. The relationships of patients

with their families and the total social environment are facilitated by social workers in more developed societies.

To handle complex types of diagnostic or therapeutic equipment, there are still other types of health personnel, especially in highly industrialized countries. We cannot consider them all, but will concentrate on the broad fields of nursing, pharmacy, medical technology, dental personnel, medical assistants, and community health workers in this chapter.

NURSING PERSONNEL AND MIDWIVES

The modern professional nurse has evolved from an untrained person, usually a woman, who took care of patients in bed. Over the years, many types and levels of nurse have developed. If all of these are counted, nursing is usually the most populous category of health personnel in a country.

Historical Background

In ancient Greece, the Aesculapian temples, to which the sick went for prayers, might be considered the antecedents of hospitals. In these structures there were priests or assistant priests to take care of the sick patients. In the Roman empire, there were also *valetudinaria* for the care of injured soldiers and slaves. The caretakers were usually male slaves.

From the earliest times, however, in a family's home, the women took care of sick relatives. When the Christian Church showed its charity and mercy by building structures for the sick poor, it chose women close to the

Church to work in them. Middle-aged women, who were widows, were the preferred attendants. The structures for the destitute and sick were often built near a monastery or a cathedral. These evolved into hospitals, with the nurses coming from various nursing orders. By the later decades of the Roman Empire, the hospital with nurses working in it as caretakers gradually became an established institution.

The middle-aged women caretakers became nuns. These women had no formal training, but they brought food to the bedside and tried to keep patients clean and make them comfortable.

In the eighteenth century, as hospitals in the major European cities became crowded with derelicts and the chronic sick, nursing duties fell to any poor or homeless woman willing to do the work in return for food and shelter. Some church leaders in the seventeenth century had called for deliberate training of nurses, but this was not undertaken until much later.

In 1836, the hospital in Kaiserwerth, Germany established a semireligious but formal training school for nurses. It was here that an upper class English lady, Florence Nightingale, received the training that enabled her in 1870 to found the first wholly secular nursing school at St. Thomas's Hospital in London. The idea soon spread to other cities in Europe and America, and eventually nursing schools were established by most large hospitals, if only to supply their own need for nurses. The first nursing school in the United States was started in 1873 at Bellevue Hospital, a municipal institution in New York City. As nursing schools proliferated, their educational programs varied, and a need for higher and uniform standards became recognized. In 1916, therefore, Great Britain created a governmental Registry of Nurses; for entry on the Registry the nurse had to pass official examinations.

With the rapid expansion of hospitals in developed countries in the early twentieth century, fully prepared and "state-registered nurses" (typically with 3 years of hospital training) were insufficient to meet the demand. Public health agencies, visiting nurse associations, and even physicians in private offices were making demands for more nurses. The

working life of professional nurses, moreover, was often ended by early marriage and childbearing. New and larger classes of young women, trained to become registered nurses, were necessary to keep up with the needs.

In the colonies of European powers in Asia and Africa, the education of women was extremely limited. The relatively few literate upper class women would seldom wish to engage in the "lowly" manual tasks of attending patients in bed. Nursing duties in these colonies, therefore, were usually undertaken by young men. In later years, after national independence, these male nurses, or *dressers,* or *hospital assistants* became the nucleus of a new type of semiindependent "medical assistant," discussed later.

In the less developed countries of Latin America, that had won their independence much earlier (they were severed from Europe around 1820) the development of nursing was different. The Catholic Church of Spain had played a large part in the colonization of South America, and in the seventeenth century, religious brotherhoods from Europe devoted themselves to caring for the sick. By the nineteenth century they were replaced by sisterhoods of nuns. The first trained nurses came from Great Britain to Argentina, leading to the first Latin American school of nursing in Buenos Aires in 1897. Other nursing schools were also founded in Argentina in 1908 and 1920.

External influence from the United States led also to a nursing school in Havana, Cuba in 1899. Other nursing schools had indigenous origins—in Chile (1905), Peru (1910), Brazil (1917), Ecuador (1927), and elsewhere; it took great effort and courage to start each of these schools, and their output was relatively small. A nursing career was not attractive to educated young women, when a conventional notion in middle or upper class families was that the training would only convert them into "mere servants in white."

After about 1910, with the spectacular growth of hospitals and the heightened standards of patient care in industrialized countries, the output of graduate nurses from hospital-based training schools failed to keep up with the demands. At first, almost any woman would be hired to assist the trained nurses with the simple chores of patient care—cleaning rooms, serving meals, and so on. Around 1920, some larger hospitals began training women for a few months as *practical nurses.* Eventually a training schedule for such nurses, lasting 1 year, became widely adopted.

For these nursing auxiliaries, less prior education was required, and it was expected that much of their skill would come from prior experience. In the United States these personnel were sometimes called vocational nurses, and in 1938 New York State established official curriculum and examination standards for "licensed vocational nurses" (LVNs). In many countries, less than fully trained nurses have been designated as *nursing assistants* or *assistant nurses.* Beyond these, in most countries, hospitals and other health facilities still employ women, and sometimes men, who learn their duties entirely on the job. They may be called nurses' aides, nursing auxiliaries, or (if men) orderlies.

Modern Nursing Education

Until about 1940, nursing education for all levels of nurse was conducted almost exclusively in hospitals. Since the nursing student rendered a great deal of patient care during training, the educational program was relatively inexpensive. This pattern remains predominant throughout the world, although in North America and a few other high income regions nursing education has been transferred largely to academic settings. These may be in "associate degree" programs of community colleges or through regular baccalaureate degree programs in universities. Some nurses, with administrative or teaching goals, may obtain still higher academic degrees. Clinical exercises are still carried out in hospitals or other health facilities.

In many developing countries, nursing auxiliaries or assistant nurses, intended for service in rural health units, may be trained entirely in a rural health center. To enter this training they are expected to be young and healthy and to have completed only 4 to 6 years of elementary school. The period of training is seldom more than 1 year and often is less. The emphasis is on the surveillance of infants and prena-

tal women. The auxiliaries often learn a little also about treatment of common ailments, so that their functions may, in fact, overlap with those of *community health workers.*

The transfer of nursing education to academic settings in the United States has been especially striking. Between 1952 and 1982 the spectrum of settings for professional nursing education has changed completely; the U.S. trends have been as follows:

Educational Setting	Percentage	
	1952	1982
Hospital schools	92.1	15.8
Community colleges	1.0	51.7
Universities	6.9	32.5
All settings	100.0	100.0

Thus over the 30-year period ending in 1982, professional nurse preparation in the United States moved from being 92.1 percent in hospitals to 84.2 percent in academic settings. In other English-speaking countries, such as Canada and Australia, the same transformation of nursing schools has occurred, but at a later period. In the welfare-oriented health systems of these countries, the physical setting of nursing schools remains typically close to hospitals, but the teaching program is administratively and financially separate.

This change of educational setting occurred at different times in the 10 provinces of Canada and the 6 states of Australia. The first college-linked education of basic registered nurses in Australia was started only in 1974. In Belgium, both the French and the Flemish speaking schools were changed to academic settings also only in the 1970s. The physical—though not administrative—linkage to hospitals is found also in the universal health system of Norway and the former-socialist system of Poland.

The entire concept of higher education in junior or community colleges—so appropriate for basic nursing education—has not been implemented very much in low-income developing countries. In such countries of both transitional and very poor economic levels, nursing schools are still mainly within the structure of large public hospitals.

The most obvious consequence of change in the setting of nursing education has been that hospitals could no longer rely on the free service of student nurses. Additional registered nurses and second-level nurses were required. In Australia, training of *enrolled* or second-level nurses was upgraded to enable them to provide the care formerly given by student nurses working under supervision. In Canada, it was found that nurses trained in community college programs had somewhat lesser skills initially than nurses trained in hospital-based programs. These clinical skills were acquired after 6 months of experience, but hospitals had to be prepared to provide this additional training.

Furnishing the clinical component of nursing education in hospitals, administratively and financially separate from nursing schools, required new relationships among faculty, students, and hospital nursing supervisors. Although the principal responsibility for supervision of the clinical work of students rests with hospital nurses, there seems to be a trend in several countries toward having the academic instructors participate in the clinical component of training as well.

The shift in locale of nursing education also affects its financing. No longer part of the hospital budget, nursing education is not financed from patient care funds but rather from education funds. Since the education of health manpower generally in all these countries is financed largely or completely by government, this source puts the financing of nursing education on a par with that of educational programs for other health personnel.

National Supplies of Nurses

The training of various levels and types of nurses in different countries has been so diversified that international agencies have chosen to cluster all categories as *nursing persons*. The tabulations used by the World Health Organization and the World Bank combine graduate professional nurses with practical nurses, assistant nurses, and other nursing auxiliaries. The mix of total "nursing persons" tends to contain greater proportions of graduate-level nurses in higher income countries and greater

shares of assistant or auxiliary nurses in lower income countries. But the aggregate totals of nursing persons are strongly related to a country's economic level, regardless of the policy characteristics of its health system. This is evident in the countries illustrative of different health systems, indicated in Table 2.1.

It is evident in Table 2.1 that the overall stock of all types of nurse in countries is roughly proportional to the country's economic level. This is true in all four types of health system reviewed in this book (Volume I). Within any one level of economic development, the overall nurse–population ratios have no special relationship to the type of health system. The proportion of graduate or professional nurses in the higher income countries, moreover, is greater than in the lower income countries. Thus, in the United States the pro-

Table 2.1. National Supplies of "Nursing Persons" per 100,000 People, by the Country's Economic Level and Its Type of Health System, c. 1981

Types of Health Systems	Economic Level		
	Affluent	Transitional	Very Poor
Entrepreneurial United States	556		
South Korea		286	
South Africa		204	
Kenya			21.4
Indonesia			43.5
Welfare oriented Belgium	769		
Canada	833		
Brazil		87.7	
Turkey		80.6	
India			21.4
Liberia			34.2
Comprehensive Great Britain	833		
Sweden	1000		
Costa Rica		159	
Nicaragua		170	
Sri Lanka			79.4
Tanzania			—
Socialist Soviet Union	357		
Yugoslavia	333		
Cuba		270	
Albania		182	
Vietnam			79.4
Mozambique			17.8

Source: World Bank, *World Development Report 1988.* Washington: The Bank, 1988, pp. 278–279.

portion of total nurses who in 1986 were fully qualified (R.N. designation) was 69 percent, whereas in the Philippines (1980) it was 37 percent. Likewise, in the welfare-oriented health systems of Canada and Japan, these proportions were 84.3 and 53.1 percent, respectively. In the welfare-oriented Brazilian health system in 1982, professional nurses were only 16.2 percent and in Egypt 39 percent of the total supply.

In very poor countries with entrepreneurial health systems, such as Zaire or Pakistan, the professional nurse supply in 1981 constituted 22 and 41 percent of the total. In welfare-oriented India (1986) and Zimbabwe (1980), such professional nurses were 39.4 and 29.6 percent of the total. In these low-income countries, the relatively few women who complete secondary school seldom wish to study nursing. To provide nursing service, therefore, it is necessary to train large numbers of elementary school graduates (4 to 6 years) as auxiliary nurses.

On the other hand, countries with a relatively large supply of nurses are the Netherlands and Great Britain, with 588 and 833 nurses per 100,000, respectively. These supplies are maintained, despite high turnover, only by training large proportions of assistant nurses—68 and 54 percent, respectively. Poland also had a substantial supply of nurses in 1981, with 435 per 100,000; of these, 89.5 percent were fully qualified and only 10.5 percent were auxiliary. Poland at this time did not have a large reserve of unemployed women, who ordinarily constitute the applicants for training as assistant nurses.

The stock of professional nurses and their ratio to physicians, of course, varies greatly among countries. Thus in the United States in the late 1970s there were 961,000 professional nurses and 361,400 physicians—a ratio of 2.66 nurses per doctor. Professional nurses were also more numerous than trained auxiliary nurses; the latter numbered 489,000 or 0.51 for each professional nurse. In Great Britain the relative stocks of doctors and nurses were similar: 74,500 physicians and 145,400 professional nurses or nearly two (1.95) nurses per doctor. Auxiliary nurses numbered 59,400 or 0.41 per professional nurse.

In developing countries the proportions among different types of nurse and their ratios to doctors are quite different. In Colombia, for example, in the late 1970s there were only 3,325 professional nurses in relation to 12,720 physicians, or 0.26 nurses per doctor. Auxiliary nurses, however, were much more plentiful than professional nurses, numbering 16,645 or 5.0 for each professional nurse. Likewise in Kenya in the late 1970s there were 1,320 professional nurses, in relation to an almost equal number of doctors (1,270), or a ratio of 1.04 nurses per doctor. But auxiliary nurses again were much more plentiful than professional nurses, numbering 4,250 or 3.2 per professional nurse.

The output of nurses, nevertheless, has been increasing quite steadily in nearly all countries, in spite of the impression of a "nurse shortage" almost everywhere. In the industrialized countries between 1965 and 1975, the ratio to population (density) of professional nurses and midwives increased by 26.7 percent. For auxiliary nursing personnel, the density increased by 30.2 percent. In the developing countries over the same decade, the density of professional nurses and midwives increased by 11.5 percent, and for equivalent auxiliary nursing personnel it increased by 20.0 percent. At times of general unemployment in any economy, of course, previously inactive nurses often return to work.

The failure of nursing schools to turn out more professional nurses, in the face of increasing demands for their service, has led to corrective responses in many countries. Better salaries have brought inactive nurses back to work, but these older women are more likely to serve as nursing administrators or educators. Part-time work has been arranged. The proposal for a "registered care technologist" by the American Medical Association—to substitute for trained nurses—has generated only negative responses. In spite of an ever-increasing world supply of nurses at all levels, these essential personnel are perceived as being much less abundant than needed.

The shortages are most widely recognized in the more affluent industrialized countries, but the problem is evident also in the poorest countries. Sri Lanka estimates a shortage of 5,600 nurses and India of 35,000. Egypt in

1985 required 9,300 more nurses. Pakistan speaks of excessive doctors, with a shortage of nurses at both graduate and auxiliary levels. Australia also perceives a shortage of both its first-level and second-level nurses. The Republic of Korea (South) anticipates a shortage of 18,000 nurses by the year 2000.

In almost all countries, the largest shares of nurses of all levels and educational backgrounds are employed in hospitals. The percentage of nurses in hospital employment is probably highest in industrialized countries, where hospitals are most highly developed. The bed–population ratios and the intensity of care (reflected in hospital personnel per occupied bed) are both involved. In developing countries hospital employment also absorbs the lion's share of professional nurses, but auxiliary nurses are divided about equally between hospitals and community health programs.

In the early twentieth century, when hospitals were only modestly developed even in the affluent countries, a significant fraction of bedside nursing care in those countries was given by nurses employed directly by patients. These *private duty* nurses were engaged to serve patients of high or even moderate income. As hospitals have become financed for better staffing, and as people have come to expect more service from hospitals, fewer private duty nurses are seen; hospital nurses now perform the tasks formerly done only by private duty nurses. The trend implies an increased availability and democratization of nursing care in hospitals.

The geographic distribution of nurses in a nation corresponds generally to the location and size of hospitals and ambulatory care centers. Insofar as these facilities are established in rural areas, nurses are ordinarily employed in them. As noted earlier, auxiliary nurses in developing countries are frequently recruited from and trained in a rural district, where they are sensitive to local culture and attitudes. In some isolated rural posts, these auxiliary personnel may be given very broad responsibilities, but they often find themselves confronted with disease problems that they cannot handle. Theoretically they should refer difficult cases to an appropriate facility, but this may be blocked by poverty and inadequate transportation.

Specialized Nurses

After their basic training in a hospital or an academic setting, nurses in many countries may undertake further training to become specialized. This may be in several subdivisions of clinical medicine—such as surgery, pediatrics, obstetrics and gynecology, and gastroenterology. Advanced training for these nursing specialties takes place ordinarily in a large hospital, with departments in the various medical and surgical specialties. These specialties are found mainly in the industrialized countries.

Outside of general hospitals, nurses may become specialized in several fields. To serve in a factory or mine, as an industrial nurse, the nurse works for a period under supervision. The first such specialization was undertaken in England in 1878; the employees of a firm organized a "self-help medical club," to which they made small monthly payments for a nurse and physician. The idea spread slowly to the United States and other countries. After World War I large companies proceeded to appoint industrial nurses for first-aid and care of minor health problems. Equivalent nurses in public schools, to cope with sick or injured children, were appointed in New York City in 1902. School nursing has spread throughout the schools of Europe, America, and elsewhere.

Public health or *district nursing* was also launched in England, by a Liverpool merchant ship owner in 1859. In 1860, a training school and residence for district nurses—to visit the poor in their homes—was established at the Royal Liverpool Infirmary. By 1867, Liverpool had 18 districts served by trained nurses. In 1874, Florence Nightingale wrote an influential pamphlet on *Suggestions for Improving the Nursing Service for the Sick Poor.*

District nurses initially gave bedside care to the sick poor at home, as well as care to isolated cases of communicable disease. Gradually, emphasis shifted to the education of mothers about the care of newborn infants. Preventively oriented maternal and child health (MCH) service became the major function of most public health nurses. This emphasis has persisted, even as infectious disease has declined. In many national health systems, the public health nurse is regarded as a specialist in MCH services.

Another specialization of nursing is in the field of psychiatry. An understanding of the condition of psychotic patients in hospitals requires preparation of a special type. The use of tranquilizing drugs and the *therapeutic community* in mental hospitals, after World War II, led to a greatly increased rate of discharge of psychotic patients and a more active role for the psychiatric nurse. In Great Britain, France, Belgium, and several provinces of Canada, "psychiatric nurses" have been trained from the outset through a curriculum different from that for general registered nurses. In other countries, such as Iceland and the Netherlands, specialized training is given for nurses who serve the mentally handicapped or retarded. Registered nurses may also undertake extra training in psychiatric nursing.

Changing Role of Nurses

Over the years, the scope of functions that nurses have been expected to perform has steadily broadened. The great majority of professional (fully educated) nurses in all countries work in hospitals, and here their technical services have increased with advances in medical diagnosis and treatment. Intensive care units (ICUs) in large hospitals require many more highly trained nurses than the general wards, and such ICU units are increasing. The aging of the population, as people survive into the later decades of life, contributes to this increase. In addition, more institutional beds in almost all countries are being reserved for patients needing long-term care. Although much of this care is given by assistant nurses, regulations and custom demand their supervision by professional nurses.

As more health services are utilized by an increasingly educated population—with economic support from various social sources—the physician passes more tasks along to the nurse. In surgical and medical cases, nurses start and monitor intravenous infusions, catheterizations, the dressing of wounds, and other matters. Under broad surveillance, they administer anesthesia, as a nurse anesthetist. They help with childbirths, even though they may not be trained in midwifery. They also operate X-ray, electrocardiograph, and laboratory equipment.

Outside the hospital, increasing numbers of nurses are demanded by public health agencies and visiting nurse associations. With elderly and chronically ill patients at home, they are called on to give home care through various programs. Industries expand their nursing service, to meet the pressures of factory employment. Nurses are sought by physicians or dentists as office attendants. (This less demanding work may serve as an alternative to the heavy requirements of bedside nursing or supervision.) To staff hospital outpatient departments (OPDs), more extensively trained *nurse practitioners* may be employed—with varying degrees of medical supervision. Along with the "physician assistant," the nurse practitioner was developed in the United States, as a specially qualified nurse, capable of performing many medical and surgical procedures.

In the face of all this heightened demand, the entry of young women into professional nursing in most countries has declined in the 1980s. More women are completing secondary school, but their prospects for training have increased in many other fields, such as medicine, law, management, engineering, higher education, and the clergy. The opportunities for talented women have greatly multiplied, and are no longer so limited to "women's work" as in the past. Even elevated salaries have only partially compensated for the rigors and subordinate social status of the nurse.

Recognizing this reduced attractiveness of professional nursing, many countries have again modified their mixtures of registered and auxiliary nurses. In Great Britain and the Netherlands, this has been noted in the data presented earlier. It is even more apparent in the lower income countries, such as the Philippines, Brazil, Egypt, Zaire, Pakistan, India, or Zimbabwe.

In developing countries generally, professional nurses are often the most highly qualified health care providers available. With the worldwide movement for primary health care, they are called on to provide countless tasks that, in affluent countries, would be done only by physicians.

Midwives

From ancient times, the childbirth process has been attended by older women, who have had many babies of their own, and have helped other women in the delivery process. In classical Greece and Rome, these women had some formal training, but during Medieval times, as medical science declined, midwives learned their skills only from experience. In the sixteenth century, the delivery of babies became an accepted function of physicians—in obstetrics. In 1580, a law in Germany prevented unskilled shepherds and herdsmen from attending childbirth. Normal cases were typically attended by midwives.

Around 1700, a Dutch physician, Hendrick van Deventer, practiced obstetrics and orthopedics in the Hague. He has been called the "father of modern midwifery" because of his book on the structure and functions of the female pelvis in childbirth. Another Dutch physician performed Cesarian sections. These obstetricians did much to improve the education and status of midwives. The Netherlands, Denmark, and Great Britain are countries that have had a strong tradition of trained midwives and nurse-midwives.

Schools for training professional midwives were established in the eighteenth and nineteenth centuries in many European countries, including Sweden, Finland, Norway, and Germany. Japan and New Zealand also train midwives. Customarily, the midwife attended childbirths in the home, but as this process took place increasingly in hospitals in the twentieth century, midwives became employed by hospitals, along with nurses. They carry out most normal deliveries in hospitals, referring complicated cases to physicians.

In Great Britain (1988), more than 20,000 trained midwives worked in the National Health Service, and 81 percent of them were employed within hospitals. They handled (under indirect medical supervision) three-quarters of the childbirths, regarded as normal, and referred complicated cases to a physician. The remaining 19 percent of British midwives work in the general community, providing prenatal and postpartum care in the home, in clinics, and in physician's offices. It is notable that in countries with the lowest infant and maternal mortality rates, the great majority of childbirths are attended by trained midwives. Legislation in several countries (Sweden, Norway, Portugal, and Ireland) requires that midwives be trained first as registered nurses. In most European countries, however, midwife education is parallel with but separate from that for general nurses.

In developing countries that were formerly British colonies, such as India or Burma, many programs for training professional midwives have been established. These curricula are similar in length (3 years after secondary school) to that for nurses, but different in content. There are also 4-year programs for the combined professional nurse-midwife. To work in rural areas, stationed at health centers or health posts, auxiliary midwives are also trained for 1 year after elementary or middle school. Young auxiliary midwives are prepared also in Thailand, the Sudan, and other low-income or middle-income developing countries.

The United States and Canada are unusual in their failure to develop and use the trained midwife. In these countries, the image of midwives as "superstitious and unsanitary old women" has persisted in most states and provinces. Only certain jurisdictions have authorized the training and licensure of professional midwives or nurse-midwives. Nevertheless, as part of the women's liberation movement, the trained midwife is gaining recognition in some excellent medical centers.

In most developing countries of Asia, Africa, and Latin America, the majority of childbirths occur in the mother's home, under the care of *traditional birth attendants* (TBAs). (This term is used to distinguish these empirical women from professionally trained midwives.) TBAs work in rural villages, and win the confidence of women for their skills and understanding. They are abundant in India, the Philippines, Brazil, Nigeria, and elsewhere. The policy of many ministries of health is to recognize reality and to give training in hygiene to the TBA. This also encourages their registration with the government, their supervision, and their co-operation in programs to extend family planning (contraception).

One of the few national surveys of TBAs was conducted in the Philippines in 1974. At least one TBA was found in each of 32,400 *barrios,* yielding an estimated total of 38,000. There was one TBA for about 200 women of child-bearing age. Some 92 percent of them were in rural communities, where 70 percent of the population lived. In the cities, with 30 percent of the population, about 8 percent of the TBAs were located. Almost 100 percent of TBAs were married or widowed. The number of childbirths attended ranged from 1 to 9 per year by 39 percent of TBAs to 30 or more by 16 percent. Nearly 70 percent of the TBAs had learned about attending births from relatives or neighbors; only 19 percent had taken instruction from the Ministry of Health.

Policy toward TBAs in Thailand is like that found in several developing countries, especially if they have an entrepreneurial type of health system. In 1976 there were an estimated 17,000 TBAs in Thailand, or about one for each three villages. In the later 1970s, as part of a national family planning (birth control) program, about 6,400 of these were given a 35-hour course, spread usually over 2 weeks. Their work was then "supervised" by auxiliary midwives in the Ministry of Health network of commune health centers (each serving about 10 villages). In Thailand and similar developing countries, some 60 to 80 percent of babies were delivered by TBAs in 1980, and studies suggest that training them reduces the rate of maternal and neonatal mortality. TBAs are essentially weakly qualified private practitioners, who serve as village mothers. In a few developing countries, such as Cuba, TBAs have been legally suppressed, and childbirths occur mainly in hospitals, attended by physicians. In Nicaragua and most developing countries, however, policy has favored recognizing TBAs, upgrading their performance with training,

and regarding them as part of the private sector of health service delivery.

PHARMACISTS

The preparation and dispensing of drugs—substances for the treatment of disease—go back to ancient times, but the origins of the modern pharmacist can probably be traced to Arabic culture around 1200. Products of vegetable, animal, or mineral origin were imported from Persia and the Orient, and they were kept in highly decorated jars on the shelves of pharmacy shops. Closely linked to the pharmacy shop and its inventory of various drugs is the expert on these matters, the apothecary or pharmacist.

Historic Background

Toward the late thirteenth century, pharmacies appeared in Italy. They followed the Arabian model and first developed in the richer monasteries, then in the royal courts. Later pharmacies appeared under private ownership in the towns. The pharmacist of the fourteenth century was often an astrologer or an alchemist, to whom people attributed magical powers. At this time they had status similar to physicians and in Venice, from 1258 A.D., the two were in the same guild. Later pharmacists and physicians formed separate guilds. Not until the late eighteenth century was a scientific institute for the analysis of drugs established in Germany, bringing a new dignity to pharmacy.

The separation of pharmacy from medicine can be traced, in a sense, to the thirteenth-century edict of Emperor Frederick II, requiring the licensing of physicians. At the same time, pharmaceutical practice was authorized, and business relationships between physician and pharmacist were forbidden. Government supervision of pharmacies, to protect the population, was also established, although we do not know how carefully it was carried out.

With the Renaissance in northern Europe, drug therapy developed along more rational lines. Paracelsus (1493–1541) led a movement to replace Greek humoral pathology with a concept of therapy with various chemicals—particularly of mineral origin. This work and that of the followers of Paracelsus, while done by physicians, helped to establish pharmacy as a special discipline. The pharmacist or, as more often called, the apothecary had special skills with drugs. Yet, he had no formal education, except by apprenticeship. In Venice in 1565, he was required to serve 5 years as an apprentice, 3 years as a clerk, and then pass an examination. During the later Middle Ages, the apothecaries, the barber-surgeons, and also the physicians formed guilds to protect their interests, and to set standards for admission to the guild.

In the meantime, the universities had been turning out physicians for several centuries. The university-trained doctor usually dispensed his own medications and was essentially in competition with the apothecary. The fees charged by the apothecary were usually lower, so that he naturally attracted low-income patients. It was this competition between the two groups that led to the founding of the first *dispensary* by physicians in France around 1640 (later in England). The physician set up places, unconnected with hospitals, for dispensing drugs at low prices, so that the poor would not consult apothecaries. Yet, it was well recognized both in Great Britain and on the continent that the apothecary served as the principal doctor for the poor, especially for the treatment of common ailments. Adam Smith had written at the end of the eighteenth century that the apothecary "is the physician to the poor at all times, and to the rich whenever the distress or danger is not great."

In nineteenth century Britain, apothecaries as well as surgeon–apothecaries were often regarded as general practitioners. Many people were concerned, nevertheless, that they were not subject to any official requirements in education, except the customary apprenticeships. In 1813, therefore, a bill was introduced in the British Parliament "for regulating the practice of Apothecaries, Surgeon-Apothecaries, Practitioners in Midwifery, and Compounders and Dispensers of Medicine throughout England and Wales." This proposal generated a great

deal of controversy, but with numerous modifications it became law in 1815.

One of the changes most disagreeable to the apothecaries was a clause compelling them to compound and dispense prescriptions submitted by physicians. In some ways, this was the beginning of the end for the apothecary, for, as time passed and the numbers of physicians increased along with the emergence of purely pharmaceutical chemists and druggists, more time had to be devoted to compounding and dispensing the doctor's prescriptions, and less could be spent on the independent diagnosis and treatment of patients. This change in role, however, was a slow process that took at least a century to run its course.

In the late eighteenth and early nineteenth centuries, national associations of pharmacists were formed in several countries, and open controversies broke out among physicians about the proper role of each group—particularly those in France and England. Physicians did not want pharmacists to be permitted to diagnose and treat disease, and pharmacists did not want physicians to dispense drugs. Nevertheless, both practices continued throughout the nineteenth century.

From as early as the fourteenth century in Europe, pharmacists had dispensed drug compounds prescribed by physicians, but this did not stop the pharmacists from dispensing other drugs on their own initiative. As both medicine and pharmacy developed technically and socially throughout the nineteenth century, the tendency evolved for physicians to practice medicine, along with dispensing of simpler drugs, and pharmacists to practice pharmacy, along with doing limited diagnosis and treatment. Pharmacists also served as wholesalers, from whom physicians purchased the drugs that they dispensed. In early nineteenth-century America, some physicians operated general pharmacies.

Differentiation between apothecaries, as experts in drugs, and physicians as experts in diagnosing disease, remained unclear until the dawn of the twentieth century, or even later in some countries. Much confusion surrounded terminology. As late as 1933, a British law (the Pharmacy and Poisons Act) recognized the right to sell drugs by: pharmaceutical chemists, pharmaceutists, chemists and druggists, and chemists. There were distinctions among these based on the right to sell poisons, but all had the authority to prepare compounds prescribed by a physician, as well as to dispense their own concoctions.

The first formal education of pharmacists in Europe originated by way of isolated courses in France in the sixteenth century. Education of pharmacists in a university was not required until Austria passed legislation in 1778, and this policy evolved later in other European countries. Physician opposition to university education for pharmacists was effective in France until 1803, and later similar opposition existed in Germany and England. The first pharmacy school in the United States was started in Philadelphia in 1821. In some countries, university graduates were designated as *first class* pharmacists, who could own and operate a pharmacy, whereas those who had learned by apprenticeship were *second class.* It was well into the twentieth century before current standards of university education (typically four or five years of study following secondary school) were generally applied in countries.

In England, the Pharmacy Act of 1868 marked a major turning point; it declared that registration as a *chemist and druggist* required passing an examination of the British Pharmaceutical Society (founded in 1841). This act did not limit the authority of chemists to filling out prescriptions from physicians, although in practice this policy gradually evolved as scientific medicine gained greater popular acceptance. A great lore of secrecy was associated with sickness remedies, guarded zealously by particular apothecaries, pharmacists, or even doctors.

The American Pharmaceutical Association was founded in 1852; elsewhere in Europe local or regional pharmacy societies had been started much earlier, but national associations came later. The various associations attempted to promulgate codes of ethics—opposing quackery, false claims, and adulteration of drugs. Although these codes did not specifically require pharmacists to carry out physi-

cians' orders, they had a similar effect. "Ethical" pharmacists would be expected to carry out functions for which they had been systematically trained.

Other legislation also affected the development of pharmacy, particularly laws concerning the inspection of pharmacy shops. In Paris, the faculty of medicine was charged with the inspection of pharmacies, and only later in 1863 was this authority entrusted to a commission containing three pharmacists and two physicians; mixed commissions of this type (with both physicians and pharmacists) continued in France until 1908. Similar joint medical and pharmaceutical commissions inspected pharmacies in Germany, starting in 1842 and continuing to the present time. In Great Britain, the relevant legislation concerned not the inspection of pharmacies, but the licensure of chemists in 1868, noted above. Similar laws were passed in the states of the United States in the same period, following the Civil War (1861–1865).

It was the growth of a pharmaceutical manufacturing industry in the late nineteenth century, along with the rising effectiveness and status of the medical profession, that led gradually to the disappearance of the apothecary and to the emergence of the pharmacist as the expert in dispensing drugs prescribed by physicians. By 1880, there were already 592 drug companies in the United States and hundreds in Europe. Because their prepackaged products were beyond the average physician's capacity to handle properly, the pharmacist clearly became the expert in storing and dispensing them, as well as understanding their uses. In addition, the pharmacist was the expert in compounding prescriptions for those physicians who were not satisfied with a totally prefabricated product. Mass pharmaceutical production was also facilitated by the replacement of natural substances with synthesized compounds.

This transition of the pharmacist from a competitor to an ally of the doctor came first in the larger cities. Not only were there more patients to serve in the cities, but there were more doctors, with whom the pharmacist naturally wanted to maintain friendly relationships. In rural areas, where pharmacies were rare, physicians continued to maintain their own stock of drugs for dispensing—as they still do in many rural regions today. The same applies, of course, to the rural health center, that has its own small pharmacy (without which it attracts few patients). Pharmacies at any location still sell directly to the patient drugs that— at least in principle under the nation's laws— do not require a medical prescription.

Pharmacists in the Late Twentieth Century

Even today many patients—particularly those of low income—go directly to pharmacists for some medication to reduce their symptoms. In the more developed countries, such drugs available without a medical prescription are defined by law; they may be dispensed *over the counter* (OTC) or directly. In the less developed countries, drug regulation and its enforcement tend to be weaker, and almost any type of drug (except narcotics) may be dispensed OTC for the asking. On the other hand, in rural districts of all types of country, rich and poor, where pharmacies are scarce or lacking, the private doctor may dispense drugs as part of the medical service. Organized health centers for ambulatory care also typically maintain their own drug supplies for dispensing to patients.

The education of pharmacists, in general, is provided in a university setting, and the graduate must be licensed by a governmental authority. In many developing countries, however, where the supply of university-trained pharmacists is low, drugs are handled and dispensed by very briefly trained *dispensers* or *dispensary assistants.* In all types of country, large pharmacies are staffed by various pharmacy clerks as well as professional pharmacists.

The supply of professional pharmacists differs tremendously between the industrialized and the developing countries. In the mid-1970s, their density per 100,000 population in six industrialized and six developing countries was as follows:

Industrialized Countries		Developing Countries	
Norway	33	Afghanistan	0.20
Poland	43	Haiti	0.23
Canada	53	Liberia	0.42
Belgium	68	Malaysia	0.43
United States	71	Indonesia	1.30
Australia	99	Paraguay	2.27

The stock of pharmacists in industrialized countries appears to reflect national health system policy on drugs. The relatively modest ratio in Norway (33 per 100,000 people) was associated with rigorous limitations on the import of pharmaceuticals to that country. The work of the pharmacist is confined essentially to the storage and dispensing of drugs. The much greater supply in Belgium (68 per 100,000) was associated with a welfare-oriented health system that, nevertheless, had a long tradition of free private enterprise. Pharmacy shops may be opened almost anywhere. The very great abundance of pharmacists in Australia (99 per 100,000) was probably linked to that country's enactment of a "Pharmaceutical Benefits Scheme" in 1950—financing from federal tax revenue almost all necessary drugs prescribed for any resident. With so many pharmacists in Australia, at one stage of that country's national health insurance saga, these personnel had been assigned the unusual role of collecting voluntary insurance premiums.

The ample stock of professional pharmacists in the United States (71 per 100,000 people) probably had other meanings. The entrepreneurial U.S. health system has permitted the education of far larger numbers of pharmacists than were required for the dispensing of drugs. The need for skilled pharmacists to *compound* drugs, furthermore, steadily declined. The vast majority of pharmaceuticals in use were prepared and packaged directly by the manufacturers. Thus, pharmacists are seeking roles beyond the maintenance and dispensing of various drugs.

The commonest solution in the United States and also in Canada has been the operation of *drugstores*—shops that sell cosmetics, candy, toothpaste, and so on, as well as drugs. Less frequently pharmacists may perform simple diagnostic tests (such as urinalysis for glucose) and distribute health educational materials. In hospitals, where the institutional pharmacist can monitor the array of drugs prescribed for each patient, he/she can identify the possible hazards of drug interactions—reporting these to physicians. The community pharmacist often seeks to establish the drugstore as a neighborhood center for various health service campaigns.

In developing countries, with diverse types of health systems, the supply of professional pharmacists is obviously small—less than 5 per 100,000. This is in spite of the fact that a relatively large proportion of national health expenditures in these countries goes to purchase drugs. Most of these drugs are dispensed without a prescription by drug sellers with little or no training. In the early 1980s, university-trained pharmacists numbered 4 per 100,000 in Nigeria, 2 per 100,000 in Senegal, and only 0.3 per 100,000 in Kenya. Drug dispensing in Kenya, however, was handled mainly by assistant pharmacists amounting to 2 per 100,000. Developing countries of a transitional economic level, with more welfare-oriented health systems, had more fully trained pharmacists in the 1980s, such as 22 per 100,000 in Peru or 28 per 100,000 in Costa Rica.

In Asian countries, such as Indonesia (with an entrepreneurial health system) or Malaysia (with a welfare-oriented system), many drug shops are operated by traditional Chinese herbalists. These small shops are not usually regarded as pharmacies, under law, nor are their proprietors licensed as pharmacists. They are registered simply as "small businesses." Indonesia had only 2 fully trained pharmacists per 100,000 in the 1980s, but 14 assistant pharmacists.

In some Latin American countries, the rare pharmacist may give drug injections to patients, who otherwise would have a long trip to a physician or health facility. In the formerly socialist countries of Eastern Europe pharmacists ranged from 22 per 100,000 in the German Democratic Republic to 47 per 100,000

(with another 43 assistant pharmacists) in Bulgaria. In summary, the supply of professional pharmacists or even "assistant pharmacists" in developing countries is typically much smaller than the need; in the industrialized countries (especially those with more entrepreneurial health systems), the supply of pharmacists is actually excessive and these personnel are seeking new roles in the delivery of health service.

DENTISTS AND ALLIED DENTAL PERSONNEL

The professional dentist (sometimes, stomatologist) and various types of auxiliary dental personnel are of relatively recent origin. For centuries in the Middle Ages the treatment of diseased teeth consisted essentially of extractions by almost any friendly neighbor. Barbers, travelling artisans (tooth-pullers), and others also did these extractions, when they were not done ingeniously by relatives or friends. By the eighteenth century physicians extracted diseased and painful teeth, using a suitable grasping instrument.

The first school of dentistry was organized in Germany in 1824, but the discipline did not really develop in Europe. Unlike the other health professions, dentistry developed scientifically and technologically mainly in the United States, after the first dental school was launched in Baltimore in 1840. The first university-based school was founded at Harvard in 1867. It was to America that students from Europe and elsewhere flocked for education on the restoration of carious teeth and the replacement of lost teeth with dental prostheses.

Advances in the prosthetic replacement of teeth in the United States led naturally to the training of various skilled technicians. The objective of prevention and dental health promotion was also put forward in America; dental hygienists were trained to educate school children and to clean the teeth or do *prophylaxes* in both children and adults. Motor-driven dental equipment, particularly high-speed drilling instruments, brought great technological progress to modern dentistry, and led to the use of various aides and assistants at the dental chairside. These capabilities raised the professional status of dentists, but did not reduce their resistance to the rationalization of dental tasks—equivalent to the delegation to nurses of many formerly medical tasks.

In relation to dental need, there is a serious shortage of dental personnel throughout the world. Even in the wealthiest nations, there are not enough dentists to meet the basic needs. A high proportion of American children, for example, do not see a dentist once during the year, even though the United States has a relatively high supply of dentists—about 59 per 100,000 people in 1984. Sweden has probably the highest national supply of dentists—about 110 per 100,000 in 1984. In the countries of Africa, the dentist–population ratio was about 1 per 100,000 or fewer in the 1980s. In countries of Asia dentists also numbered only 1 or 2 per 100,000 in the 1980s. Even in Western Europe, outside the Scandinavian countries, fully qualified dentists were fewer than 75 per 100,000. The socialist countries of Eastern Europe had greater supplies of stomatologists and *dentistas,* two levels of professional dentist.

The most practical and effective approach to the problem of dental care has been pioneered by New Zealand. In 1920, this small country in the South Pacific started a program of training *dental nurses* to work in the schools and give complete dental care to children. Dental nurses receive two years of training in a special center, following high school. Yet their functions are far broader than those performed by the dental hygientist, first trained in America in 1916, and found now in Europe and elsewhere. The hygienist's work is largely confined to cleaning teeth and educating on dental hygiene, whereas the dental nurse does fillings, extractions (rarely necessary), and of course prophylactic work under the only occasional supervision of a dentist. With equipment located in the schools, dental nurses are able to serve large numbers of children efficiently. World Health Organization observers have found the quality of their work to be highly satisfactory, even though it is done more slowly than that of the professional dentist. In some countries this form of dental worker is known

as a *dental therapist* or *dental auxiliary,* but the functions are equivalent.

Although the concept of the dental nurse has been highly controversial in many countries, it has been emulated enthusiastically in about 20 nations; these are mainly in the British Commonwealth (e.g. in Malaysia), most recently in several provinces of Canada. The 2-year training program of dental nurses is, of course, far less costly than the 5- to 8-year university training required for professional dentists. Dental nurses are remunerated at a much more modest level than are dentists, whether paid by fees or salary. Moreover, it has simply not been possible to attract enough dentists into work with children. According to WHO, in 1975 these operating dental auxiliaries numbered 9 per 100,000 in the industrialized countries and only one per 100,000 in the developing countries.

Although the ratio of dentists to population has not been increasing at the same rate as that of physicians, and in some countries has even declined, the net output of dental service has increased almost everywhere. The reason is a much expanded use of chairside dental assistants and the availability of more efficient equipment, such as high-speed drills. For many years dental assistants were trained on the job in dental offices or clinics, but since about 1920 special courses of 1 or 2 years have been offered; there are 23 such dental assistant training programs in the United States, where this service is most highly developed.

The dental technician or mechanic is the person who prepares dental prostheses—partial or complete dentures to replace the natural teeth. In the more developed countries, these personnel (usually men) work in dental laboratories on the basis of castings submitted by dentists. In the developing countries, however, and even to some extent in provinces of developed countries (e.g., Australia and Canada), there are "denturists" who serve patients directly and provide complete upper and/or lower dentures to persons whose teeth have been totally extracted. Essentially they are dental mechanics, to whom the population has direct access at much lower costs than through the channel of a dentist. Although not always officially licensed, the denturist is a social response to the need for major restorations of teeth in poor people.

OTHER CLINICAL HEALTH PERSONNEL

There are many other types of health personnel in national health systems, particularly in highly developed countries. Large medical centers, providing elaborate diagnostic and treatment service, may employ scores of types of special technicians, therapists, and aides.

Diagnostic and Therapeutic Technicians

The numbers and ratios of diagnostic technicians in a country are a good reflection of the technological development of its health system. In developing countries, laboratory technicians numbered only 2 per 100,000 population in 1975, compared with 43 per 100,000 in the industrialized countries. For radiological technicians the comparison in 1975 was 2 per 100,000 in the developing countries and 19 in the industrialized countries. These great disparities may even understate the real differences, insofar as the industrialized countries have a great deal of automated equipment that even augments the productivity of technicians. (These comparisons, of course, should not imply that developing countries ought to try to reach the technological level of industrialized countries, which may well be excessive even for their own needs.)

Among these diagnostic technicians in affluent countries there may also be subspecialties—for example, technicians skilled in biochemical tests, as against bacteriological work. In a few affluent countries, these technicians may be trained in university courses, but in most they are prepared in technical institutes for 1 or 2 years after secondary school.

Before the twentieth century, examinations of urine or blood or body exudates were performed by physicians or pharmacists, who had some understanding of chemistry. With the discovery of bacteria and the greatly extended use of microscopy in the nineteenth century, hygienic laboratories—for examining specimens for infectious organisms—had been established. The first hygienic laboratory for this

explicit purpose was set up in Munich, Germany in 1866.

The great bacteriological discoveries came from Europe, but their application was more rapidly developed in America. In 1888, public health laboratories were organized in Rhode Island by C. V. Chapin and in Michigan by Victor Vaughan. A larger diagnostic laboratory service was established in New York City by Hermann Biggs in 1893, following a scare from the cholera epidemic in Germany. The initial purpose was simply to identify bacterial causes of disease. A federal Hygienic Laboratory was set up in Washington, D.C. in 1902.

In the early twentieth century, large hospitals developed diagnostic laboratories for the same bacteriological purpose. Many patients had infectious diseases, that required identification by microscopic examination. As noninfectious diseases, such as diabetes or nephritis, became better understood, crucial chemical tests of the urine or blood were developed. Hospital laboratories for *clinical pathology* (in contrast to public health or hygienic laboratories) were initially operated by hospital physicians on a part-time basis. As the volume of work increased, hospitals trained young high school graduates, usually women, to perform various tests. With further advancement of organ pathology, these technicians learned to stain tissue specimens and examine them microscopically.

Around 1920, large hospitals both in Europe and America began to set up formal training programs for laboratory technicians. As more knowledge was acquired, the course of training became longer, and in some countries hospital-based training was linked with university education in the basic sciences. Eventually technicians or technologists were trained in specialized fields, such as microbiology, chemical analyses, and tissue pathology. In the less developed countries, various types of *assistant technician* were trained in hospitals for special tasks, such as examination of blood smears for malaria parasites or of sputum for tubercle bacilli.

Other technological developments gave rise to still other specialized personnel. The rapid development of radiography after 1900 gave rise to the trained X-ray technician, and the development of electrocardiography generated the ECG technician. Various types of rehabilitation therapist were trained to help the large numbers of disabled soldiers (and also civilians) after World War I and World War II. Schools for the education and rehabilitation of crippled children can be traced to institutions in Germany and Italy in the early nineteenth century, but formal training of physiotherapists and occupational therapists came much later. Advances in nutrition in the twentieth century gave rise to the nutritionist and, on a more practical level, the dietician.

As public health developed, still other specialized personnel were formally prepared. In the early twentieth century, for environmental protection various types of sanitary inspector or sanitarian were trained—usually in public health agencies (in a few countries, at universities). Health education became a special public health discipline after World War II. The maintenance of records and statistics in public health programs, as well as in hospitals, generated the specialist in health records and later in *health information systems.* As national health systems become more complex, sophisticated administrative skills are required. Physicians are often assigned supervisory roles in hospitals and health programs, but the value of trained *health administrators* or *health managers* has become increasingly recognized. The technical or professional level to which all these types of personnel are trained varies greatly among countries; it tends to be higher in the affluent industrialized countries and lower in the less developed countries.

On the therapeutic side, there are technicians skilled in operating renal dialysis machines and similar equipment. Inhalation therapists and plaster cast technicians are other personnel categories. Rehabilitation of patients with serious physical disabilities includes *therapists* for physical, occupational, and speech therapy. These personnel help the patient to regain body functions through carefully planned exercises and the use of special equipment. Some patients may require braces, artificial limbs, or other prosthetic appliances, which are prepared by other personnel. Very few of these rehabilitation workers, however, are available outside the industrialized countries. After World War II, with thousands of crippled people in Europe, Japan, and America, these countries naturally promoted the development of rehabilitation services. Special rehabilitation facilities sometimes housed these several types of personnel, but they gradually became absorbed into the staffs of general hospitals, especially large ones. The skills required for testing hearing have become the domain of audiologists in highly developed countries, and the selection and adjustment of prosthetic hearing aids are done by other special personnel.

Still other types of specialized health personnel may be available outside hospital settings, as well as in them. The clinical psychologist does psychometric testing in schools and clinics, and in many countries participates in treating emotionally disturbed patients. The social worker, in the outpatient department of hospitals or in ambulatory care units, tries to help patients adjust to their environment or to change the environment for the patient's welfare. All these specialized personnel are most frequently available in the highly developed countries. In developing countries, the functions of these personnel may be performed by nurses or others.

In some countries the roles of two categories of specialized personnel may be combined into one. In France, there are *social assistants* (assistantes sociales) who are trained to do the work of both social worker and public health nurse. In rural prairie regions of Canada, small hospitals have *combined technicians* who carry out both laboratory and radiological procedures. On an informal basis in developing countries such multipurpose roles are doubtless commonly assumed by doctors, nurses, and general health auxiliaries.

Specialized Community Practitioners

Beyond technicians, working directly or indirectly under medical supervision, there are specialized community practitioners, who are not physicians but who diagnose and treat common disorders of certain body organs— particularly the eyes and the feet. Patients ordinarily seek care from them directly, without necessarily any referral from a physician.

Visual refractions in many industrialized countries are provided by optometrists or *dispensing opticians.* Their course of training varies greatly among countries; in the United States it is university based and leads to an academic degreee, but in most countries it involves a vocational course of about 2 years after secondary school. The legally authorized scope of optometrists is strictly limited to prescribing eyeglasses for correction of refractive errors, and excludes the treatment of any other disorders of the eye. It is expected that patients with other eye conditions (e.g., infections or cataracts) will be referred to ophthalmologists.

The grinding of lenses and preparation of eyeglasses or spectacles are tasks done by opticians or optical companies. In most developing countries and in some industrialized countries, only opticians (and not optometrists) are available, since all refractions are done by medical ophthalmologists. It is not a secret that in many countries ophthalmologists (also called oculists) have effectively blocked the development of optometry, to reduce competition. As populations become more educated and interested in reading, the need for personnel, skilled in visual refractions, increases. With high demands for eyeglasses, it is obviously wasteful for physicians to do refractive work that can be done well by optometrists.

The care of the foot has also generated a special type of health personnel—the podiatrist or chiropodist. These personnel are limited essentially to the affluent industrialized countries; elsewhere the treatment of superficial foot conditions (bunions, dermatitis, etc.) is done by physicians. In the industrialized countries, of course, the nearly universal wearing of shoes, often poorly fitted, gives rise to these foot problems—especially in the elderly. Podiatrists in most countries that have them are trained for 2 years in a technical school. In the United States, with its tendency to upgrade all health occupations, podiatry requires a 4-year university course.

Finally in the sphere of community health work, there are various types of personnel concerned with environmental controls. In most countries they are known as sanitary inspectors, health inspectors, or sanitarians. Their preparation usually requires a year or two of technical studies after secondary school, but for directing environmental sanitation in a region, university education may be required. For detection of hazards at the workplace and promotion of occupational health and safety, there are industrial hygienists whose educational preparation is extensive. In developing countries auxiliary health personnel trained for only a few weeks may do vector-control work, such as DDT spraying of houses to combat malaria. Community health work may also require personnel for other restricted tasks, such as vaccinators, family-planning advisors, or venereal disease investigators.

PUBLIC HEALTH ADMINISTRATORS

Perhaps the most recently recognized category of support personnel in the health services throughout the world is the specialist in health service administration. For centuries, it was assumed that the top administrative authority in any organized health program, either within institutional walls or on a community basis, had to be a physician. The physician might be assisted by fiscal or other administrative aides, but final authority rested with the doctor. This policy still prevails in many countries, especially the poorer ones where the market for private medical services has not been as great. It was in the United States that the first formal training programs developed for public health administrators, and later hospital and other administrators, who were not necessarily physicians.

When the U.S. school of public health was first pioneered (jointly by Harvard University and the Massachusetts Institute of Technology) in 1916, and the first school of hospital administration was established (at the University of Chicago) in 1934, the focus was primarily to train physicians for these administrative responsibilities. Gradually, as the demands for effective administrators increased more rapidly than the supply of physicians who chose to enter this work (in the face of the generally more lucrative rewards of private practice), persons with other academic backgrounds were welcomed into these schools. These included nurses and other health professionals, as well as graduates in engineering, social sciences, general administration, and so on. Gradually, especially since World War II, schools of public health have been established on every continent. Some of these are still oriented mainly to the postgraduate training of physicians, but most offer training to nutritionists, public health nurses, statisticians, health educators, environmentalists, health planners, and various types of administrators.

Since 1948, the World Health Organization has compiled information on postgraduate education in public health throughout the world. The trend in such training programs has been as follows:

Year	Countries	Schools
1968	42	100
1972	44	121
1985	54	216

The trend in growth of these schools undoubtedly reflects a response to the increasingly recognized need for trained public health personnel, but one must ask whether the response has been proportional to the needs.

Of the 216 centers for higher education in public health, as of 1985, 78 were independent colleges and 138 were departments in a medical school that offered some postgraduate training (as well as teaching undergraduate medical students). These latter included 20 departments in formerly socialist countries, which were part of postgraduate medical institutes, that had no undergraduate medical students.

Most of these educational programs were sponsored by universities. Of the 78 independent schools, 50 were in universities and 28 were within the jurisdiction of Ministries of Health. Of the 138 centers that were departments of medical faculties, 104 were sponsored by the parent university and 34 were sponsored by Ministries of Health.

Student enrollment for postgraduate training in public health throughout the world is surprisingly small. WHO asked the schools to report on the number of students in the basic public health degree or diploma course— wording intended to rule out undergraduate

medical or related students, as well as graduate students in fields of study other than public health. The world total for the early 1980s was 19,533 students. This comes to about 90 students per training center.

The distribution of students is heavily skewed toward the independent schools. These schools, constituting 36 percent of the total, had 12,459 students enrolled or 64 percent of all the students. (In fact, 77 percent of these or 9,549 were in the 23 independent schools of the United States.) The remaining students who were in departments of medical faculties were divided between 4,096 in postgraduate medical institutes of socialist countries and 2,978 in the 118 medical schools where the teaching staff is mainly occupied with undergraduate medical students. Thus the average enrollment of postgraduate public health students in customary medical schools is about 25 (the median being much smaller), compared to an average enrollment in the independent schools of public health of 160 students. This contrast in enrollment is significant. It undoubtedly reflects the relative potentials for growth of schools that are independent or free standing, compared with those that are part of medical faculties, dominated inevitably by clinicians and laboratory-based scientists.

The advantages of independent status for schools of public health may explain why they tend generally to be stronger institutions. Aside from larger average student enrollments, their faculty resources are also much greater— an average of 41 full-time staff in the independent schools and 17 in the medical school departments. Both types of school make great use of part-time faculty. More important, the 17 teachers in the average medical school department must also spend a great share of their time with undergraduate medical students, whereas the 41 teachers in the average independent school can devote their entire time to postgraduate teaching and research.

Of the departments that constitute a medical school, the department for preventive and social medicine or public health tends to have the lowest rank. In the world of biomedical science, oriented to sick individual patients, an orientation to populations commands little respect. This translates into a lean allocation of resources for faculty posts, space, curriculum time, books and equipment, and for all the resources essential to effective education. Ultimately one must ask whether public health is, indeed, a branch of medicine? Modern public health is a highly interdisciplinary field, to which medical science makes some contribution among many others. In 1953, Yale University Professor C.-E. A. Winslow wrote, "Public health is not a branch of medicine or engineering, but a profession dedicated to a community service which involves cooperative effort of a dozen different disciplines."

The count of disciplines today is clearly higher, and most of them would probably be closer to the social than to the biomedical sciences.

One other feature of higher education in public health warrants emphasis, if one sets out to compare the two types of academic setting. With some exceptions, the departments of medical schools admit only physicians for postgraduate study. The great majority of the independent schools admit public health personnel of diverse backgrounds—nurses, pharmacists, economists, sociologists, statisticians, engineers, architects, nutritionists, psychologists, business or public administrators, laboratory technologists, physiotherapists, record analysts, educators, sanitarians, and many others, in addition to physicians. Patterns of instruction vary. In some schools there are special academic "tracks" for persons of a particular background. In others, all students are enrolled in classes together. The constant interchange of ideas that this mixture of students makes possible is regarded by many as adding a special value to the educational experience.

MEDICAL ASSISTANTS AND COMMUNITY HEALTH WORKERS

Because of their mounting importance in modern health systems, we should examine the background of health care auxiliaries. There are two types: (1) *medical assistants,* who are trained for 2 or 3 years as doctor substitutes, and (2) *community health workers,* who are trained for only a few months to pro-

vide primary health care. Neither of these is to be confused with the traditional practitioner, who is descended from the prescientific era. Both medical assistant and community health worker provide services as part of an organized framework.

The earliest medical assistant, trained to work in a scientific medical setting was probably associated with the barber–surgeons attached to European armies as early as the fifteenth century. In the armies of Peter the Great, Czar of Russia in the seventeeth century, field-barbers were used extensively, because the military forces were so large and trained physicians so few. They were identified by the German term *feldsher,* and their military use continued into the nineteenth century. In 1861 serfdom was abolished in Russia, and in 1864 a scheme of local government was introduced by Czar Alexander II. The local district assembly, representing mainly landowners, was known as the *zemstvo* and had responsibility for health services. The zemstvo health service, however, had very few doctors, and the personnel solution was to appoint military feldshers, retired from the armed forces.

In 1864, five schools for feldshers were opened to prepare them more appropriately for work in rural areas. By 1900, these had grown to 32 schools, and graduate feldshers outnumbered physicians by two-to-one in Russia. By then, women were also being trained as *feldsher-midwives,* and these were extensively used at health posts in the vast rural stretches of Czarist Russia. By the time of the Russian Revolution in 1917, there were 65 feldsher or feldsher-midwife schools, and the course had been extended to 4 years.

Despite the feldsher's training, the prevailing philosophy of Czarist Russia was that he was "good enough for the peasants," whose ailments were considered "simpler" than those of city-dwellers; besides, feldshers were much less expensive to support than physicians, even if the latter could be persuaded to work in rural areas. It is easy to understand, therefore, why after the Revolution, feldsher training was discontinued as "second-class medicine." Training enough physicians to serve both the rural and urban populations, however, was an enormous task. The government then decided, therefore, to retain the feldsher, give him more systematic training, and back him up with reliable medical supervision. Not until recent years, when the supply of physicians in the Soviet Union became very great, was the policy on feldshers changed again. In thinly settled rural areas, feldsher-midwife posts are still important, but most feldshers are assigned to specialized tasks in industrial hygiene, school health work, emergency service, laboratory technology, or environmental sanitation.

In the nineteenth century an entirely different path of development toward health auxiliaries arose from colonialism, dominated by European powers. Medical missionaries were often the first scientifically trained physicians to come to Africa and Asia, and in the small stations or even hospitals that they established, local men would be hired to serve as "dressers" or medical aides; their only training at first was by observation on the job. David Livingstone, who in 1840 was one of the first European explorers of central Africa, was also a medical missionary.

One of the earliest programs for formal training of these auxiliary health personnel was in Jamaica, which had been taken over by the British in 1665. In 1845, a network of dispensaries and rural hospital outposts was established; these were staffed by native *dispensers,* who had learned a little from British doctors in sugar and banana estate "hospitals." Finally in 1878 a program was organized for formal training of dispensers. If these medical assistants passed an examination, given by government physicians, they were allowed to sell herbal preparations as private practitioners in rural areas. Slavery was abolished in Jamaica in 1838 (well before such action in the United States), but Jamaica gained independence from the British only in 1962. A modern medical school had been established in 1954, and the new chapter in the training and use of health auxiliaries began in the 1970s.

Another approach—the use and training of explicitly "second class" surgeons and physicians from indigenous people—was applied in India. The Indian Medical Service may be traced to British medical missionaries who came to India with the East India Company after 1700. A directory of medical personnel serving the company was issued in 1764, and in that year accounts about Bengal, Madras, Bombay, and Calcutta made reference to *head surgeons* and *surgeon's mates.* Later, the engagement of local men led to designations of *subordinate* and *assistant surgeons.* These lower level doctors were apparently trained at regular medical schools, such as Madras University Medical School, but the passing grade was set at 33 percent (for the regular student it was 50 percent), and the duration of study was 3 instead of 5 years. Later, separate colleges for assistant surgeons were established with a 4-year curriculum. These Indian policies of training lower level doctors, rather than explicit medical assistants, influenced other colonial health systems.

In 1878, for example, the Fiji School of Medicine was founded for training vaccinators, and in 1886 it became a school for preparing "assistant medical officers" in a 3-year course. Only around 1970 did it become a duly recognized medical school for training physicians. Similar developments occurred in Africa after 1918—in Nigeria, Tanzania, Sudan, and even in independent Ethiopia. At the beginning, the schools in all these and other African countries offered an abridged type of medical education, with limited basic science, weak teaching staff, simplified examinations, and a generally "vocational" rather than scientific orientation. Only after World War II did the schools evolve from units for training second-class or "assistant doctors" to full-fledged medical schools producing licensed physicians.

Sometimes, as in the Sudan, formal training of medical auxiliaries was the avowed motive at the outset. Here in 1924, a school of medical assistants required only 4 years of elementary education for entry, and the training course lasted 18 months. Later in 1940, another school required 6 years of elementary school plus several years of auxiliary nursing experience for entry. The curriculum lasted 2 years, but the graduates were still less than fully qualified physicians. In Uganda, the later well-recognized medical school at Makerere had started in 1927 as a school for "senior African medical assistants." It evolved into the Makerere University Medical College only after 1952, when a school specifically for training medical assistants was established elsewhere. Developments in Kenya broadly paralleled those in Uganda, with eventual development of decentralized schools for medical assistants in several provinces.

In former French colonies, after the First World War, schools for medical assistants were established, and they continued to serve this purpose. In Hanoi, Indochina a school for both civilian and military medical auxilaries was established in 1924. The course lasted for 4 years—including both theoretical and clinical studies—but the graduates were always designated as *assistant doctors.* Similar policies were applied in the French colonies of Africa; the training, however, was shorter. In Senegal, a basic course lasting 1 year was offered; those who performed poorly became aides, whereas those who did well could study for an additional year to become "basic auxiliary health workers." After several years of experience, these personnel could become *technical health agents* and staff the dispensaries and health centers.

After World War II, and the achievement of national independence by nearly all the former European colonies in Africa and Asia, at first the health policies of the previous colonial power were continued. Soon, however, regular medical schools for preparing physicians were organized almost everywhere, and at the same time the training of medical assistants was generally increased. Additional schools were established, and the content of their teaching programs was often strengthened. Although the various types of medical assistant were theoretically supposed to work under medical supervision, physicians were so few, outside the hospitals, that their work was largely performed independently. In the interests of turning out greater numbers of health personnel, the duration of training of various new types of health auxiliaries was frequently quite short.

In the 1940s, Ethiopia—one of the few African countries that was, in fact, not a colony—started a training program at the town of Gondar for medical assistants and dressers. In 1950 a "rural health demonstration program and teaching center" was operating in the Philippines, with World Health Organization sponsorship; in addition to practical nurses and assistant doctors, *village health workers* were trained here. In 1953 a "Rural Health Services Scheme" was launched in Malaysia, including a brief 1-year training program for *assistant nurses* and *assistant midwives;* although their functions were initially limited to maternal and child health service, they were later broadened to general primary health care. Treatment of the sick at Malaysian rural health centers, however, is still done by the preindependence *hospital assistant* (always male), whose training has been extended to 3 years after secondary school. In Sri Lanka, the "apothecaries" from the colonial days were upgraded after independence to *assistant medical practitioners,* prepared through a 2-year course after secondary school. In the later 1950s, many other developing countries—such as Iran, Somalia, Papua New Guinea, Libya, and Zanzibar—launched training programs for "assistant medical officers" or "assistant doctors." (These were all types of medical assistant.)

In Latin America, until recently, opposition from the medical profession retarded the development of both medical assistants and community health workers (CHWs). The nurse, however, as the doctor's helper, was accepted, and assistant nurses often serve as general health auxiliaries in rural villages. Although these were usually young village women, in some Latin American countries men, trained originally as sanitary inspectors, were given some clinical orientation and sent out to staff rural health posts in the same way. Since about 1970 several Latin American countries have developed the *promotore de salud* or health promoter. Pioneered in Venezuela under the slogan of "simplified medicine" ("medicina simplificada") this community health worker was deliberately trained for clinical duties, without the pretense of serving as a nurse. Elementary school (six grades) completion is usually required and the training program lasts about 6 months. U.S. Peace Corps nurses and doctors have also trained rural health promoters in some countries, such as Ecuador. In Guatemala a program for training *rural health technicians (technicos de salud rural* or TSRs) was launched in the 1970s, requiring completion of secondary school and 2 years of training.

Even in a very developed country, such as the United States, the extremely high degree of medical specialization resulted in a shortage of general practitioners for primary medical care. In the 1960s, when this issue became critical, medical corpsmen were returning home from the Vietnam War, and several training centers recognized their potential as medical auxiliaries in areas of doctor shortage. They were given supplemental training to serve as *physician's assistants,* and provide general primary care under medical supervision. As noted earlier, nurses soon recognized the opportunity for these broadened functions, and became trained, typically in 1-year special courses, as nurse practitioners. This concept, however, was not adopted in Western Europe, where general practitioners were more plentiful and where national health financing programs assured everyone legal entitlement to attention by physicians.

In 1965, a dramatic change occurred in the concept of health auxiliaries. Only 16 years after its revolution, China had widespread social and political disturbances, known as the "Great Proletarian Cultural Revolution." As part of this, the deficiencies of rural health services were vehemently condemned. In response, a new type of community health worker was trained. Peasants from the agricultural communes were briefly trained in a health center or hospital—for 3 to 6 months. They were then expected to continue work in the fields, and serve part-time as the general health auxiliary to a *production brigade* of 400 to 600 people. These community health workers were called *barefoot doctors* and hundreds of thousands were rapidly prepared; each year they were required to take additional instruction for 2 or 3 weeks. By 1980, well over one million barefoot doctors were at work in China, and the sheer magnitude of this accomplishment impressed the entire world.

Around 1970 a major spurt occurred in the recognition by countries of the value of community health workers. Policies of the World Health Organization, to achieve much greater health care coverage of rural areas in developing countries, doubtless contributed to this.

Accomplishments of the vast program for training and using *barefoot doctors* in China were doubtless another influence. These community health workers were reported to be reaching, with elementary primary care, the immense rural population in China's agricultural communes. More and more countries established or expanded CHW training programs. In 1978 the Conference on Primary Health Care, sponsored by WHO and UNICEF in Alma Ata (USSR), gave a dramatic boost to the CHW concept as a practical strategy for rapidly attaining health care coverage of rural populations in developing countries. As its historical development reflects, the exact meaning of community health worker—his/her training, supervision, functions, and so on—differs widely today among countries.

After the Alma Ata Conference, many developing countries undertook training of community health workers with new enthusiasm. The greatest initiatives were shown by countries of Asia and Africa. Large CHW training programs were launched in India, Burma, Nepal, Bangladesh, and Sudan. Zimbabwe developed a strong program, as did Tanzania. Since CHWs at the outset were often not paid, they were called *community health volunteers,* although eventually some small remuneration was usually given. The quality of CHW performance, however, has often been found deficient because of weak supervision.

The schedules of training, the functions, the degree of supervision, and other features of both medical assistants and CHWs display bewildering variations around the world. In developing countries—particularly those with low levels of literacy—the expectation of basic education prerequisites is usually very modest; often four grades of elementary school are considered enough. The CHW training course tends to be very short—around 3–9 months—with great reliance placed on learning through experience. In the more highly developed countries, where the population's general level of education and literacy is high, admission to training as a medical assistant may require completion of 8 to 12 years of basic education. The training course tends to require a minimum of 1 year or more often 2 or 3.

Because of this great diversity, and the lack

of a satisfactory scheme of classification, there are few national or international data on the numbers or ratios to population of these auxiliary personnel. One can say only that many countries of all types are showing increasing appreciation of the value of medical assistants and CHWs. Even the United States, with all its health personnel, developed physician's assistants (followed by nurse practitioners) as recently as the 1970s, in compensation for insufficient general medical practitioners. Most industrialized countries recognize the value of auxiliaries mainly for reasons of economy. The high cost of physicians leads naturally to the search for other less costly personnel who can perform certain functions perfectly well. So long as various personnel work as a team—a concept fully accepted for inpatient hospital care—health tasks can be divided among team members with no loss of quality.

In developing countries, the increasing use of community health workers is partly due to economic considerations, but principally a response to the urgent problems of achieving primary health care coverage for large rural populations. As noted earlier, medical schools have multiplied in developing countries, especially since 1945, and thousands of new doctors have been turned out. Except for temporary periods of mandatory rural service, however, the vast majority of these physicians settle in the larger cities. Most countries are not willing to make medical care a basic public service, with all physicians employed by government and stationed where needed. A "free trade" concept in medicine has left the rural areas in virtually all developing countries seriously underserved. Community health workers are the logical and feasible solution for the present.

In perhaps one respect, it is possible to generalize about CHW personnel. Their training is almost always provided in settings and under sponsorships outside the nation's general educational system. It is not given in either universities, polytechnical institutes, vocational schools, or other training units coming under the supervision of a Ministry of Education. Even hospitals, where nurses and various technicians are trained, play only a small part. Community health workers are trained predominantly in rural health centers or other facilities for ambulatory care. Responsibility is typically assumed by a Ministry of Health or one of its subdivisions at provincial or local levels. CHWs are also typically employed by government and stationed in areas where the public health authority considers them most needed.

CURRENT PANORAMA OF HEALTH PERSONNEL

These sketches of the background and current features of the main types of health personnel may be enough to suggest the variety of health-related professions and occupations functioning in countries today. In affluent and industrialized countires, the disciplines are more varied and complicated than in the developing and agricultural countries. Everywhere there are physicians, regarded as the top experts in modern medical science and technology, although their numbers and ratios to population in many developing countries may be extremely low. To treat their ailments, people in some of these countries may have to rely on the help of practitioners who follow doctrines that were formulated centuries before the modern scientific era. The practitioner of traditional Chinese medicine and the Ayurvedic doctor of India often learn these doctrines in formal schools. In most developing countries, however, particularly in their rural areas, people must often depend on traditional healers who have had no formal education, except perhaps by apprenticeship to an older healer.

It should be apparent that in developing countries there is a manifest delineation of health care responsibilities among allied health workers along sex lines. Personal preventive services, especially for babies and expectant mothers, are given by women at various levels of nurse, but the diagnosis and treatment of disease in any patient are usually done by men. One can hardly doubt that this policy springs from the prejudices of male-dominated societies, in which women are not entrusted with the more critical decisions of treating the sick. It is also related to the historic origins of many of the doctor substitutes from the military services—such as the original nineteenth-century Russian feldsher, some African dressers, or the latter-day American *Medex* from the Vietnam War. When emancipation or liberation of women has become a top national priority, as it did in the postrevolutionary Soviet Union, or in modern Cuba, this policy abruptly changes. Not only are many of the Soviet feldshers women, but more than half of the new physicians in Cuba and the Soviet Union are likewise women. The same applies in China.

In contrast to both physicians and traditional healers, who attempt to treat every type of illness, in many affluent countries there are various secondary practitioners, often formally trained, to whom the population has direct access for special health conditions. Among such practitioners are optometrists (in some countries call opticians) for visual refractions, podiatrists (or chiropodists) for cure of superficial foot conditions, and midwives or nurse-midwives for care of pregnant women and delivery of babies. Midwives may be formally trained or they may be untrained and older village women, somewhat equivalent to the traditional healers who are generally men. These practitioners are not to be confused with cultists (often legally recognized), who attempt to treat all disorders with one technique, such as manipulation of the spine by chiropractors.

Nurses, broadly defined, are the most abundant type of health worker in most countries. The term *nurse* emcompasses fully trained professional nurses, as well as a variety of auxiliary nurses with much less training and basic education. In most industrialized countries, professional nurses are the largest share of the total, but in developing countries various types of auxiliary nurse are usually the most numerous. The scope of functions authorized for each type of nurse differs greatly between countries and sometimes between the urban and rural districts within one country.

Auxiliary to the doctor for special tasks is a diversity of other health personnel, more of them being found in the highly developed countries. There are technicians for laboratory examination of body fluids, excreta, or tissues; radiographic or radiological technicians to operate X-ray machines; a specialized ECG tech-

nician for the electrocardiograph; and a dietician who is the technical expert in food selection and preparation for the sick and the well. For various modalities in rehabilitation there are physical therapists, occupational therapists, and speech therapists. For testing hearing there may be audiologists. In addition to the psychiatrist, there may be psychologists and psychiatric social workers. Similarly, a general medical social worker may assist any type of doctor in helping the patient to cope with sickness and make use of all community resources. Moreover, ancillary to all these health workers may be a second echelon of auxiliary personnel, such as the laboratory assistant or the physical therapy assistant.

With the expanding organization of health services, both curative and preventive, a whole spectrum of public health personnel has come to be necessary. These may be specialists in medicine, nursing, and other fields, or they may be wholly different types of health workers such as environmental sanitarians (sometimes called inspectors), sanitary engineers, nutritionists, health educators, or vaccinators. Health administrators may have technical competence in a clinical field or they may be trained specifically for administration of hospitals, clinics, or other health care organizations.

As new technologies develop, still further classes of health worker are trained. The inhalation therapist, a recent example, is trained in the special problems of administering oxygen or doing procedures for treating lung disease. The hearing aid technician, the family planning (contraception) specialist, and the emergency ambulance paramedic are further types of personnel developing in response to new modalities or emphases in the health services.

With all these personnel skilled in diverse aspects of the health services, it is apparent that the individual doctor, the solo medical practitioner of old, can no longer render modern comprehensive health care alone. A whole team of doctors, nurses, secondary practitioners, auxiliary health workers, and others is required. Even if this array of health personnel does not work together in a coordinated framework, there must be some informal relationships among them. The demands of efficiency and effectiveness, however, are increasingly leading the many types of personnel to work together systematically, as a team in the conventional sense. The objective of integrating prevention with treatment is giving further impetus to the health team idea.

In this overview, we have purposely not categorized health professions, as against paraprofessional personnel or health occupations. Everyone seems to agree that the doctor is the prototype of a professional person, with many implications for social autonomy. The status of other health personnel is the subject of controversy, which takes various forms in different countries. In large measure, although not entirely, professional status depends on the length of educational preparation, and it entitles a person to make important decisions independently. Beyond doctors, however, there are arguments, both substantive and semantic, about the extent of professionalism in most health fields. Almost all health workers seek upward social mobility, higher earnings, and greater social prestige. They also seek more interesting work and greater responsibility. It is probably wisest to avoid the profession-versus-occupation argument, and simply recognize that many types of personnel are needed to render comprehensive health service in any country.

All the organization of health services, required by the scores of types of health personnel, has generated criticism from many people. Bureaucratic patterns are said to destroy a sympathetic doctor–patient relationship. The rules required in any organized program cause inflexibilities that may belittle the individual. Sentimental recollections of a devoted family doctor, with his little black bag, are the conventional contrast. In other ways the same criticism applies to pharmacists, nurses, and other personnel.

But the objective fact is that modern health service is complicated. Populations have needs that existing resources often cannot satisfy. If public or even private funds are insufficient, any health care encounter must be all too brief. Quality is obviously difficult to maintain.

The challenge is to design and manage health services that make the most rational use of all personnel available. Whatever the manpower resources, their performance must never lose sight of the human needs of the individual.

REFERENCES

Nursing

Aiken, L. H. (Editor), *Nursing in the 1980s: Crises, Opportunities, Challenges.* Philadelphia: Lippincott, 1982.

Biscoe, Gillian, "Too Few Nurses?" *World Health,* 14–15, April 1988.

Brown, Esther Lucile, *Nursing Reconsidered—A Study of Change,* Part 2. Philadelphia: Lippincott, 1971.

Bullough, Bonnie (Editor), *The Law and the Expanding Nursing Role.* New York: Appleton-Century-Crofts, 1975.

Bullough, Bonnie, and Vern Bullough, *Expanding Horizons for Nurses.* New York: Springer, 1977.

Bullough, Vern L., and Bonnie Bullough, *The Emergence of Modern Nursing,* 2nd ed. New York: Macmillian, 1969.

Delevan, Sybil M., and Sandra Z. Koff, "The Nursing Shortage and Provider Attitudes: A Political Perspective." *Journal of Public Health Policy,* 11(1):62–80, Spring 1990.

Friss, Lois, "Simultaneous Strategies for Solving the Nursing Shortage." *Health Care Management Review,* 13:71–80, 1988.

Harrington, C., "A Policy Agenda for the Nursing Shortage." *Nursing Outlook,* 36:118–119, 153–154, 1988.

Iglehart, J. K., "Problems Facing the Nursing Profession." *New England Journal of Medicine* 317:646–651, 1987.

International Council of Nurses, *Health Care for All, Challenge for Nursing.* Geneva: ICN, 1983.

Roemer, Milton I., and Ruth Roemer, *Health Care Systems and Comparative Manpower Policies.* New York: Marcel Dekker, 1981.

Sand René, *The Advance to Social Medicine.* London: Staples Press, 1962.

Midwifery

Brennan, Barbara, and Joan R. Heilman, *The Complete Book of Midwifery.* New York: Dutton, 1977.

Mangay-Maglacas, A., and H. Pizurki, *The Traditional Birth Attendant in Seven Countries: Case Studies in Utilization and Training.* Geneva: World Health Organization (Public Health Papers No. 75), 1981.

Parfitt, Rebecca R., *The Birth Primer.* Philadelphia: Running Press, 1977.

Sullivan, Deborah A., and Rose Weitz, *Labor Pains-Modern Midwives and Home Birth.* Ann Arbor: Braun-Brumfield, 1988.

World Health Organization, European Region, *Legislation Concerning Nursing/Midwifery Services and Education.* Copenhagen (Euro Reports and Studies 45), 1981.

World Health Organization, South-East Asia Region, *Survey on Nursing and Midwifery Education and Personnel in the South-East Asia Region of WHO.* New Delhi: WHO, 19 March 1976.

Pharmacists

Ackerknecht, Erwin H., *A Short History of Medicine,* rev. ed. Baltimore, MD: Johns Hopkins University Press, 1982.

Adams, F. W., "The Pharmacy Act, 1968—a Turning Point." *The Pharmaceutical Journal* (London, Edition), 205:40–41, 4 July 1970.

Boussel, P., H. Bonnemain, and F. J. Bove, *History of Pharmacy and the Pharmaceutical Industry.* Paris: Asklepios Press, 1983.

DeWar, Thomas, "A Hundred Years of Pharmaceutical Legislation." *The Pharmaceutical Journal* (London, England), 146:126–129, 12 April 1941.

Gish, Oscar, and Loretta Lee Feller, *Planning Pharmaceuticals for Primary Health Care: The Supply and Utilization of Drugs in the Third World.* Washington, D.C.: American Public Health Association, 1979.

Hamarneh, S. K., *Origins of Pharmacy and Therapy in the Near East.* Tokyo: Naito Foundation, 1973.

Kremers, E., and G. Urdang, *History of Pharmacy,* 4th ed. Phildelphia: J. B. Lippincott, 1976.

Silverman, M., and P. R. Lee, *Pills, Profits, and Politics.* Berkeley, CA: University of California Press, 1974.

Srivastava, G. P., *History of Indian Pharmacy.* Banaras (India): Banaras Hindu University Press, 1954.

Thompson, C.J.S., *The Mystery and Art of the Apothecary.* London: John Lane and the Bodley Head, 1929.

Trease, George Edward, *Pharmacy and History.* London: Bailliere, Tindall, and Cox, 1964.

Urdant, George, *Pharmacy's Part in Society.* Madison, WI: American Institute of the History of Pharmacy, 1959.

West, Sheila K., "Pharmacy Manpower in the United States: A Wasted Resource." *International Journal of Health Services,* 4(1):181–187, 1974.

Wootton, A. C., *Chronicles of Pharmacy,* Vol. 1. London: Macmillian, 1910.

Other Health Personnel

Bui, Dang Ha Doan, "Statistical Analysis of the World Health Manpower Situation circa 1975." *World Health Statistics,* 33(2):127–150, 1980.

Dandare, M., and U. Shah, "Community Health Workers: What Is Their Real Value?" *World Health Forum,* 4:200–201, 1983.

de Zoysa, Isabelle, and Susan Cole-King, "Remuneration of the Community Health Worker: What Are the Options?" *World Health Forum,* 4:125–130, 1983.

Fendall, N.R.E., "The Medical Assistant in Africa." *Journal of Tropical Medicine and Hygiene,* 71:83–95, April 1968.

Fendall, N.R.E., *Auxiliaries in Health Care.* Baltimore: Johns Hopkins Press, 1972.

Fulop, Tamas, and Milton I. Roemer, *International Development of Health Manpower Policy.* Geneva: World Health Organization, 1982.

Fulton, J. T., *Experiment in Dental Care: Results of New Zealand's Use of School Dental Nurses.* Geneva: World Health Organization (Monograph Series No. 4), 1951.

Gilson, Lucy, G. Walt, K. Heggenhougen, O. O. Lucas, M. Perera, D. Ross, and L. Salazar, "National Community Health Worker Programs: How Can They Be Strengthened?" *Journal of Public Health Policy,* 10(4):518–532, Winter 1989.

Ministry of Public Health and Association of Medical Schools of Colombia, *Study of Health Manpower and Medical Education in Colombia: Preliminary Findings.* Washington, D.C.: Pan-American Health Organization, 1967.

Newell, K. W. (Editor), *Health by the People.* Geneva: World Health Organization, 1975.

Ofusu–Amaah, V., *National Experience in the Use of Community Health Workers: A Review of Current Issues and Problems.* Geneva: World Health Organization (Offset Pub. No. 71), 1983.

Pitcairn, D. M., and D. Flahault (Editors), *The Medical Assistant: An Intermediate Level of Health Care Personnel.* Geneva: World Health Organization (Public Health Papers No. 60), 1974.

Roemer, Milton I., "Primary Care and Physician Extenders in Affluent Countries." *International Journal of Health Services,* 7:545–555, Fall 1977.

Roemer, Milton I., "Innovative Functions of Health Personnel in Other Countries: Lessons for U.S. Health Planners." *Inquiry,* 16(3):259–263, 1979.

Roemer, Ruth, "The Legal Scope of Dental Hygienists in the United States and Other Countries." *Public Health Reports,* 85(11):941–948, November 1970.

Sidel, Victor, "Feldshers and Feldsherism: The Role and Training of the Feldsher in the USSR." *New England Journal of Medicine,* 278(17): 934–939, 218(18):987–992, 1968.

Sigerist, Henry E., "Developments and Trends in Dentistry." *Washington University Dental Journal,* 7:131–141, May 1941.

Skeet, Muriel, "Community Health Workers: Promoters or Inhibitors of Primary Health Care?" *World Health Forum,* 5:291–295, 1984.

Skeet, Muriel, and Katherine Elliott (Editors), *Health Auxiliaries and the Health Team.* London: Croom Helm, 1978.

Storms, Doris M., *Training and Use of Auxiliary Health Workers: Lessons from Developing Countries.* Washington, D.C.: American Public Health Association, 1979.

Vederese, M. L., and L. M. Turnbull, *The Traditional Birth Attendant in Maternal and Child Health and Family Planning.* Geneva: World Health Organization (Offset Pub. No. 18), 1975.

Wang, Virginia Li, "Training of the Barefoot Doctor in the People's Republic of China: From Pre-ventive to Curative Service." *International Journal of Health Services,* 5:475–488, 1975.

Werner, David, *Where There Is No Doctor.* Palo Alto, CA: Hesperian Foundation, 1977.

World Health Organization, *The Training and Utilization of Feldshers in the USSR.* Geneva: WHO (Public Health Papers No. 56), 1974.

World Health Organization, *World Directory of Schools of Public Health and Postgraduate Training Programmes in Public Health.* Geneva: WHO, 1985.

World Health Organization, *Strengthening the Performance of Community Health Workers in Primary Health Care.* Geneva: WHO (Technical Report Series 780), 1989.

CHAPTER THREE

Health Facilities

In addition to health personnel, there are three other types of health resource—facilities, commodities, and knowledge—in all national health systems. This chapter will examine health facilities in the world scene. Among these facilities, the oldest type in every country is the hospital.

HOSPITALS

The early development of physical structures in which to care for the seriously sick and provide certain other services is tied more closely to social and religious circumstances than to scientific technology.

History of Hospitals

The origins of modern hospitals are usually traced to places of refuge for the sick poor established by the Christian Church in the Middle Ages. The links between these places of shelter and religion are certainly clear, but the essential idea arose much earlier than Christianity. According to some interpretations of the Ancient Papyrus Ebers, several thousand years before Christ there were temples in Egypt where the sick were brought for religious healing.

Early Origins. As early as the sixth century B.C., Aesculapius was a legendary Greek physician who became deified as the god of medicine. In subsequent centuries, temples were built in his honor, and patients would come to them for prayer as well as for massages and baths. At about the same time Buddhist temples were built in India, and patients came to them in search of religious cures. Given the close ties between medicine and religion, these

were essentially the earliest hospitals, to which seriously sick patients came for help. Chinese medicine of this period had an elaborate pharmacopeia, but evidently made no use of hospitals. Later, when Buddhism spread to China, Chinese Buddhist monks traveled to India, and about 400 A.D. one of them described with admiration the "medicine houses" sheltering the poor and treating the sick.

Later at the height of the Roman Empire, there were improvised military hospitals or *valetudinaria* for wounded or sick soldiers. Likewise, large landowners with hundreds of slaves had infirmaries for sick or disabled slaves; a slave who died was a lost investment.

The first Christian hospitals were established under Constantine, the Roman Emperor who converted to Christianity. These facilities were built in the fourth and fifth centuries in and around Constantinople (now Istanbul). Many became associated with monasteries. As institutions for merciful care of the poor, the aged, and the sick, they were not very well developed until the twelfth century A.D. After about 1145, they were rapidly established throughout Europe, usually near a large cathedral.

The Crusades from Western Europe to the East also played a part in the evolution of hospitals. One group of crusaders organized the Hospitalers of the Order of St. John, which in 1099 established a facility to acccommodate 2,000 patients in the Holy Land. (This order survives today in England as the St. John's Ambulance Corps.) The first English hospital, in fact, was St. John's built at York in 1084. In Berlin, the Hospital of the Holy Ghost was built in 1070, followed by many other hospitals of the same religious order.

Until the late twelfth century, however, hospitals in both Eastern (Byzantine) and Western Europe were mainly custodial, religious, and charitable institutions. Provisions for medical care began to develop on some systematic basis only in the thirteenth century, when the hospital's administration was gradually withdrawn from the full control of religious orders and put into the hands of civil, ordinarily municipal, authorities. This was usually brought about by the need for larger hospital capacities, beyond the financial means of the church, and requiring support from public revenues.

The spread of leprosy throughout Europe in the twelfth and thirteenth centuries also contributed to the growth of facilities for the sick—*lazarettos* or *lazar houses,* as they were called. Although they segregated these suffering patients under crude conditions—usually outside the main cities—they helped free Europe from this disabling chronic disease.

Examples of hospitals combining ecclesiastical and municipal management were St. Bartholomew's, built in London in 1137, and the Hotel Dieu in Paris, which opened at about the same time (although an "inn for the poor" was said to have occupied this site since 600 A.D.). These institutions had directors and various departments for preparing food, doing laundry, and bathing patients. Each large bed in the open wards accommodated two or three patients—usually without any awareness of the hazards of cross-infection. If any "medical" treatment was given, it was by monks and clerics. Nursing was the task of the nuns or sisters.

Not until the Renaissance, with the growth of cities and the flowering of universities—including the education of physicians—did hospitals begin to acquire a valid medical and therapeutic character. The rebirth of classical knowledge and culture began in Italy in the fourteenth century, and somewhat later in northern Europe and England. The leper houses were gradually converted into hospitals, and physicians were appointed to make regular visits to all the patients—"male and female," as the ancient records specifically indicate. But the story of European hospitals is not one of uninterrupted progress. During the tumultuous days of the Protestant Reformation, many hospitals tied to the Catholic Church were closed down and deprived of financial support from both religious and civil authorities.

Hospital patients in the fourteenth and fifteenth centuries were still restricted largely to the very poor. Some limited medical care was given, sometimes by a Municipal Physician. A somewhat similar development of charitable hostels or hospitals occurred also in the Moslem world, with religious inspiration, but less directly linked to a church.

After the Renaissance, medical services in hospitals improved slightly, with drugs being prescribed and limited nursing services given by religious sisters. The hygienic conditions and general atmosphere, however, remained grim; only the most destitute and homeless of people would agree to be admitted to a ward. A patient with any resources would prefer to stay at home. With the gradual advances of medical science in the sixteenth and seventeenth centuries, hospitals expanded under both religious and secular authorities, the latter acquiring increasing importance.

With the much greater social and scientific advances of the eighteenth century, the period of Enlightenment in the Western World, many new hospitals were built. By 1732 there were 115 hospitals in England, although many were still combinations of almshouses and medical institutions. A few hospitals in London—such as Guy's, endowed by a philanthropist (not by the church or municipality) in 1724—even admitted paying patients. In Dublin a lying-in hospital for maternity cases was founded in 1745. In Vienna, the famous *Allgemeines Krankenhaus,* destined to contribute significantly to advances in medical science, was opened in 1795.

Background of Diverse Sponsorships. Larger political events inevitably influenced the ownership and control of hospitals. The French Revolution in 1789 and the Mexican Revolution in 1910 led to governmental supervision of church activities in civil life. The many church-sponsored hospitals in those countries were taken over completely by government, and usually put under the administration of cities or provinces. The relative balance between church and state, however, varied among countries. The several socialist revolutions later in the twentieth century led to sweeping conversion of pluralistic hospital ownership into national networks of public institutions.

In the Western Hemisphere, the Spanish Conquistador, Cortez, built a sturdy hospital for his soldiers and settlers in 1524, and a Catholic hospital was built in Quebec in 1639. In Latin America, colonized mainly by Spain and Portugal (where the Christian Church was very strong), religious sponsorship was carried over, with the funding of numerous charitable or *beneficencia* hospitals. In the British and French colonies of Asia and Africa, the hospitals under colonial authorities were mainly governmental.

In the British colonies that were to become the United States, the precursor of a hospital, a public almshouse, was founded in Philadelphia for Quakers in 1713, followed by the Pennsylvania Hospital in 1752. It was regularly attended by physicians, without pay, including Dr. Benjamin Rush, one of the signers of the U.S. Declaration of Independence.

In the early nineteenth century, a new type of hospital sponsorship emerged in Europe: the *voluntary nonsectarian* institution. A group of citizens, often led by one or two large benefactors, would establish a general hospital without involvement of either church or state. Financial support would come from charitable donations and later from government subsidy; with nonindigent patients beginning to use hospitals, private fees would also be collected. This pattern became prominent in England and in British colonies overseas, including North America, Australia, and India.

In the late nineteenth and early twentieth century, the rise of social insurance (discussed later) began to influence hospitals. This source of relatively stable economic support for medical care of workers and often their dependents led to the financial strengthening of hospitals in several countries. Polyclinics (for specialized medicine) were constructed directly by social insurance bodies, and later these added their own beds. Special hospitals for tuberculosis were built by the insurance funds in Europe. In Latin America after 1939, many general hospitals were built by social security agencies exclusively for insured workers.

Events in the later nineteenth century, with the explosive urban and productive development of the Industrial Revolution, laid the technological groundwork for the modern hospital. Findings in physiology, histology, and chemistry in the first half of the nineteenth century provided the basis for the sensational applications in bacteriology (Pasteur) and organ pathology (Virchow) in the second half. With the discovery of anesthesia and recognition of the benefits of antisepsis, then asepsis, the entire character of hospitals changed. Previously feared, as places in which to die, hospitals began to become places for the preferred treatment of serious illness—both medically and surgically. After Florence Nightingale's pioneering in nursing education in 1860, trained nurses gradually replaced nuns as attendants of the sick. Patients became customarily kept one to a bed, and efforts were made to keep the wards clean. Each hospital had its laboratory (or perhaps a laboratory for each main department), a pharmacy, a kitchen, and laundry. Medical schools became increasingly affiliated with large hospitals, and sometimes such schools were even founded by hospitals.

Recognition of the infectiousness of tuberculosis and the possibilities of cure through prolonged bed rest gave rise to the sanitorium. But to be economical, these usually had to be quite large; hence, the most practical type of sponsorship came from larger units of government—the province or the central national authority. The same applied in the nineteenth century to asylums for the mentally ill, after they were freed from imprisonment with criminals.

The development of several types of specialized personnel for mental illness has been intimately linked to the entire history of mental hospitals or, as they were once called, "insane asylums." The first such asylum exclusively for the mentally disturbed was established in Spain in 1408, but the treatment of its inmates centered around magic, prayer, and punishment far more than use of any medical procedure. In Europe and elsewhere seriously disturbed mental patients were often kept in jails, with criminals, for want of any other facilities. The French Revolution (around 1792) was a turning point, with the courageous work of Dr. Philippe Pinel, who succeeded in having the chains removed from the miserable psychotics and replacing restraint with sympathetic *moral treatment*. An equivalent crusade to establish treatment-oriented mental hospitals was led in America by a retired school teacher, Dorothea Dix, around 1840. It was the late nineteenth century, however, before therapeutically oriented mental hospitals developed widely in Europe or America, and it was the early twentieth century before the *mental hygiene* movement arose, with its orientation toward treatment of mental and emotionally disturbed patients at early stages, in community clinics.

Since the fifteenth century, European governments had established national hospitals for military personnel and sometimes police. Merchant mariners were also provided special hospitals at the main ports of England in the eighteenth century, and the same was done in the United States after 1798. Later in the nineteenth century, some governments that built railroads set up hospitals for the railroad workers. In the twentieth century, especially in the less developed countries, other government employees were provided care in special hospitals.

Private industry in the late nineteenth and early twentieth centuries also built hospitals for workers at isolated enterprises, such as mining and lumbering. In the less developed countries of Latin America, Asia, and Africa, small hospitals were established at sugar plantations, tea or rubber estates, and other agricultural enterprises. Medical care for sick workers was important to maximize their productivity, and care was often given to family members for the sake of morale. Industrial injury compensation laws after 1885 also encouraged hospital construction, when employers were obligated to meet the medical costs of work injuries.

European cities had very old hospital buildings, but in the United States, most hospital construction could start anew. The proliferation of hospitals, in general, is illustrated by trends in the United States, where in 1872 the total number of hospitals amounted to 178 and by 1910 had become more than 4,300. Most of these were small facilities, averaging fewer than 100 beds; unlike policies in Europe or elsewhere, these units were not staffed by a small elite group of prestigious physicians. Al-

most any local physician, reasonably qualified, was free to admit his private patients and become a member of the hospital's medical staff. The same practices developed in Canada— that is, the *open staff* hospital in contrast to the *closed staff* hospitals everywhere else. General hospitals became regarded as necessary adjuncts of private medical practice.

In the colonies of Asia and Africa, local government was weak or nonexistent, so that the hospitals built were controlled by the central government—first in the colonial capitals, then in other cities. When these European colonies became emancipated, the strong central control of public hospitals was usually maintained. Religious missions from Europe and America also established some rural hospitals, and later these were sometimes integrated into national hospital systems.

Finally, in the later twentieth century, some hospitals have been established as purely commercial enterprises. Often with the combined support of private physicians and wealthy families, these *proprietary* facilities have been built to serve relatively affluent or insured people. Typically, these units are small but well provided with nursing personnel and modern equipment. In the United States, private corporations have acquired control of *chains* of such hospitals throughout the country and abroad.

After 1920, hospitals in all industrialized countries increased in number, average size, and complexity. The commonest types became general hospitals, serving almost all types of patients, although usually in separate departments or wards for medical cases, surgical cases, maternity care, children, infectious disease patients, and so on. The range of functions in general hospitals has broadened steadily over the centuries. Originally places of merciful shelter for the destitute and the sick, they evolved into places for advanced medical and surgical therapy. When medical education became formalized, they served as places to teach medical students methods of diagnosis and treatment. Eventually they served as schools for training nurses and later other types of medical personnel. Only in the late nineteenth and early twentieth century did they develop *outpatient departments* for helping ambulatory patients who did not require admission to a bed. As medical science advanced, they became centers for clinical research, and sometimes even basic science research. As preventive medicine has developed, hospitals have offered preventive services—immunizations, early case-finding (through routine diagnostic tests), and health education.

Hospital Sponsorship

From this historical review, we can see how modern hospitals have come to be under diverse forms of sponsorship or ownership. It is now customary to classify the ownership or sponsorship of hospitals in a country into three general categories: governmental, voluntary nonprofit, and proprietary. Governmental includes sponsorship by any level of government—local (municipal or other local jurisdiction), provincial, or national. Governmental sponsorship in the industrialized countries is predominantly by local governments, and in developing countries it is mainly by central government. There may be different agencies of government: not only ministries of health but also authorities concerned with military affairs, social welfare, transportation (railroads or airlines), public lands, rural community development, and so on. Social security agencies, often within ministries of labor, are important sponsors of hospitals in many countries.

Voluntary nonprofit hospitals include the many institutions founded by religious bodies. Although historically meant for patients of the same faith, this is no longer the policy. There may be some tendency, however, to appoint to the hospital staff physicians and others of the sponsoring religious group. On a world scale the Catholic Church is a major sponsor of hospitals, doubtless because of the important part it played in the origin of hospitals in medieval Europe. Other voluntary nonprofit hospitals are under the sponsorship of nonsectarian groups; these often take shape around a philanthropic donor of funds to build the structure. In Latin America, settlers from a particular European country have established nonprofit institutions—hence, the Italian hospital, the French Hospital, and so on. Voluntary hospitals may also be sponsored by charitable organizations, such as the Red Cross, or

societies fighting certain diseases, such as leagues against cancer or tuberculosis. Associations promoting the welfare of mothers or children sponsor maternity or children's hospitals.

Hospitals under proprietary sponsorship may be built under varying circumstances. Sometimes a group of physicians constructs a facility for their own patients. Some proprietary hospitals are developed in a community because the initiative has not been taken by government or by a nonprofit group. Such hospitals may even serve as resources under a governmental program financing hospital care. Still other proprietary hospitals are intended specifically for private patients seeking hospital care outside of a public system, such as in England with its National Health Service. Hospitals built and operated for employees by a business enterprise must also be counted under proprietary sponsorship.

On a world scale, most hospital beds are in institutions sponsored by units of government. The predominance of governmental beds characterizes countries on all the continents, except North America. In Western Europe, Sweden, for example, had in 1980 an exceptionally high complement of hospital beds (15 per 1,000 population), of which 94.3 percent were in governmental facilities. In the formerly socialist countries of Eastern Europe, as elsewhere, 100 percent of hospital beds were governmental. In Asia, 89.0 percent of hospital beds in Thailand (1980) were in governmental facilities, although most patients must pay for services in them. Peru in South America had only 1.8 beds per 1,000 people in 1977, of which 81 percent were in government hospitals. In Africa, the hospital beds of Ghana were 76.1 percent governmental in 1979.

Nongovernmental hospital beds, of course, are divided between voluntary and proprietary sponsorships. In some countries, voluntary institutions predominate over the proprietary ones; in others the relationship is the converse. Thus, in the United States, 64.4 percent of total beds in 1987 were in voluntary nonprofit hospitals and 10.1 percent in proprietary hospitals. Likewise in Ghana, the corresponding figures (in 1979) were 22.3 and 1.6 percent, respectively. In Sweden, on the other hand, where overall nongovernmental beds are few, the voluntary hospitals sponsored in 1980 only 0.8 percent of the beds, compared with 4.9 percent in proprietary units. In the Philippine Republic, voluntary nonprofit hospitals (1980) had 14.5 percent of the beds, compared with 25.3 percent in proprietary facilities. Japan is unusual in having several rural hospitals operated by agricultural cooperatives.

These varying mixtures of hospital sponsorships in countries have many implications for the planning and operation of hospitals. Planning the location and size of hospitals, in reasonable relationship to the distribution of populations, has become recognized as sound social policy in most countries. Such planning is much easier to carry out with governmental hospitals than with those under private sponsorship. The latter are, of course, subject to regulatory controls, but these may be complex and difficult to apply; many countries, furthermore, do not adopt regulatory measures for various political reasons.

Hospitals under governmental sponsorship are more likely to apply uniform standards in their operation; voluntary and proprietary hospitals are more likely to show greater diversity. In spite of this, one finds great variations among hospitals, even in highly centralized nations, where local imagination or initiative appears. National standards tend to set a floor but not necessarily a ceiling on hospital practices. The technological development of governmental hospitals is likely to be greater than that of private hospitals in most countries. In a few countries, such as the United States or Japan, the staffing and equipment of voluntary nonprofit hospitals are often highly sophisticated. In Europe, however, and in most developing countries, the most advanced technology is found in public hospitals; private hospitals cater to patients with relatively uncomplicated ailments.

Public and privately sponsored hospitals differ in many other respects. In general, public institutions are open to all patients; they admit cases on the basis of medical need. Voluntary and proprietary hospitals may restrict admissions on the basis of the patient's ability to pay for care or other considerations. A hospital's bed capacity, of course, sets limits on the number of patients admitted, but throughout the world one sees public hospitals that are greatly overcrowded, with the patient-beds put in the corridors; this is seldom done in private hospitals. It is not uncommon for beds in a public hospital to be filled to more than capacity—sometimes with two patients in one bed—while in a nearby voluntary or proprietary hospital the occupancy is low. With relatively easier cases, moreover, the private hospital nursing staff can give patients very solicitous care, whereas the public hospital nurses find it difficult to give even minimal care. Admission of a patient to a hospital bed depends everywhere on the decision of a doctor on the hospital staff, but the structure of this staff, as we will see, differs with hospital sponsorship.

The administrative structure of hospitals differs considerably among countries, even for hospitals of the same type of sponsorship. In general, however, government hospitals are under the direction of some official agency, through a conventional pyramidal chain of command. Thus, the top administrator of the hospital ordinarily reports to a governmental authority at the next higher echelon, without any intervening *board of directors.* Sometimes there is a hospital board, but its members may consist of public officials or persons appointed by a public body. Similarly, all personnel working in the hospital may have to be appointed through the channels of a government *civil service* or similar process. These procedures, which are intended to guard against favoritism in public employment, may in fact cause delays and other difficulties in the administration of the hospital.

Voluntary nonprofit hospitals almost always have boards of directors, composed usually of the major donors who financed the hospital construction and representatives of other relevant groups. This board is self-perpetuating, insofar as it selects its own successors. The board is the highest authority in governing the hospital, unless the facility is part of a network of voluntary institutions under a superior body such as in a Catholic sisterhood. The board typically appoints the hospital administrator, who is then responsible for day-to-day operations. The medical staff members are also usually appointed by the board or a special committee to which this power is delegated. Proprietary hospitals seldom have a board of directors in the conventional sense, although

Table 3.1. Hospital Sponsorship: Percentage of Hospital Beds under Governmental and Private Sponsorship, Industrialized Countries in the 1980s

Country	Government	Private
Japan	5.1	94.9
Canada	35	65
Belgium	37	63
United States	38.3	61.7
Israel	41.4	58.6
Germany	52.3	47.7
Spain	67	33
France	69	31
Australia	73.3	26.7
New Zealand	79	21
Denmark	90	10
Norway	90	10
Great Britain	92	8
Sweden	94.5	5.5
Soviet Union	100	0.0

Source: World Health Organization, World Health Statistics Annual. Geneva: WHO, 1983.

Table 3.2. Hospital Sponsorship: Percentage of Hospital Beds under Governmental and Private Sponsorship, Developing Countries in the 1980s

Country	Government	Private
South Korea	18.6	81.4
Brazil	26.1	73.9
Philippines	45.4	54.6
Kenya	46.3	53.7
Zaire	48.8	51.2
Liberia	56	44
Zimbabwe	60.1	39.9
Indonesia	65	35
Tanzania	66	34
Argentina	68.6	31.4
India	69.8	30.2
Ghana	76.1	23.9
Venezuela	76.2	23.8
Peru	80.3	19.7
Pakistan	81	19
Ecuador	85	15
Malaysia	88.9	11.1
Thailand	89.1	10.9
Kuwait	90	10
Egypt	93.8	6.2
Barbados	95	5
Turkey	95.9	4.1
Burma	98	2
Iraq	98	2
Libya	98	2
Costa Rica	98.1	1.9
China	100	0

Source: World Health Organization, World Health Statistics Annual. Geneva: WHO, 1983.

the owner or owners may constitute a *board* nominally. The organizational structures within hospitals, involving departments, sections, and so on, are discussed further in Chapter 13.

Considering hospital sponsorship simply as government or private (including proprietary), the proportions in the 1980s are presented in Table 3.1 for industrialized countries and in Table 3.2 for developing countries.

Hospital Bed Resources

It is evident from Table 3.3 that, in general, the supply of hospital beds in a country (per 100,000 population) is roughly proportional to the country's economic level. Variation of hospital bed supply with the type of national health system is less consistent. At a given economic level, the more welfare-oriented health systems may or may not have greater bed supplies than the more entrepreneurial systems, but the numbers depend on special political circumstances in each country. Thus the comprehensive health system of Sweden has a larger bed supply than does the entrepreneurial system of the United States, and the hospital beds in socialist Cuba exceed those in entrepreneurial South Korea. Socialist Mozambique, however, has fewer beds than entrepreneurial Kenya, the result undoubtedly of the prolonged hostilities in the west African country. After peace was achieved in socialist Vietnam, its hospital bed supply became much greater than that in entrepreneurial Indonesia.

Larger hospital bed supplies tend to be found in countries in which hospital sponsorship is predominantly public rather than private. The abundant stock of beds in Scandinavian countries is associated with the predominant control of hospitals by local governmental bodies, whereas the more modest stock of beds in the United States or Canada is associated with the substantial control of hospitals by nongovernmental bodies (75 percent of beds in the United States and 65 percent of beds in Canada).

The technological equipment and the various amenities for patient care are strikingly different in the hospitals of affluent countries compared with those of lower income coun-

Table 3.3. National Supplies of Hospital Beds per 100,000 People, by the Country's Economic Level and Its Type of Health System, c. 1981

Type of Health System	Economic Level		
	Affluent	Transitional	Very Poor
Entrepreneurial			
United States	526		
South Korea		178	
South Africa		345	
Kenya			149
Indonesia			65
Welfare oriented			
Belgium	909		
Canada	714		
Brazil		400	
Turkey		208	
India			81.3
Liberia			154
Comprehensive			
Great Britain	714		
Sweden	2000		
Costa Rica		227	
Nicaragua		164	
Sri Lanka			278
Tanzania			106
Socialist			
Soviet Union	1250		
Yugoslavia	625		
Cuba		526	
Albania		588	
Vietnam			233
Mozambique			90.9

Source: World Health Organization, *World Health Statistics Annual.* Geneva WHO, 1983. Also: World Bank, *Social Indicators of Development 1989.* Washington: The Bank, 1989.

tries. General hospital beds are set up in rooms with only four or six beds in the affluent countries, whereas in those of lower income, large wards of 16 or 20 beds or more are still rather common.

Equipment for laboratory analyses, X-ray diagnosis and treatment, rehabilitation, and diverse other services are often rudimentary in the hospitals of Asia, Africa, and Latin America. A large multibedded ward may have only a single toilet, in place of plumbing for every private or semiprivate room. Corresponding differences are found in hospital pharmacies, kitchens, laundries, and other hospital facilities. The space devoted to care of outpatients in older hospital structures is often much below the need. Surgical operating and deliv-

ery rooms may be meagerly equipped, as are emergency services and departments for physical rehabilitation. Older hospital buildings are often spread out in separate pavilions, whereas modern structures are more often unified in a high structure, with numerous elevators.

In general the staffing of hospitals is related to their size; larger facilities have more complex equipment and more numerous nurses and other personnel per bed, and smaller hospitals have fewer capabilities and smaller complements of staff. Because of their greater staffing, the hospitals of affluent countries have a relatively rapid turnover of patients (every 7 to 14 days), whereas average lengths of stay in hospitals of lower income countries are typically longer—2 or 3 weeks. (This is further discussed in Chapter 13.)

In the more affluent industrialized countries, where 10 percent or more of the population are in the older age groups (65 years and over), there are usually long-term care facilities for less intensive care. In Europe, both Western and Eastern, these nursing homes are sponsored mainly by local units of government, but in the United States their sponsorship is mainly proprietary. With hospital service becoming increasingly expensive in most countries, the resort to lower-cost extended-care facilities is mounting. (This subject is further discussed in Chapter 13.)

The optimal supply of hospital beds needed by each country, for planning purposes, has been a subject of study and debate everywhere. If there is an assured payment system, it seems that almost any additional hospital beds provided will tend to be used, up to a ceiling not yet determined. The ideal bed–population ratio obviously depends on the prevalence of disease or injury and the characteristics of the whole health system. In many affluent countries, rising medical care costs have led in recent years to a judgment that the bed supply is excessive. In the poorer countries, the bed supply is still clearly less than the needs—even though improved transportation and education are usually required to enable the people to make better use of the beds available.

Because of its ancient origins and also its provision of highly advanced medical technology, the modern hospital is regarded by many people as the center, physically and ideologically, of all health services in a region or province. In recent years, however, a more health-oriented rather than disease-oriented viewpoint has developed in many national health systems. This has led to a greater appreciation of organized facilities for health services provided to the ambulatory person. These facilities may be known as clinics, health stations, polyclinics, health centers, or by other terms. Their development has been quite different from that of hospitals.

AMBULATORY CARE FACILITIES

Unlike hospitals, started by religious or municipal bodies, the origin of facilities for organized care of the ambulatory person was not linked to other social institutions. From the earliest times, care of the ailing but ambulatory patient was given by individual healers or later physicians. The patient came to the quarters of the doctor or the doctor was called to the patient's home.

Historic Development

Provision of such ambulatory care by a group of personnel in an organized facility was a great departure from tradition. Such an innovation arose far later than did hospitals. Not being linked to established authorities, religious or governmental, the idea generated great opposition. Even though the first *dispensaries,* as they were called, were intended only for the poor, they constituted a threat to individual medical practitioners, and were bitterly opposed.

The first organized ambulatory medical service was established in Paris in 1632 by a wealthy and humanitarian physician, who was also General Overseer of the Poor. It started as a consultation center, from which the patient would be referred to a physician, surgeon, or apothecary, who had agreed to treat these people without charge. The facility was in a rented house and had no connection with any hospital. The Medical Faculty of the University of Paris raised numerous objections, attacked the unit in a parliamentary court, and eventually forced it to close. Soon after, however, the

same court ordered the Medical Faculty to set up a similar "system of charitable consultations to the poor," and by 1707 such charitable dispensaries had to be established at all schools of medicine throughout France.

In 1675, the idea of a dispensary for ambulatory service to the poor was proposed by the Royal College of Physicians in London. Opposition here came from the Society of Apothecaries, who did not wish to dispense drugs to the poor at low prices, since such poor people were their customary patients. A vendetta continued between physicians and apothecaries until 1697, when a dispensary was finally regularized at a house leased by the Royal College of Physicians.

By the mid-eighteenth century, dispensaries for the poor had become an accepted idea throughout Europe and the New World. The first American dispensary was founded in Philadelphia in 1786, but it had no connection with the pioneer Pennsylvania Hospital. By the mid-nineteenth century, dispensaries were serving the poor in all the main cities of Europe and America. Not until the late nineteenth century did hospitals customarily establish outpatient departments, leading to the decline of the dispensary. Even when inpatient beds became open to paying patients, and were located in private or semiprivate rooms, hospital outpatient departments in North America continued to be restricted to the poor. They were staffed *gratis* by doctors, who received fees from their private inpatients. In Europe and elsewhere the hospital outpatient clinic became a major resource for ambulatory care to people of all income levels, as discussed below.

In the late nineteenth century, with maturing humanitarianism and the epochal discoveries of bacteriology and hygiene, a new type of organized ambulatory unit developed in France—the infant welfare station. (A similar innovation in London a century earlier had not spread widely.) Nursing mothers were provided with clean cow's milk and education on infant hygiene and diet. Around 1900, the idea diffused to America, where it was first adopted by charitable voluntary agencies and then by local departments of public health. The same sequence of voluntary action, soon followed by special public health agency units, occurred with clinics for tuberculosis, for venereal disease (social hygiene), for dental examinations of school children, and for immunizations. In contrast to the work of dispensaries, these services were all notably preventive, although they were intended mainly for the poor.

Around 1900, private industries with more than 100 employees began to set up clinics for first aid to injured workers—a movement accelerated in industrialized countries by worker's compensation laws for such injuries. *Industrial medicine* policies, however, usually emphasized referral to outside physicians for any treatment of a condition beyond first aid. Public schools in affluent countries also organized school health units, staffed by nurses and sometimes physicians, for detecting communicable disease in children. Universities and colleges in many countries came to offer comprehensive ambulatory services (and sometimes hospital or *infirmary* care) for students, especially when they were living away from home.

With these many special-purpose and preventively oriented clinics developing, soon after World War I, social workers in the United States (who had organized *settlement houses* for immigrants in low-income urban neighborhoods) proposed that these diverse services be brought together under one roof. In 1919, the American Red Cross backed the idea, advocating the establishment of multipurpose *health centers.* The Red Cross did a national survey in 1920 and reported 72 such health centers in 49 U.S. cities. Their services were kept strictly preventive, to avoid criticism from the private medical profession.

At this time, a Consultative Council on Medical and Allied Services, attached to the British Ministry of Health, proposed that all ambulatory services, both preventive and therapeutic, be provided to the general population through a network of primary and secondary health centers constructed throughout the British isles. They would be staffed by private physicians, supported by nurses, social workers, technicians, and other allied personnel, who would be salaried by the local government. Although the Dawson Report (1920), as it was known from the name of the Council's Chair-

man, was initially supported by the British Medical Association, it was later opposed. The recent revolution in Russia had created an atmosphere of anxiety about *socialized medicine,* and in the end nothing was done.

In 1920, the same concept of integrated (both preventive and therapeutic) health centers for organized ambulatory services was introduced by public health officials in the United States, first in New York and then in California. But these proposals met the same fate as the Dawson Report, because of opposition from private physicians who now carried a great deal of political weight.

Even when the health center concept was implemented in a British colony—at Kalutara, Ceylon (now Sri Lanka) in 1916—its functions were confined to preventive services. Here, there was no competitive opposition from private doctors, but the policy adopted was for sick patients to be referred to the nearest hospital, as outpatients or inpatients.

Actual implementation of the Dawson idea, to provide integrated preventive and treatment services together in health centers for ambulatory patients, was first carried out in the Soviet Union, after its 1917 revolution. With an explicit socialist policy to establish complete health services as a function of government, the most efficient pattern was to engage doctors as government employees and station them both in hospitals and ambulatory care units on salaries. In the rural areas, where a single doctor would work with feldshers (medical assistants) and nurses, the facilities were called health centers. In the cities, where teams of doctors in different specialties worked together, they were usually called polyclinics.

In North America, where *open medical staff* hospitals were the norm, specialists did not develop the teamwork found in European *closed staff* hospitals. In the American environment, specialists in private offices would sometimes join each other in a *private group practice.* The Mayo brothers in a small town, Rochester, Minnesota, established such a pattern in the 1880s, and it extended slowly to other somewhat rural regions of the United States. After World War I (1914–1918) and then very rapidly after World War II (1939–1945), private group practice clinics spread throughout the United States and Canada. Ater 1950, these multispecialty clinics were complemented by many group practices of a single specialty. By 1984, there were almost 15,000 such group practice clinics in the United States, each containing three or more doctors sharing their work and income in some way; this was nearly half of all doctors in ambulatory practice. Some of the larger medical groups, such as Kaiser-Permanente, include hundreds of specialists and are linked to health insurance programs. These have come to be known as *health maintenance organizations* (HMOs), and will be discussed later.

After World War II and the emancipation of most of the world's colonies, the inhibitions against establishing health centers for comprehensive ambulatory care largely (but not completely) disappeared. In India, the Bhore Report (1946) recommended the coverage of this large nation with primary health centers; a succession of reports elaborated on the idea and—although not yet completely achieved—the health center is India's conventional public facility for ambulatory care. The same applies throughout other countries of Asia and Africa. In Latin America, influence from the United States kept the health centers restricted to prevention for some years, but by the late 1950s here too comprehensive ambulatory care became the general policy.

In Great Britain, the initial plans for the comprehensive National Health Service in 1946 contemplated revival of the Dawson concept of a nationwide network of health centers, but because of intense medical opposition the idea was dropped. Not until the 1960s, did local health authorities venture to construct health centers and invite general practitioners to rent space in them. The arrangement was an immediate success, and integrated community health centers multiplied to accommodate about 33 percent of British general practitioners; these facilities were staffed with nurses and numerous other health personnel. Most of Britain's remaining general practitioners are in private *group practices* that in many ways are similar to small health centers.

In the United States, the 1960s also brought many changes in the facilities for ambulatory health care. With a sort of rediscovery of poverty, the federal government launched a national network of *neighborhood health centers* in urban slum areas. In spite of much opposition from the medical profession, hundreds of these and similar ambulatory care units were established by different branches of federal and state governments and also by voluntary groups of people. Young men and women, deliberately objecting to governmental health services as bureaucratic and insensitive, organized *free clinics* in large cities throughout the nation for contraceptive advice, treatment of venereal disease, and the ambulatory care of any ailment.

Health Centers After 1980

With these historical developments, health centers providing organized ambulatory health services have spread to all countries. Their extent, however, and the scope of services offered vary with the general health policy of the country. Their overall importance, furthermore, is greater in the economically less developed countries.

Industrialized Countries. In the entrepreneurial health system of the United States, the commonest type of health center is simply a structure to house the local public health agency and several of its preventively oriented clinics. The special "neighborhood health centers" for the poor, and similar facilities started in the 1960s, grew and then declined to less than 1,000 in the 1980s. Private group medical practice clinics were much more numerous, as were clinics attached to industrial enterprises or schools; these will be discussed in Chapter 12.

In the welfare-oriented health systems of western Europe, the private medical profession usually has a strong voice, so that health centers have been limited essentially to preventive services; treatment is the province of private physicians. In France, Belgium, and Germany, local sickness insurance funds and also municipal governments have established health centers for maternal and child health services, immunizations, and other preventive services; these are staffed by salaried physicians and nurses. The same is true in Japan, where the Ministry of Health has constructed a nationwide network of health centers exclusively for prevention. In Australia, some community health centers have gone beyond preventive services to include primary medical care, but this is only for persons of very low income.

In the industrialized countries with comprehensive health systems, health centers have offered a much broader scope of services. We have noted the extensive construction of such facilities in Great Britain since the 1960s; these units house general practitioners serving the general population. At the same time, nurses, dieticians, and others—salaried by the local health authorities—provide preventive services. In Norway and Sweden health centers for general ambulatory care of everyone are much more extensive. In Norway, outside of the main cities, the majority of general practitioners are located in health centers and are paid both by fees and by salary. In Sweden and Finland health centers with salaried medical personnel are the predominant resource for ambulatory care of everyone. Municipal governments establish the health centers, although the medical salaries are paid by the national health service program. In Italy, as the coverage of its National Health Service is extended, health centers are becoming the standard setting for local primary medical care.

In the Soviet Union and other European countries that were, until recently, socialist, ambulatory care was provided through organized facilities as the national norm. Just as bed patients were treated in hospitals, ambulatory patients were diagnosed and treated in polyclinics. The standard staffing for a general polyclinic consisted of teams of a general practitioner, a pediatrician, and an obstetrician-gynecologist—supported by nurses and others. Each team was expected to serve about 4,000 people, so that a polyclinic covering 20,000 would have five such teams. In rural areas, the facility was called a health center, and might be staffed only by a general practitioner and a feldsher-midwife. After 1989, as the socialist economic systems in Europe were slowly transformed, some of the economic support for health services was transferred from general revenues to social insurance. Conditions differ, however, in the several Eastern European countries. In Poland, for example, social insurance for health care had not even been estab-

lished by 1992. In Hungary, where privatization has long been implemented, the great majority of services are still obtained in governmental health facilities. Private practice is only slightly developed, since few patients can affort it.

Transitional Countries. In developing countries, with the problems of poverty and rurality, health centers play the major role in providing the general poplation with ambulatory care. At the transitional economic level, the health system of Thailand illustrates entrepreneurial policies with a very strong private sector. Even so, health centers have been constructed throughout the country. There are some 5,600 communes, each consisting of a cluster of about 10 villages, and more than three-quarters of these have health centers. They are staffed by nurses and auxiliary personnel, who offer both preventive and treatment services. Serious cases are referred to a district hospital where a doctor may be consulted.

In the Philippines, also entrepreneurial, the Ministry of Health, with some help from local governments, has created a national network of some 2,000 health centers, each of which is supposed to have a medical health officer. These units are intended to serve 20,000 to 30,000 people, but medical vacancies are common and the utilization rate has been low. Services are inclusive of treatment of simple ailments, but the major emphasis is preventive. For any continuing care needed, the patient is referred to a private physician or a hospital outpatient department. South Korea is another transitional country with an entrepreneurial health system, where health center development has been relatively modest. Only about 200 have been built for a national population of 40,000,000. With insurance enabling most people to see private physicians, health centers are used essentially for preventive services.

In the welfare-oriented health systems of transitional countries, health centers have come to play increasingly important roles. In Brazil, for example, there are thousands of health centers in small towns and villages, offering primary health care; although emphasizing prevention, they are medically staffed and provide treatment. In addition there are large polyclinics in all the main cities, providing ambulatory specialist care; these are for the 80 percent of the Brazilian population covered by social security. In both health centers and polyclinics the doctors are salaried, along with the other personnel. Insured workers and dependents visit private doctors only exceptionally, since this requires personal copayments and polyclinic care is without charge.

Egypt also has hundreds of health centers in cities and rural areas, although the latter are called *rural health units.* All facilities are staffed with at least one physician, and provide a full range of primary health care, both therapeutic and preventive. Since Egyptian health policy favors the training of large numbers of physicians (and not medical assistants), there are very few medical vacancies. Most of these physicians, however, spend many hours each day in private practice. In Malaysia, the health system makes a major distinction between the cities and rural areas. Private medical practice clearly predominates in the cities, but in the rural areas health centers, subcenters, and primary care clinics are the main resources. A physician is at the main health centers, but at subcenters and clinics, preventive services are given by nurses and assistant nurses, and treatment is given by medical assistants (with three years of training after high school). A large share of ambulatory service to rural people is given at the outpatient departments of district hospitals.

Costa Rica is a transitional level country with a comprehensive health system, protecting the entire population. Health centers in the cities are operated mainly by the social security program and in the rural areas mainly by the Ministry of Health. Both types are medically staffed and provide most of the ambulatory care received by the general population. In addition there are rural health posts staffed by auxiliaries for preventive services.

Israel is a unique transitional country, with its nongovernmental health insurance scheme, covering 90 percent of the population and providing ambulatory services through organized health centers. Hundreds of organized clinics are located in every agricultural settlement, town, and urban neighborhood for insured persons and their families. Even noninsured persons may use these clinics by payment of fees. In addition, the Ministry of Health maintains hundreds of family health stations for preventive services to mothers and children. Doctors salaried by the health insurance funds and by the government are free to engage in private practice after their official working hours, but the vast majority of ambulatory health services in Israel are rendered in the health centers and clinics.

Cuba is a transitional level country with a fully socialist health system that has retained its socialized character, even while the rest of the socialist world has moved away from this model. Ambulatory health services in Cuba are provided by some 400 polyclinics, each serving about 25,000 people and strategically located throughout the country. As in the previous Soviet pattern, there are teams consisting of a general internist, a pediatrician, and a gynecologist for about each 4,000 or 5,000 people. In addition since 1985, small teams of a family practitioner and a nurse have been set up around most polyclinics, to serve as few as 700 people for primary health care. Accordingly the back-up for family practitioners is the polyclinic, and for polyclinics it is the district hospital. All these personnel are salaried by the Ministry of Health, and private practice is rare.

Very Poor Countries. In the very poor countries with almost any type of health policies, health centers are the predominant pattern for delivering ambulatory care. Even in entrepreneurial health systems, as in Kenya and Ghana, the Ministries of Health have planned networks of health centers to cover the country. The achievements, however, have usually been much less than the plans. The staffing of health centers is by *clinical officers* and other auxiliary personnel; doctors are found only in the hospitals. Small fees are charged for treatment services and, with frequent shortages of drugs, the utilization rate is not high.

Indonesia is another very poor country with an entrepreneurial type of health system, where health centers have been widely established. In 1986 there were about 5,000 health centers, each of which was expected to serve 30,000 to 40,000 people. About half of these had a full-time or part-time physician. The utilization rate, however, was very low, so that their coverage was estimated to reach no more than 14 percent of the highly dispersed national population. Pakistan also planned nationwide coverage with rural health centers and smaller *basic health units,* each of which would have at least one physician. But again, coverage reached only about one-quarter of the people and utilization was generally light.

The health system of India is welfare oriented and a hierarchical network of health centers has been developed quite steadily since national independence in 1947. The earliest plans called for primary health centers, each staffed by one or two physicians (one male and one female), and expected to serve as many as 100,000 people. Soon this large a population coverage became recognized as unrealistic, and its was reduced gradually to 30,000; some 8,000 such primary health centers were built. More important, around each primary center, several subcenters were set up to give elementary primary health care to 5,000 people. The latter were staffed only by auxiliary health personnel, and the number of these structures exceeded 100,000—to reach two-thirds of India's large population. On a much smaller scale, Zimbabwe established rural health centers throughout its 55 districts. For the district population, averaging about 100,000 people, there were 3 to 5 health centers; these were staffed with professional nurse-midwives and auxiliary personnel for general prevention and general primary medical care.

Comprehensive health systems in very poor countries are found in Sri Lanka and Tanzania. In Sri Lanka, the coverage with a hierarchical framework of health centers is remarkably complete. The island has 25 districts, each with a district hospital. The district has about 10 divisions, averaging 60,000 people, and each division has around three subdivisions. All divisions and subdivisions have health centers staffed by auxiliary health personnel; important among these are *assistant medical practitioners* trained for 2 years. Despite its great poverty, Tanzania has made primary health care available to almost everyone through a national network of rural health centers and dispensaries. Unlike other African

countries, expenditures for ambulatory care have exceeded those for hospitals. Key personnel in the health centers are medical assistants, with 3 years of practical training after secondary school.

Among very poor countries, the health system of China is the most important demonstration of socialist ideology. Socialist concepts are seen in the pattern of provision of health services by governmental authorities, although not in their economic support. Preventive services are financed by government, but not medical treatment, which must be supported by insurance or personal payments.

Ambulatory medical care in China is provided in health centers, established throughout this large country's 2,300 counties and, within them, some 27,000 townships. In each township (formerly communes), there is at least one health center for primary health care, preventive and curative. In the cities the health centers are staffed by both western and traditional Chinese doctors, but in rural townships they might have only assistant doctors (medical assistants) and other auxiliary personnel. In the villages there are thousands of small health stations or clinics, staffed by briefly trained village doctors (successors to the "barefoot doctors"). In 1985–1986, the number of health stations exceeded 126,000, and of health centers it exceeded 48,000. There are also clinics at large industrial enterprises, at government agencies, and universities.

Thus, the trend throughout the world is toward the construction and use of health centers as the setting for delivery of ambulatory health services. In some industrialized countries, the long-established pattern of private medical practice remains strong, and health centers are limited mainly to the poor or restricted to preventive services. But this has changed in countries with comprehensive or with socialist health systems.

Considering health facilities as a whole, we may note the vitality in the development of both ambulatory facilities and hospitals. As the older type of facility, hospitals have acquired enormous importance in all countries over the centuries. As the newer type of facility, health centers and polyclinics have grown most rapidly in the latest century. The worldwide emphasis on primary health care contributed substantially to this development in recent decades.

In all countries, of course, hospitals provide the technological back-up to primary care. To play this role in developing countries, more hospitals are still needed. In most industrialized countries, hospital bed supplies have been deemed to reach an adequate plateau, but further improvements in quality of care are always being sought.

The growth and development of organized health facilities for ambulatory care have been somewhat stronger than that of hospitals in recent decades. Growth has clearly been greatest in the developing countries. In the industrialized countries it has been weaker (except for Scandinavia), but is changing.

Thus, the two streams of development—hospitals and health centers—proceed side by side, with contrasting characteristics in developing and industrialized countries. The type of health system also makes a difference, with greater general growth of both types of facility in the comprehensive and welfare-oriented systems. It is likely that growth will continue, as needed, in both health centers and hospitals, to provide the basic resources for comprehensive health services.

REFERENCES

Hospitals

Bridgman, R. F., and M. I. Roemer, *Hospital Legislation and Hospital Systems.* Geneva: World Health Organization (Public Health Papers No. 50), 1973.

International Hospital Federation, *The Changing Role of the Hospital in a Changing World.* London, 1963.

MacEachern, Malcolm T., *Hospital Organization and Management.* Berwyn, IL: Physician's Record, 1962, pp. 1–28.

Miller, Timothy S., *The Birth of the Hospital in the Byzantine Empire.* Baltimore, MD: Johns Hopkins University Press, 1985.

Roemer, Milton I., *Doctors in Hospitals.* Baltimore, MD: Johns Hopkins University Press, 1971.

Rosen, George, "The Hospital: Historical Sociology." In *From Medical Police to Social Medicine: Essays on the History of Health Care.* New York: Science History Publications, 1974.

Rosenberg, Charles E., "Inward Vision and Outward Glance: The Shaping of the American Hospital, 1880–1914." *Bulletin of the History of Medicine,* 53:345–391, 1979.

Sigerist, Henry E., "An Outline of the Development of the Hospital." *Bulletin of the Institute of the History of Medicine,* 4:573–581, 1936.

Thompson, J., and G. Goldin, *The Hospital: A Social and Architectural History.* New Haven: Yale University Press, 1975.

Ambulatory Care Facilities

Clark, George, *A History of the Royal College of Physicians of London,* Volume Two. Oxford: Clarendon Press, 1966.

Curwen, M., and B. Brookes, "Health Centres: Facts and Figures." *Lancet,* 2:945–948, 1969.

Davis, Michael M., *Clinics, Hospitals, and Health Centers.* New York: Harper, 1927.

Loudon, Irvine, *Medical Care and the General Practitioner, 1750–1850.* Oxford: Clarendon Press, 1986.

Ministry of Health, Consultative Council on Medical and Allied Services, *Interim Report on the Future Provision of Medical and Allied Services* (Dawson Report). London: His Majesty's Stationery Office, 1920.

Roemer, Milton I., *Evaluation of Community Health Centres.* Geneva: World Health Organization, 1972.

Roemer, Milton I., *Ambulatory Health Services in America Past, Present, and Future.* Rockville, MD: Aspen, 1981.

Rosenberg, Albert, "The London Dispensary for the Sick Poor." *Journal of the History of Medicine and Allied Sciences,* 14:41–56, January 1959.

Rosenberg, Charles E., "Social Class and Medical Care in Nineteenth Century America: The Rise and Fall of the Dispensary." *Journal of the History of Medicine and Allied Sciences,* 29:32–54, January 1974.

Sand, René, *The Advance to Social Medicine.* London: Staples Press, 1952.

Schorr, Lisbeth B., and Joseph T. English, "Background, Context, and Significant Issues in Neighborhood Health Center Programs." *Milbank Memorial Fund Quarterly,* 66:289–296, July 1968.

Solomon, Howard M., *Public Welfare, Science, and Propaganda in Seventeenth Century France: The Innovations of Thèophraste Renaudot.* Princeton, NJ: Princeton University Press, 1972.

Terris, Milton, "Hermann Biggs' Contribution to the Modern Concept of the Health Center." *Bulletin of the History of Medicine,* 20:387–412, 1946.

CHAPTER FOUR

Health Commodities and Knowledge

Health commodities and knowledge in the health sciences are the final resources in every national health system, and their production and distribution are examined in this chapter.

DRUGS AND EQUIPMENT

Numerous commodities are required in every health system for the treatment or prevention of disease. Most widely needed are drugs and vaccines, but in addition countless types of supplies, instruments, and medical equipment are used for diagnostic or therapeutic purposes. The development of the production of drugs has the longest and most complex history, which should be reviewed.

History of Drugs

Since ancient preliterate times, natural products from plants or animals have been used for the treatment of disease. There might be little distinction between drugs and foods, and the intended effect was usually based on magical concepts more than empiricism. Each primitive healer made his own concoctions, and his manner of doing so was considered crucial.

In ancient Egypt, there is evidence that a special type of artisan was skilled in the preparatio of drug products, as well as cosmetics and perfumes. This was done in special laboratories, and the products were kept in certain storerooms. Later in the classical world of Greece and Rome, there were also artisans skilled in making drugs from plants, especially from their roots—hence, called *root cutters.* Hippocratic medicine made relatively little use of drugs, except in connection with special diets. Itinerant Greek physicians, nevertheless, carried a supply of drugs that they had collected from various sources. A Greek bowl from the sixth century B.C. pictures a drug-packing activity. Medicinal tablets were made from a special clay *(terra sigillita)* on the island of Lemnos and sold throughout the entire classical world.

The drugs used by the practitioners of ancient China and India (Ayurveda), two thousand years before Christ, were customarily made by the doctor himself. A separate drug-producing function did not exist. In both of these ancient schools of medicine, drugs were the major form of therapy, and their preparation, as well as dispensing, was the principal task of the physician.

It was in the eighth century that Arabian medicine, keeping alive the classical tradition, gave rise to alchemy—the effort to create gold from the baser metals. In the course of the search for "potable gold" came the discovery of "aqua regia" (a mixture of nitric and hydrochloric acids), which gave rise to chemical pharmaceutics. Around the tenth century there emerged in Cairo and also in Persia a separate class of artisans, skilled in the preparation of compounds from both organic and inorganic materials—the apothecaries. These artisans would sell their concoctions directly to patients.

In the twelfth and thirteenth centuries, drugs were compounded and sold in the Arab world of North Africa. Each vendor, however, probably made his own products. The first organized production of a drug, which was sold to physicians and others for dispensing, has been traced to medieval Italy. In 1294 A.D., a small entrepreneur in Venice made a preparation from vipers, which was claimed to be an antidote to snake bites and various poisons; this was exported widely. Venetians likewise produced and exported cinnabar, borax, soap, lead, talc, and turpentine. Certain monasteries in Italy also made and sold compounds claimed to have therapeutic value.

From the fourteenth to the seventeenth centuries, the production of drugs was largely in the hands of individual apothecaries or physicians. Sometimes a physician would purchase drugs wholesale from an apothecary, but would dispense them directly to his own patients. Drugs were typically compounded in a back room behind the one in which the doctor or apothecary saw the patient. Some oriental drugs, along with spices, were also transported to Europe in Dutch and Portuguese ships in the sixteenth century. The first part of this century was the period when Paracelsus (1493–1541) did much to establish the principle that certain metals or other chemicals were effective in the treatment of specific diseases, such as mercury for syphilis.

In England, the London Society of Apothecaries started a cooperative drug manufacturing enterprise in 1623. This business sold drugs to physicians and to individual apothecaries until the nineteenth century. The first individual pharmacist to develop a manufacturing plant for wholesale production of drugs was Antoine Baume of France. This was in the eighteenth century, and a price list published by Baume in 1775 contained 2,400 specific items, among which were 400 preparations obtained through chemical processes (rather than from natural plant or animal sources). Because of the magnitude and diversity of this activity, Baume has been considered "the father of the modern pharmaceutical industry."

It was in Germany that the roots of the modern drug industry took hold. In 1668 Friedrick Jacob Merck acquired a small apothecary shop in Darmstadt. He began to manufacture a few drugs for general sale to others, and this business grew until, in 1816, it had evolved into a pharmaceutical factory headed by Heinrich E. Merck. The initial concentration was on the preparation of pure alkaloids—morphine in 1827, codeine in 1836, and cocaine in 1862. In 1887, another Merck descendant opened a branch in America.

The German dyestuffs industry contributed chemical techniques that facilitated the manufacture of drugs. The Schering Company grew out of an apothecary shop in Berlin started in 1852. Friedrich Bayer and Company was started in 1863, and in 1899 produced a synthetic remedy, aspirin (acetylsalicylic acid) that eventually became the most widely used pain reliever in modern medicine. Another German pharmacist or chemist, Freidrich Wohler, in 1828 achieved, for the first time a laboratory synthesis of an organic substance, urea, normally produced in the animal body.

The sequence of retail apothecary shop, to wholesale production of a few compounds, to larger factory, to pharmaceutical corporation was repeated scores of times in Germany, France, Britain, and Italy. In the United States the same story was illustrated by the Abbott Laboratories, starting as a one-man drugstore in Ravenswood, Illinois in 1866, and growing to a corporation with 31,500 employees, selling drugs to 130 countries a century later. Another such development was started by Eli Lilly, who began to manufacture drugs with two employees in Indianapolis in 1876; by 1976 there were 23,000 employees and annual sales of over $1 billion.

Since the late nineteenth century, the preparation of drugs in the industrialized countries has been a steady evolution of the process from compounding by the individual pharmacist, on the prescription of a doctor, to the manufacture and packaging of completed drug compounds by large companies. Around 1900, there must have been thousands of individual pharmacies, small companies, and large companies producing countless drugs in Europe and America. In the U.S. scene, where free enterprise was particularly unfettered, the abuses of false therapeutic claims for various "patent medicines" were rampant. This has led to increasingly rigorous legislation discussed below.

A major regulatory objective in almost all countries has been the delineation of drugs that may be dispensed only with a doctor's prescription, in contrast to those—such as aspirin or vitamins—that may be sold directly to people "over the counter." In the industrialized, affluent countries of all political types, these requirements are rather strictly followed. With respect to narcotics, there are serious problems of illicit sales and consumption, but for the great majority of drug products, pharmacy regulation has been effective in regulating drug distribution. In most developing countries, however, both the transitional and the poorest ones, the enforcement of regulations on drug distribution (which may be in the official statutes) is notoriously weak. Almost any medication may be purchased in a pharmacy, on request, with or without a prescription. This is quite aside from the dispensing of items by unlicensed "drug sellers."

When Paul Ehrlich discovered arsphenamine in Germany for the treatment of syphilis in 1909, the search for similar "magic bullets" for curing each and every disease began in earnest. Thousands of chemical compounds were developed through research in medical centers as well as pharmaceutical companies. The discovery of insulin in 1922 by Banting and Best in Canada was a major breakthrough, although it was an animal product rather than a synthetic chemical. In 1935, when Domagk in Germany developed sulfanilamide, and a few years later when Fleming in England discovered penicillin, a wholly new era was opened for conquering bacterial infections—the era of *chemotherapy.*

Pharmaceutical production has become increasingly linked to the chemical industry. Sophisticated technologies have been successful in mass production of tablets, capsules, fluids, and other preparations, along with their packaging for direct sale in pharmacies or dispensing by physicians. With the protection of patent laws, a monopoly is granted for many years, so that drug prices can be relatively high and profits are large. Drugs are so important in the treatment of disease that their purchase has come to consume a large share of the health budget in every country, particularly the less developed countries dependent on imports.

Governments have usually played a relatively small part in the production of drugs, except in the completely socialist countries, in contrast to their large roles in the training of personnel and the construction of health facilities. The major exception has been in the initial preparation of vaccines and other biologicals derived from animals. The large scale of production in many private pharmaceutical companies, however, has eventually enabled them to produce most vaccines more economically than governmental health agencies. Certain relatively simple drugs—such as oral rehydration salts, intravenous infusions, aspirin, or antiseptics—are packaged by government agencies from materials that have been purchased commercially.

To reduce the cost and ensure the quality of drugs, some welfare-oriented countries have established pharmaceutical enterprises under government. Shortly after its independence (1947), India developed a plant for manufacturing penicillin. Egypt has established quasi-governmental enterprises for preparing drugs on the basis of importation of the necessary chemical compounds. In the fully socialist countries, drug production and distribution have been undertaken almost entirely by the central government. When constituent chemicals must be imported, this is done, but as much as possible use is made of raw chemicals from within the country, and the fabrication of pills, solutions, and so on is done in domestic factories.

A high proportion of drugs consumed in developing countries, of course, are not "modern" in the sense of having been manufactured and sold by pharmaceutical companies. They are natural products, usually from plants but sometimes from animals or minerals, prepared and sold by a traditional practitioner or herbalist. Some of these herbal preparations are, no doubt, of value, and much research is being done in China and elsewhere to determine which materials have therapuetic effects and which do not. One must not forget that in previous centuries, practically all drugs were "natural" with "synthetic" preparations being relatively recent. Some of the most widely used drugs are still obtained—through various chemical purification processes—from natural plants, such as digitalis from the foxglove plant, morphine from the opium poppy, or atropine from the *atropa belladona* plant. As chemical knowledge has increased, it has been possible to extract the constituent substance in these plants, with the active pharmacological material, and sometimes the entire drug can be synthesized. Some 25 percent of modern drugs, nevertheless, are still produced directly or indirectly from organic materials obtained from plants or animals. Three-quarters are synthesized from petrochemical or fermentation processes.

The actions and effects of different drugs are highly variable. Some are preventive, such as diphtheria toxoid vaccine; some are curative, such as penicillin in the treatment of pneumonia; some are therapeutic—in the sense of treating the disease though not eliminating it—such as insulin for diabetes or digitalis for heart disease; and some are only palliative, such as aspirin for reduction of pain or paregoric for easing of diarrhea. In any event, drugs of different types are virtually indispensable in the provision of health care. Because of their often rapid palliative effect, they may be overused, and much medical care may be of poor quality when the doctor or other healer hastily gives or prescribes a drug in place of a careful examination of the patient, a proper diagnosis, and prudent therapy. Because they are often abused, however, the great value of drugs must not be denigrated. The efficient discovery, testing, production, and distribution of drugs are essential requirements of every health system.

Development of Medical Equipment

Simple medical supplies, such as bandages to stop bleeding or warm water to clean soiled skin, must have been used since the earliest times. Soap, as a cleasing agent, was known in ancient Rome, but it was not manufactured outside Italy until about 1200 A.D. in France. The first English patent granted to a soap maker was in the seventeenth century. Later, as chemistry developed, various antiseptics were prepared to kill microorganisms in human tissue. By the eighteenth century, these materials were manufactured and sold for medical and especially surgical purposes. Countless types of supplies for surgical treatment, for setting fractures, for laboratory tests, and for X-ray examinations came to be manufactured in the nineteenth century. Modern surgery requires countless instruments and devices. Ophthalmology, cardiology, gynecology, obstetrics, urology, and neurology each has its own special instrumentation.

Equipment for the diagnosis and treatment of disease depended more directly on careful scientific discovery, demonstrating its value. The French physician, René T. H. Laennec,

invented the stethoscope in 1817, permitting identification of abnormalities in the chest through auscultation to hear internal sounds. Various forms of stethoscope soon came to be manufactured in Europe and America, and sold to doctors. Today this simple instrument, to magnify internal body sounds, has become virtually the symbol of a physician, and sometimes of a nurse. Not until the discovery of X-rays by Roentgen in 1895 was there a significant further advance in equipment to facilitate the diagnosis of internal disorders.

The origins of the microscope are not entirely clear, but are often attributed to the English philosopher and scientist, Roger Bacon, in the thirteenth century. Galileo, who invented the telescope in 1609, is also credited with developing a microscope about the same time. It was not until many years later, however, that practical medical use of the microscope was made by Antoni van Leeuwenhoek of Holland. van Leeuwenhoek was able to demonstrate the presence of red blood corpuscles, microorganisms, spermatozoa, and so on in 1683, although the human significance of these tiny living things was not recognized until later. In the nineteenth century, as the demand for microscopes became widespread, it was manufactured by optical instrument companies, particularly in Germany. With constant improvement in its powers, the compound microscope has become a necessity in medical and hospital laboratories everywhere. It must be purchased from companies in Germany, United States, Japan, and a few other countries. Even greater magnification, useful in basic biological research, was made possible by the electron microscope, invented in Germany around 1932.

The discovery of X-rays, and the invention of the special vacuum X-ray tube by Wilhelm Roentgen in 1895, opened up a chain of increasingly sophisticated diagnostic equipment that has had major impacts on hospitals and medical practice throughout the world. Commercial companies, first in Germany, then in Holland, Great Britain, the United States, Japan, Switzerland, and elsewhere, developed further refinements in the use of X-rays for examination of various body organs. Soon after 1900, the destructive effect of X-rays on young tissue cells (such as in the gonads) was recognized, leading to radiological treatment of cancer. The pace of appearance of new radiographic inventions, coming principally from the laboratories of commercial firms, has steadily accelerated, leading to increased medical capabilities and also higher costs.

The invention of computerized tomography (CT) scanning by an English company in the late 1960s constituted a quantum leap in the capability of localizing internal lesions, especially in the head. The cost of the CT scanner, however, is extremely high, so that it has become generally available only in very affluent countries. In the less developed countries, these instruments may not be available at all or only in one or two hospitals; this creates serious ethical issues regarding the patients on whom it will be used. In the 1980s, furthermore, a private U.S. firm invented another machine for imaging internal organs even more sharply—by nuclear magnetic resonance (NMR)—at still higher costs. The task of calculating cost–benefit ratios of these various advanced technologies has become a special challenge to health economists. Policy issues are especially serious in countries that want at least one NMR or MRI (magnetic resonance imaging) machine in the national capital, when scores of rural health stations lack even essential drugs or scales for weighing small babies.

Prostheses

The commonest prostheses in a national health system are probably eyeglasses. Recognition of visual defects can be traced to the time of Plato and also ancient Chinese medicine, but the invention of spectacles or eyeglasses is generally considered to have come in the thirteenth century. Roger Bacon (1214–1294) was a Franciscan monk who became a professor at Oxford University in England; he described in his writings convex lenses, which enlarged small letters so that elderly monks could read them. The word was spread to monasteries in Italy and Germany. Another monk, Allasandre de la Spina, is often credited with the arrangement of lenses in frames, to be worn as spectacles in the early fourteenth century.

The invention of printing around 1440 gave a great impetus to the production of eyeglasses, and soon after 1440 spectacle making became an established craft in Germany, with guilds in the field. By 1500, there were spectacle-makers' guilds in Germany, France, England, Italy, and Holland. Methods of more rapid production of spectacles were developed in Germany and England, from where the products were sold everywhere, including the American colonies. In the eighteenth century, it was Benjamin Franklin who conceived the idea of bifocal eyeglass lenses, which were actually ground in England.

The production of eyeglasses did not become organized on a commercial scale until the nineteenth century. In 1833, a small shop in Southbridge, Massachusetts employed four spectacle makers, turning out relatively large numbers of eyeglasses; people would choose among them, by trial-and-error, to find the one that was most helpful to their vision. One of these artisans, George Wells, founded in 1869 the American Optical Company. This firm developed many techniques for more efficient mass production of refractive lenses. By the end of the nineteenth century, many other firms for the manufacture of spectacle lenses, frames, and other products had arisen in America and Europe.

Optometry, the measurement and correction of refractive errors of vision, arose as a skilled profession in the late nineteenth century; the American Optometric Association was organized in 1904 and promoted university education in this skill. Similar professional status for optometrists (or dispensing opticians) has developed in Great Britain, Australia, New Zealand, and Canada—less so in Germany, Denmark, and Switzerland. In France, Holland, Belgium, and other industrialized countries, visual refraction is regarded as a skilled trade or craft. In most developing countries, a few optometrists—trained abroad—are found in the main cities. Most optometrists work in small independent shops, but in some affluent countries they are associated with medical specialists in ophthalmology.

Aside from eyeglasses, many other prostheses are available in some national health systems. In affluent countries there are prostheses for the physically handicapped, crutches and wheelchairs, and all sorts of orthopedic shoes. Hearing aids have become increasingly effective. In less developed countries, such aids to daily living may be ingeniously improvised.

Drug Production and Consumption

The production of modern pharmaceutical products, which are mainly synthesized from various chemical compounds, is heavily concentrated in a relatively few countries. In 1985, world pharmaceutical production was valued at $95,600,000,000 at current prices, and more than half of these products were from two countries—the United States and Japan. In terms of their overall share of world drug production, the major drug-producing countries in 1980 were as follows:

Country	Percent of Total Drug Production
United States	30
Japan	24
Federal Republic of Germany	13
France	9
Great Britain	6.4
Italy	6
Switzerland	4
All other countries	7.6
Total	100.0

This means that most countries must obtain their drugs mainly by importation from a small number of highly industrialized countries.

The consumption of drugs is also concentrated in a relatively few large countries. Two-thirds of all modern drug consumption in 1985 was in the following eight countries:

Country	Percent of Total Drug Consumption
United States	28.1
Japan	14.9
Federal Republic of Germany	6.4
China	5.0
France	4.7
Italy	3.9
Great Britain	2.5
India	1.9
All other countries	32.6
Total	100.0

On a per capita basis, the drug consumption of people in industrialized countries was much higher than in developing countries. Expressed in U.S. dollars, the per capita value of drug consumption in the more developed and less developed regions of the world in 1985 was as follows:

More Developed Regions	Value per Capita ($)
Japan	116.3
North America	106.3
Western Europe	54.5
All developed	62.1

Less Developed Regions	Value per Capita ($)
Latin America	13.8
Africa	4.9
Asia	4.2
All developing	5.4

Examining drug consumption in individual countries, the expenditures in the five countries with greatest drug consumption ($80 per capita or more) in 1985 may be compared with those in countries with low consumption (under $20 per capita). These amounts were as follows in U.S. dollars during 1985:

High Consumption Countries	Amount per Capita ($)
Japan	116.2
United States	110.5
Federal Republic of Germany	98.2
Switzerland	92.6
France	80.9

Low Consumption Countries	Amount per Capita ($)
Mexico	15.7
Egypt	15.0
Brazil	10.3
China	4.4
India	2.3

Within these national drug expenditures, those made in the high consumption countries come largely from public sector sources, whereas those made in the low consumption countries come largely from private sector sources.

Regarding individual pharmaceutical companies, a relatively small number sell the lion's share of all products. Although the total drug industry comprises some 10,000 companies, only 15 of these, in the United States, West Germany, Switzerland, and Great Britain, account for 80 percent of world shipments. The two largest drug-selling companies in the world (Merck and Company and American Home Products) are both based in the United States. This was true of 7 of the top 10 companies in 1985. The subsidiaries of these 7 firms accounted for 50 percent of their total sales in the late 1980s.

In the 1950s and 1960s, the world pharmaceutical industry shifted from producing mainly over-the-counter to mainly medical prescription drugs, so that physicians became the major targets for drug promotion. Competition among firms, therefore, was based on product differentiation, patents, and brand names. To capture larger shares of the drug market, pharmaceutical companies in the United States increased their expenditure for research from 3.70 percent of sales income in 1951 to 12.53 percent in 1985. Analysis of 508 new drugs, introduced between 1974 and 1985, however, disclosed that only 29.5 percent of them yielded any therapeutic improvement over older drugs.

Legislation on drug patents is intended to establish a period of years, during which the innovating company is allowed to enjoy a monopoly on the production of the new drug. In the United States, this protected period is 17 years, but it is 20 years in most European countries. Such patent protection has the effect of preventing local manufacturers in developing countries from making similar less costly products. Expenditures on the marketing of various brand-name products to physicians involve more than 20 percent of sales revenue— much more than expenditures on research and development. Relatively little is spent, furthermore, on drug research for the control of trop-

ical diseases of greatest concern to the developing countries.

The use of drugs permeates all parts of national health systems. Pharmacology, of course, is an essential discipline in the training of doctors and nurses, and pharmacists are trained in university courses in most countries. Every organized health program must make provision for its supply and distribution of drugs; even mental health programs now count heavily on the use of psychotropic drugs. The administration of drug supplies and the regulation of drug production and marketing are major features of system management. The economic support of drugs is, of course, basic in every budgetary process. In the delivery of health care, drugs are important at primary, secondary, and tertiary levels. They are important in disease prevention, especially if we recognize that immunizing agents are a type of drug. They are important in special programs for children, for the aged, for treating tuberculosis and venereal disease, and for all types of hopsitals and health centers.

In all but the socialist and a few other developing countries, the pharmaceutical industry is almost entirely in the private sector, engaged in competitive trade and investing a great deal in advertising both to doctors and to the population generally. (In the United States, monopolistic trade agreements on drug prices have led to several governmental prosecutions.) As a result, thousands of drugs have been produced, of which many have identical pharmacological effects and only different names and prices. To clarify matters, all new drugs approved for manufacture and sold in a country are given a "generic" name—usually a simplified form of its chemical composition. When and if the drug is patented, this is always under a *brand* name (e.g., *Valium* is the brand name for the generic *diazepam*). Since the patent law prohibits any other manufacturer from producing the drug under this name (or even under another name by payment of *royalties*) for a certain length of time, the price is usually relatively high. When the patent has expired, any firm may produce and sell the drug under its generic name, but all too often this name is not well known by the doctors or others.

To reduce costs, several countries authorize

the pharmacist to substitute generic drugs for the brand-name products prescribed by the physician. (This may, however, be specifically prohibited by the physician.) The equivalence of generic and brand-name products has been a subject of controversy, but in organized health programs, generic drugs are coming to be routinely used.

To simplify the prescribing and limit the number and cost of drugs, many health programs—hospitals, governmental or insurance schemes, and so on—prepare *formularies,* which are lists of specified drugs that are kept in the pharmacies and may be prescribed by the doctors. Many of these are generic compounds, which are almost always less expensive than their brand-name equivalents. For each pharmacological action—for example, antihypertensive agents—there might be two or three different preparations in the formulary, but not 20 or 30 that exist on the market. Formularies are increasingly being used in organized health care programs.

Policy on "Essential Drugs"

To promote the more rational use of drugs, the World Health Organization has encouraged countries to adopt a restricted list of *essential drugs.* With such a list, the number of drugs used in a country can be reduced to a few hundred that have been found to be safe, effective, and reasonably priced. Since countries have differing health needs, their lists of essential drugs must differ, but they typically contain the names of about 200 to 300 products. Legislation providing for essential drugs may be of two types. It may provide for a *national formulary* that specifies which drugs may be produced, imported, and distributed in a country. Among industrialized countries, Norway is a model, with an official list of about 1,100 drugs registered for importation and use in the country. Only a few developing countries have such comprehensive regulation—the best known being Bangladesh. The second type of legislation on essential drugs applies only to those used in public sector facilities.

In 1982, the Bangladesh Ministry of Health banned the import or sale of 1,700 drugs that it regarded as "harmful or unnecessary." By

1983, more than twice as many of the 45 most essential drugs were being made, and were being sold at lower prices. With such prices, the tight budget of the Central Medical Stores went further and could serve more people. Prices were also reduced in private stores. Although the large drug companies had opposed the essential drugs policy, they did not lose in overall sales volume; their sales volumes actually increased. Similar comprehensive drug regulation has been enacted in Sri Lanka and Mozambique.

Altogether about 50 developing countries, as of 1990, have enacted legislation on essential drugs, but in the great majority the restricted list is applied only to drugs used in public facilities—in governmental hospitals and health centers. Another 40 countries have enacted certain components of an Essential Drugs Program. Of the 5,000,000,000 people in the world (1987), between 1,300,000,000 and 2,500,000,000 have little or no regular access to essential drugs. The grossly unequal distribution of drugs between developed and developing countries remains serious. In 1985, some 75 percent of the world's population accounted for less than one-quarter of total drug consumption. And mostly in the developed countries, some 25 percent of the world's population accounted for more than three-quarters of total drug consumption.

On the brighter side, in recent years the promotion of drugs in developing countries has shown greater honesty by major pharmaceutical companies. Surveys of prescription drug marketing material in 1973 and 1980 disclosed gross exaggeration of clinical claims and understatements of possible adverse reactions in developing countries. A broad survey in 1984 showed much greater accuracy in the promotional material of many pharmaceutical companies. The companies discarding a "double standard" in drug promotion—which had distorted the claims made in developing countries—were found to suffer only insignificant reduction of profits. The reliability of drug promotional claims was not found to bear any relationship to the political character of the country in which the firm was located—whether highly entrepreneurial, welfare oriented, or comprehensive. Most cases of irrational drug promotion involved domestic firms in developing countries—about 60 percent domestic companies and 40 percent multinational.

Another beneficial trend has been the greater use of generic drugs, in contrast to brand-name products, as noted above. This has occurred particularly in the United States and has led to reduction of expenditures for drugs. This has been due to the exhaustion of patent restrictions and also to the passage of laws in many U.S. states, permitting pharmacists to substitute equivalent generic products for branded ones.

Because of a long history of misleading labeling and advertising of drugs, regulation has become increasingly rigorous in nearly all industrialized countries. The first such regulatory law was enacted in England about 1875, followed by Swiss legislation in 1900. The United States enacted its first Pure Food and Drug Act in 1906, followed by more stringent laws in 1938, requiring proof of drug safety, before a new drug could be marketed. This policy led to similar drug control legislation throughout the world during the next 40 years. The tragedy of *thalidomide* (causing severely defective babies, when taken by the pregnant woman) in Europe led to further regulatory requirements on both drug safety and efficacy in 1962—initially in the United States, Norway, Sweden, and Great Britain. The concept of efficacy was new and important. By the 1980s, such regulation had become worldwide. The bureaucratic difficulties of drug regulation have generated major debates about the problems of a lag in the introduction of effective drugs, as against the benefits of assurance of drug safety. These debates have been intensified by the search for effective drugs to treat patients afflicted with AIDS. Insofar as this and other kinds of drug regulation are an aspect of health system management, they will be further discussed later.

KNOWLEDGE AS A RESOURCE

Knowledge is an indispensable resource in every health system. The history of the development of knowledge about health and disease is, of course, as long and complex as the history of mankind. Since the origins of science in the ancient world, scientific knowledge in the health-related disciplines has become increasingly abundant and complex. To cope with the enormous accumulation of facts and concepts about the diseases of human beings, how they may be treated or prevented, and how positive health may be promoted, increasingly elaborate specialization has been necessary. Not only has the magical or empirical healer been largely replaced by the scientific physician, but the domain of medicine has become subdivided into some 50 or more specialties and subspecialties, and the process of health service has been subdivided among dozens of allied health professions.

Within each of the subdivisions, research, observation, and experience are contributing new knowledge all the time. The discovery of new facts is invariably dependent on previous discoveries. The invention of the microscope was necessary before microorganisms could be identified. Then, numerous other scientific observations were necessary to demonstrate that these tiny organisms could cause disease. Still further scientific research was required to show how infectious disease might be spread from one person to another. The protection of individuals against the hazard of contracting communicable disease, of course, depended on the massive additional research necessary to elucidate immunization.

Examples of the long chains of discoveries and research that evolved to produce the cognitive groundwork of modern health services would be countless. Two or three thousand years ago, new knowledge was produced at only a few places on earth; knowledge was produced in urban centers of ancient Greece, China, India, or Egypt, but it spread very slowly—usually from the direct communication of travelers. As civilizations developed in all parts of the globe, scientific research has been carried out in hundreds of places, and new facts or at least theories about nature are communicated rapidly.

In modern times, it has become commonplace to observe that scientific knowledge has grown exponentially; in the last 50 years, it is said, there have been more discoveries than in all previous centuries. Yet recent discoveries obviously depended on the previous foundation of knowledge about man, society, and nature.

Development of Knowledge through Research

Observation and research contributing to knowledge about human health and disease have been carried out all over the world. The earliest recognition of disease as due to natural, rather than supernatural, phenomena came from classical Greece, with the work of Aristotle and Hippocrates and their followers (500–300 B.C.). In the later period of Greece and the rise of the Roman Empire, there was a vast organization of medical knowledge by Galen (131–201 A.D.). Roman medicine contributed to environmental sanitation, the advance of surgery, and the development of hospitals.

In the early Middle Ages, classical knowledge was kept alive by Arabic physicians, such as Rhazes (844–926 A.D.) and Avicenna (980–1037 A.D.). In the eleventh and twelfth centuries, medicine was elevated to a higher plane by the school founded at Salerno on the southern coast of Italy. The theories of Galen still prevailed, and this knowledge was kept alive mostly in Spain. Universities were founded at Paris in 1110, at Oxford in 1167, and at Naples in 1224. Human dissection was done at the universities in Italy, with the result that their contributions to medicine were greater than those of the universities in northern Europe.

Epidemics stimulated knowledge of contagion in the later Middle Ages. Leprosy led to leper hospitals or *lazarettos* all over Europe between 1096 and 1472. In the middle of the fourteenth century, the devastating bubonic plague was spread to Europe from Asia, by way of Constantinople. The *Black Death,* as the plague was called, finally proved the infectiousness of this disease. In 1348, the City of Venice first introduced the idea of quarantine—by requiring incoming ships to be isolated for 40 days before landing.

In 1495, syphilis appeared in Spain, on the return of Columbus's sailors from the West Indies. It spread rapidly in Europe in an acute malignant form. Mercury ointment became the routine treatment.

Fresh impetus to the study of the human body came from a school of artists in Florence, Italy, the most noted of whom was Leonardo da Vinci. Anatomical dissections were made by Vesalius (1514–1564) in Padua, Italy. Paracelsus from Switzerland (1493–1541) greatly advanced medical knowledge from the dogmas of Galen, through observation and experimentation; he introduced various chemicals for treating disease. Surgery was advanced by Ambrose Paré (1510–1590) of Paris; he introduced ligatures, rather than boiling oil, to stop surgical bleeding. His confidence in the healing power of nature was summed up in the sentence "I treated him and God cured him."

An English scientist, William Harvey (1578–1657), discovered the circulation of the blood through experimental vivisection, ligation, and perfusion. He demonstrated that the blood was of prime importance, and the heart was only a pump to keep it in motion. The great extension of knowledge through the magnifying power of a microscope was made possible by the lens grinding of Antoni van Leewenhoek, a Dutch scientist (1632–1723). Thomas Sydenham (1624–1689), a British physician, reintroduced the study of disease at the patient's bedside; he emphasized the unique natural history of each disease. Another British physician, William Petty (1623–1687) developed quantitative biostatistics, to clarify the rate of occurrence of disease and mortality rates.

The eighteenth century in Europe, known as the era of the Enlightenment, was a period of great emancipation of human thought. The religious Reformation in Christianity had occurred earlier, and led to the general demand for liberty in all political, spiritual, and intellectual matters. Human protection against smallpox, through vaccination with cowpox virus, was developed by Edward Jenner of England (1749–1823). Surgery was greatly advanced by the establishment of the Academy of Surgery in France in 1731. In London, the work of the Scottish anatomist, John Hunter (1728–1793), put surgery on a more scientific basis, leading to the founding of the Royal College of Surgeons of London in 1800.

The great American and French Revolutions toward the end of the eighteenth century brought political changes that led to urban and industrialized society. The Industrial Revolution brought productive labor-saving machinery to manufacturing, transportation, and every aspect of life. In medicine, occupational hygiene had been launched by the work of Bernardino Ramazzini in Italy (1633–1714). Broad concepts of public health were advocated in the writings of the great German physician, Johann Peter Frank (1745–1820).

The flowering of political freedom, industrial development, and scientific thinking had enormous influence on medicine and health in the nineteenth century. Darwin's *Origin of Species,* published in 1859, disposed of the concept of man as the center of the universe and contributed to the whole development of the biological sciences. Different European countries have served in various periods as centers of medical science—attracting physicians. In the early nineteenth century, it was France with its clinics and hospitals, and medical leaders such as Laennec (1781–1826) and Philippe Pinel (1745–1826).

In the middle years of the nineteenth century there were brilliant British physicians, such as Robert Graves (1796–1853), William Stokes (1804–1878), Richard Bright (1789–1858), Thomas Addison (1793–1860), Thomas Hodgkin (1798–1866), and James Parkinson (1755–1824). Their names have been applied to important disease entities that they differentiated.

In the later years of the nineteenth century, Germany was the outstanding center of medical science. Rudolf Virchow (1821–1902) was the founder of cellular pathology. Robert Koch (1843–1910) discovered the bacillus of tuberculosis. In this period Louis Pasteur of France (1822–1895) made his great contribution to bacteriology and immunology. Paul Ehrlich (1854–1915) discovered Salvarsan for the treatment of syphilis, and his concepts guided subsequent workers in the discovery of the sulfonamides and then the antibiotics. Wilhelm Roentgen (1845–1922) was the German physicist who discovered X-rays.

After World War I, the center of medical science shifted to North America. Canadians Frederick Banting and Charles Best prepared insulin from extracts of mammalian pancreas for the treatment of diabetes. Early medical education in America had started in Philadelphia at the University of Pennsylvania in 1765 and later at Harvard University and Dartmouth College. The Johns Hopkins Medical School in Baltimore demonstrated much higher standards of teaching and research after 1893. Great advances were made in the science of nutrition, with the discovery of vitamins and diseases caused by their deficiency. Joseph Goldberger (1874–1929) demonstrated that the common disease in the southern states, pellagra, was due to dietary deficiency in the B vitamin, niacin.

The shifting centers of medical science are reflected strikingly in the nationality of winners of the Nobel Prize in medicine or physiology. From 1901 to 1929, all prize winners were from Europe, except for the Canadian Frederick Banting in 1923. In 1930, Karl Landsteiner was the first scientist from the United States (although originally German) to win the Nobel Prize in medicine, and by 1950 there were 14 other American prize winners. From 1951 to 1970 there were 24 U.S. Nobel Laureates in medicine, and up to 1986 there were another 16. All the other prize winners in medicine were from Europe, except for Bernardo Houssay from Argentina in 1947. In 1987, the first Nobel Prize in medicine won by a Japanese scientist went to Susumu Tonegawa.

Modern Health Research

In the 1980s the world's greatest burden of disease and premature death was in the developing countries, but the great bulk of medical research was being done on the health problems of the industralized countries. Counted in potential years of life lost, the developing countries account for 93 percent of the world mortality burden and the industrialized countries only 7 percent. Yet of the $30 billion spent worldwide on health research in 1986, only $1.6 billion or 5 percent was devoted specifically to the health problems of developing countries, and 95 percent was for research mainly on the problems of industrialized countries.

According to the Commission on Health Research for Development, of the $30 billion expenditure on all health research in 1986, $13 billion came from private pharmaceutical companies based in industrialized countries and nearly $17 billion originated predominantly from the governments of those countries. The great concentration of health research in a few industrialized countries is reflected by the proportions of expenditures for such governmentally funded research in 1986:

Country	Percentage
United States	52.3
Japan	12.7
Federal Republic of Germany	8.8
France	5.3
Italy	3.4
Great Britain	2.6
All other countries	14.9
Total	100.0

The expenditures for health science research by pharmaceutical companies would show the same general distribution, and such support from philanthropic foundations (though relatively small) would be very heavily derived from the United States.

In most countries, health science research, whatever its source of funding, is carried out mainly in universities and their medical and related schools. In the formerly socialist countries, most research was done in separate research intitutes under governmental sponsorship. Much research everywhere is done in hospitals under different sponsorships. Pharmaceutical research is done, of course, largely by private drug companies.

Dissemination of Knowledge and Technology

Wherever health research may be conducted, its findings are widely disseminated through a worldwide network of scientific and professional journals. In this sphere, the handicaps of certain developing countries may be greater. Crucial discoveries and inventions in the twentieth century have come increasingly from a relatively few highly industrialized countries in Europe and North America, and they must be disseminated to countries on the other continents. News and reports reach the national capitals quickly, but they are not as rapidly spread to the hinterlands of the developing countries. Much more constrained than the flow of knowledge is the extension of technology based on it.

An invention, such as computerized tomography scanning, coming from Great Britain in the early 1970s, was a great breakthrough for the diagnosis of pathology in internal organs. CT scanners presented X-ray pictures of the head and body in essentially three dimensions. The invention spread rapidly to the United States and other industrialized countries. By 1979, there was 1 CT scanner per 1,000,000 population in Britain, 4.6 in Japan, and 5.7 in the United States. In some 40 developing countries surveyed in 1977, however, 85 percent of them did not have a single scanner; in the six developing countries with scanners, there might have been one or two machines for national populations of many millions.

Even for much less sophisticated technology, the application of well-established techniques is typically gravely deficient in most developing countries. Basic laboratory and X-ray equipment may have been provided to a hospital at one time, but all too frequently this equipment is in disrepair. Since spare parts must usually be imported, there are long delays for installing them. Technicians with appropriate reparative skills are often lacking. When X-ray machines are working, there may be shortages of film. Laboratory reagents are often in short supply. Drug shortages are a chronic problem in most developing countries and in several Eastern European health systems.

In one respect cross-national communications have improved in recent decades. Since the end of World War II, the English language has become very widely used in both affluent and less developed countries. Leaders in national health systems of nearly all countries can read and understand English, so that English-language books and journals may be widely distributed. Translations into Spanish,

French, Arabic, Russian, and other languages are, of course, extensive—particularly in fields covered by the international health agencies.

Many new applications of knowledge result in reduction of health system costs, whereas other applications increase costs—even though benefits may be great. The discovery of antibiotic drugs has simplified the treatment of many infectious diseases, as well as lowering the costs. Immunization against poliomyelitis has not only prevented paralytic disease but has greatly reduced the costs of its care. Low-cost oral rehydration therapy has saved countless infant lives and greatly reduced the costs of treating infantile diarrhea. Streptomycin and isoniazide have greatly lightened both the human and economic burden of tuberculosis throughout the world.

Other new technologies, however, have effects that are not so clear, with costs that are known to be high. CT scanning is one such technological advance already noted. Similar costly innovations of recent decades are renal dialysis, coronary bypass surgery, cobalt radiation therapy, and automated clinical laboratory tests. In affluent countries, such technology has been widely applied, even though proof of the benefits, in relation to the costs, has not been shown. In the United States and several Western European countries, where health system costs as a share of GNP have been rising sharply, the task of *technology assessment* has become conspicuous. In the United States, legislation in 1976 on *medical devices* required the federal Food and Drug Administration to find that new types of equipment were both safe and efficacious, before being introduced. Somewhat similar evaluations were performed in Sweden, Great Britain, France, Australia, and Germany, although these were not statutorily required.

The expansion of medical technologies, large and small, has been bewildering. The advances are dramatically reflected by a comparison of textbooks over a recent 50-year period. Cecil's *Textbook of Medicine* has been widely used throughout the world since its first edition in 1927. According to Paul Beeson, by medical standards of the 1980s, an evaluation of the recommendations proposed in this first edition found the remedies to be merely symptomatic,

dubious, or even harmful 60 percent of the time; only 3 percent were fully effective as treatment or prevention. The remedies proposed in the 1975 edition were still far from perfect, but the effective ones had increased seven-fold and the dubious ones had decreased by two-thirds.

Within the health sciences, it is fortunate that an ethics of knowledge has developed, under which open communication has become the prevailing policy. If a new treatment for some disease is discovered, it is rapidly reported in the world literature, so that it becomes available to everyone. Certain drugs or medical devices may become protected by patents, but this does not prevent their use by others, as long as the original inventor or firm is paid a royalty. Furthermore, products regarded as "natural," such as antibiotics (e.g., penicillin), are not subject to patent restrictions.

Health science disciplines have acquired a broad international character. Almost every medical specialty and allied health discipline has its international organization, which holds periodic conferences where new ideas are exchanged. The scientific and professional journals abound. An endless stream of scientists, physicians, nurses, and others from developing countries travel to the more highly developed countries for periods of study and technical training. Economic support for these international exchanges has steadily increased, although it is still far below the needs of most developing countries.

Journals for the recording and dissemination of knowledge in the health sciences have increased to the tens of thousands throughout the world. Even when a new discovery or invention is communicated rapidly throughout the world, however, its application may be impeded by lack of resources and weakness of social organization. The eradication of smallpox from all countries in 1979 was a monumental achievement, but the basic knowledge and technology had been discovered 200 years before—that is, the immunizing properties of cowpox inoculation. Two centuries were required to convince people (both doctors and community leaders) of the facts, to produce the necessary vaccine, to manage its physical shipment under specified conditions, to assemble people for the vaccination process, to develop a mechanism for reporting any cases, and to carry out other steps in the public health process leading to eradication of the smallpox virus. For each individual affected, this was a relatively inexpensive technology, whereas for certain technologies—such as renal dialysis or lithotriptic dissolution of kidney stones—the costs must be measured in thousands of dollars per case. A rich country such as the United States can, with government funds, finance the dialysis treatment of thousands of patients with end-stage kidney disease, whereas in developing countries most patients with such disease must simply be left to die.

In summary, the discovery of new knowledge through research is usually a long and costly process, and yet it is only the first step in a sequence leading to the application of a useful technology. Vast amounts of knowledge, on which health services are based, of course, have been conveyed from the past—the result of both observation and experimentation. The production of new knowledge usually requires research, although sometimes it comes from clarifying relationships between ideas not previously recognized. Second, the new fact or theory must be reported, so that others can test it and hopefully confirm it. Third, when knowledge is firmly established it must be communicated widely, if it is to bring benefits. Fourth, human and physical resources must be available, to be used for practical implementation of the new idea. Fifth must be an adequate flow of economic support to convert resources into the appropriate services. Sixth is the crucial step of application of the knowledge to derive an expected effect. Seventh is evaluation of the outcome, to determine if the whole new technology has been worthwhile.

In a world of nation-states, with very different levels of capability, this entire process usually requires many years. The speed and outreach of a new idea, embodied for example in an immunizing agent, are bound to be much greater than for an idea requiring changes in human behavior, such as smoking cigarettes. Assuring clean water proved to be a much more effective way of eliminating cholera than a policy of convincing everyone to boil the water they drank. A comparable policy on cigarettes would call for eliminating all growth of tobacco by crop substitution, but the political and economic obstacles to this would be enormous.

The excellent health record of Sweden, for example, reflected in its low infant mortality rate, is not the result of any fund of knowledge lacking in, say, India. The knowledge of nutrition, sanitation, immunization, childbirth, and infant care is essentially equal in both countries. The difference lies in the *application* of this knowledge in the daily lives of the people, their environment, and their health systems. Knowledge is indispensable in every national health system, but it is sterile unless it is applied. The application of available knowledge is the task of society in every country and the mission of its health system.

REFERENCES

Pharmaceutical Products

Bakke, Olav M., "How Many Drugs Do We Need?" *World Health Forum,* 7:252–255, 1986.

Fraser, Henry S., "Rational Use of Essential Drugs." *World Health Forum,* 6:63–66, 1985.

Gish, Oscar, and Loretta Lee Feller, *Planning Pharmaceuticals for Primary Health Care.* Washington, D.C.: American Public Health Association, 1979.

Hodes, Benjamin, "Nonprescription Drugs: An Overview." *International Journal of Health Services* 4(1):125–130, 1974.

Institute of Medicine, *Pharmaceutical Innovations and the Needs of Developing Countries.* Washington, D.C.: National Academy of Sciences, June 1979.

Jayasuriya, D. C., *Regulation of Pharmaceuticals in Developing Countries—Legal Issues and Approaches.* Geneva: World Health Organization, 1985.

Joldal, B., "Selecting Drugs on the Basis of Need." (Norway). *World Health Forum,* 6:67–69, 1985.

Lee, Philip R., and Jessica Herzstein, "International Drug Regulation." *Annual Review of Public Health 1986,* 7:217–235.

McCraine, Ned, and Martin J. Murray, "The Pharmaceutical Industry: A Further Study in Corporate Power." *International Journal of Health Services,* 8(4):573–588, 1978.

McDermott, Walsh, "Pharmaceuticals: Their Role in Developing Societies." *Science,* 209:240–245, 11 July 1980.

Rabin, David L., and Patrician J. Bush, "The Use of Medicines: Historical Trends and International Comparisons." *International Journal of Health Services,* 4(1):61–87, 1974.

Rawlins, Michael D., "The Case for Generic Substitution." *World Health Forum,* 5:329–330, 1984.

Silverman, Milton, Philip R. Lee, and Mia Lydecker, "The Drugging of the Third World." *International Journal of Health Services,* 12(4):585–596, 1982.

Silverman, Milton, P. R. Lee, and M. Lydecker, "Drug Promotion: The Third World Revisited." *International Journal of Health Services,* 16(4):659–667, 1986.

World Health Organization, *The Selection of Essential Drugs.* Geneva: WHO (Technical Report Series 615), 1977.

World Health Organization, *The World Drug Situation.* Geneva: WHO, 1988.

World Health Organization, *Action Programme on Essential Drugs and Vaccines.* Geneva: WHO Progress Report, May 1989.

Prostheses

Banerjee, Sikhar Nath (Editor), *Rehabilitation Management of Amputees.* Baltimore: Williams & Wilkins, 1982.

Cox, Maurice E., *Optometry, the Profession: Its Antecedents, Birth, and Development.* Philadelphia: Chilton Co., 1957.

Hirsch, Monroe J., and Ralph E. Wick, *The Optometric Profession.* Philadelphia: Chilton Book Co., 1968.

Shurr, Donald G., and Thomas M. Cook, *Prosthetics and Orthotics.* Norwalk, CT: Appleton & Lange, 1990.

Knowledge and Technology

Ackerknecht, Erwin H., *A Short History of Medicine.* Baltimore, MD: Johns Hopkins University Press, 1982.

Banta, H. David, and K. B. Kemp, *The Management of Health Care Technology in Nine Countries.* New York: Springer, 1982.

Basch, Paul F., *Textbook of International Health.* New York: Oxford University Press, 1990.

Beeson, P. B., "Changes in Medical Therapy during the Past Half-century." *Medicine,* 59:79–99, 1980.

Commission on Health Research for Development, *Health Research: Essential Link to Equity in Development.* New York: Oxford University Press, 1990.

Fenner, F., D. A. Henderson, et al., *Smallpox and Its Eradication.* Geneva: World Health Organization, 1988.

Piachaud, David, "The Diffusion of Medical Techniques to Less Developed Countries." *International Journal of Health Services,* 9(4):629–643, 1979.

Sigerist, Henry E., *Landmarks in the History of Hygiene.* London: Oxford University Press, 1956.

Winslow, C-E. A., *The Conquest of Epidemic Disease.* Princeton, NJ: Princeton University Press, 1943.

PART TWO

PROGRAMS

CHAPTER FIVE

Governmental Health Agencies

In all countries, government plays a substantial role in the structure and functioning of national health systems. All but the very smallest countries have several jurisdictional levels of government, passing from central to provincial to local, with other levels frequently operating between these; at each level some health activities are carried out. The distribution of authority and responsibility among the several levels, of course, differs greatly among countries, and they tend to change over time within most countries.

MINISTRIES OF HEALTH

Virtually every country has a principal governmental authority that bears the major responsibility for the health of the population. To simplify discussion, we refer to this as the *Ministry of Health,* although the agency may be described in several ways. This agency's scope may be confined to health or it may include health along with other matters. Under either arrangement, the exact scope of Ministry of Health functions has generally broadened over the years.

Evolution of Public Health Organization

Concepts of disease, its causes, and its treatment can be traced to ancient Egypt, some 3000 years before Christ. The theories were first applied to disorders in individual patients, and the concept of social action relevant to the health of groups of people arose later, in the time of classical Greece. Around 500 B.C., the Hippocratic book on *Airs, Waters, and Places* examined the relationship between the environment and human health. Ideas about *endemic* and *epidemic* disease were first de-

scribed in this work. Organized social actions to prevent disease, however, did not follow. Greek cities as early as 600 B.C. appointed municipal physicians to give medical care to the poor and to settle in the town; they were paid a basic annual salary, which could be supplemented by fees, but they did no community-oriented preventive work.

It was in classical Rome that organized preventive social action was first taken, and this was relevant to the environment. Water had been brought to Rome through aqueducts for several centuries before Christ. At the time of Augustus Caesar (63 B.C. to 14 A.D.), a public Water Board of leading citizens was appointed to maintain the water supply; hundreds of slaves were assigned to do this work. The water was intended for public baths, fountains, and public buildings; private use required a payment that could be made only by the very rich. Certain officials were responsible for cleaning the streets, supervising food markets, and maintaining the cleanliness of public baths. Public sewage to drain dirty water from the streets was also maintained by certain officials—kept in operation likewise by slaves. The *cloaca maxima* was a major drainage channel into the Tiber River, and it may still be seen in Rome.

With the decline of the Roman Empire around 300 A.D. and the rise of Christianity, Europe entered the period described by historians as the Middle Ages. The power center shifted from Rome to Constantinople (now Istanbul), which later was conquered by Arabic armies. With the Emperor Constantine (306–337 A.D.), the Christian church and the state became allied. Europe became a land of monarchs, counts, barons, and other rulers. Feudalism was a time of warring lords, whose lands were cultivated by thousands of lowly serfs. Whatever knowledge of health and hygiene survived was preserved in Christian monasteries linked to the church. Around the lord's castle, walls were built to prevent military onslaughts, and then fortification was constructed around small urban settlements.

Towns began to develop throughout Western Europe around 1000 A.D., and with the crowded settlement of people the hazards of disease increased. In most communities, special officials were appointed to look after the water supply, which was usually provided through public fountains from wells. Regulations prohibited throwing filth into streams of water. Garbage collection and disposal were difficult tasks, requiring local organization. Rural life with domestic animals continued inside the city walls and created further sanitary problems.

City life inevitably aggravated the occurrence and spread of communicable diseases. In Europe and the Mediterranean region we have evidence of diseases that are probably definable as leprosy, bubonic plague, smallpox, diphtheria, measles, scabies, anthrax, and trachoma. The contagiousness of leprosy was recognized early. By the thirteenth century there were 2,000 leprosaria in France and an estimated 19,000 in all of Europe. The isolation of lepers influenced the response of European cities to the pandemic of plague in 1348, the great scourge known as the *Black Death.* Policies on identification and isolation of cases were made by each municipal council, which also looked after the water supply and the disposal of filth. Special committees might be established at the time of epidemics, but they were later disbanded. Throughout the Middle Ages, these antecedents to public health organization existed only at the level of local communities.

Not until the late eighteenth century, with industrialization and rapid urban growth, did European cities begin to establish permanent Boards of Health. The earliest theoretical elucidation of principles of hygiene came from France when Louis René Villerme (1782–1863) wrote not only about environmental sanitation but also about the health aspects of maternity, school and factory conditions, and the hazards of infectious diseases. He showed the relationship of health to social class, housing, prostitution, prison conditions, food preparation, and so on.

Implementtion of programs to protect public hygiene was first done effectively in England. In Manchester, a series of typhus fever epidemics led to the formation in 1796 of the Manchester Board of Health, headed by a physician. The Board traced the disease to cotton mills, and recommended regulations on hours and conditions of work. In 1805, the first action was taken by a national government, when England established a Central Board of Health to guard against the entry of yellow fever from North Africa. By 1806, however, the epidemic waned and the Central Board was terminated. In 1831, facing another threat of ship-borne disease, cholera, England set up a second Central Board of Health, only to disband it again in 1832. Not until 1848 was a National Public Health Act passed in England, with long-term consequences.

In 1842, Edwin Chadwick, a courageous member of the English Poor Law Commission, published *The Sanitary Condition of the Working Population of Great Britain.* It exposed the dreadful living conditions of the urban poor, and their direct influence on health and disease. This report recommended the law enacted in 1848, which encouraged the formation of local Boards of Health. Unlike earlier laws, however, this law required the Board to appoint an *officer of health,* who had to be a legally qualified medical practitioner. By 1856, nearly 200 local Boards of Health had been established in Great Britain. These boards were a strong response to the miserable social conditions created by urbanization under early capitalism.

In 1858, the National Board of Health was again terminated, but the local Boards continued to function (under the Privy Council). In 1871, the general promotion of local Boards was transferred to the National Board of Local Government, along with the latter Board's responsibilities for enforcement of the British Poor Law. Other chapters followed in the saga leading to the birth of a permanent British Ministry of Health; most important of these was probably the enactment of national health insurance of limited scope in 1911. Then, spurred by the influenza pandemic of 1917–1918, Parliament finally took action to establish a Ministry of Health (MoH) in 1919. MoH functions were at first largely oriented to promoting local public health organization, but they included also the preparation of regulations on housing, the Poor Law administration, certain aspects of the national health insurance program, and the direct performance of research on measures concerned with the health of the population.

Similar accounts of slow and tortuous development of public health consciousness could be told for several European countries. France in 1848 enacted legislation that required an advisory public health council in each *département* and *arrondissement,* but these bodies had no executive power. In Germany similar proposals were made but not implemented with the defeat of the Revolution of 1848. In general, the movement toward protecting people against the diseases spawned by unsanitary environmental conditions arose from the exposure of the miserable housing of impoverished working-class families in the large cities. Corrective actions were called for at the local government level. The maturation of these reforms to a level yielding a national health authority or Ministry of Health did not occur widely until the second or third decades of the twentieth century.

As it happened, a British colony took action somewhat earlier to establish a permanent Ministry of Health. In 1872, New Zealand in the South Pacific Ocean responded to an outbreak of smallpox by enacting the Public Health Act of 1872. Under this law, local Boards of Health were established, and in 1876 a Central Board of Health was set up for the whole colony. This was found to be quite ineffective, however, when an epidemic of plague occurred in China in 1894, spreading to nearby Australia by 1900. This led to another New Zealand Public Health Act and establishment of a central Ministry of Health, with full-time medical officers in 1901. This Ministry has survived to the present time, and it attained great strength in 1939, when it was entrusted with responsibility for managing the medical services under New Zealand's comprehensive Social Security Act.

In the developing countries of Asia and Africa, virtually all health systems were governed by small units of the colonial governments before the end of World War II. In the colonies, health was usually regarded as an aspect of police power for government departments concerned with the *interior* or with *local affairs.* Only after independence was won in the postwar years, after 1946 in Asia and mostly in the 1960s in Africa, did these new nations establish separate Ministries of Health. Even in Thailand—one of the few Asian countries that was not a colony—public health work was a minor function of the Ministry of Interior until 1942 (see below).

In the Latin American countries, which had become independent of Spain and Portugal in the early nineteenth century, public health work had its beginnings also in the Ministries of Interior, of Local Government, or the like. Argentina won its independence in a tumultuous period between 1810 and 1827, but not until 1880 did it establish a National Department of Hygiene within its Ministry of Internal Affairs (or the equivalent). Other Latin American countries gradually did likewise—Brazil in 1897, Peru in 1903, Venezuela in 1911, Chile in 1918, up to Panama in 1926. Often these units were termed a *Direccion General de Sanidad,* but their scope was quite limited.

With World War II, the U.S. Office of Inter-American Affairs was established under President Franklin D. Roosevelt, and this agency sponsored a Cooperative Inter-American Service of Public Health (SCISP), which greatly strengthened the public health movement in many Latin American countries. Hospitals, health centers, and sanitation programs were much more widely developed. The Pan-American Sanitary Bureau, founded in 1902 with offices in Washington, D.C. (later to become part of the World Health Organization), also stimulated more public health work—especially in the control of mosquito vectors of malaria and yellow fever. In the 1940s and the postwar years (after 1945), several Latin American governments removed their General Directorates of Health from the multipurpose *interior* ministries and placed them in new cabinet-level Ministries of Health. By 1970, every government in Central and South America (and, of course, Mexico) had such a ministry. After 1930, the authority of most of these ministries had to be shared with other dynamic programs for medical care under the rubric of social security; this will be discussed below.

The Panorama of Ministries of Health

The evolution of public health organization is not exactly the same as the development of Ministries of Health, but the organization of community preventive services has everywhere been an early and basic function of such ministries. In many countries, the scope of MoHs has been extended well beyond the sphere of preventive services, which then permits these agencies to play much larger roles in the operation of national health systems. A common organization of MoHs currently classifies their functions as (1) preventive, (2) curative, (3) training, and (4) other, but there are endless variations. These may be considered in relation to the political character of overall national health systems.

Entrepreneurial Health Systems. In the affluent *United States,* there is a vast multiplicity of public and private health agencies. Relative to the total health system, the scope of the United States Public Health Service is rather limited. Its greatest powers involve establishing standards for preventive health services and granting funds to the States for providing these. The U.S. Public Health Service also provides grant support for training the health professions and conducting health-related research. The largest programs of medical care, however—Medicare for the elderly and Medicaid for the poor—are administered by a separate Health Care Financing Administration within the same federal Department (equivalent to a ministry) of Health and Human Services. Other major health programs come under the U.S. Veterans Administration, the Departments of Labor, of Commerce, of Agriculture, and so on. Moreover, as a federated country of 50 states and 3100 counties, major health responsibilities are carried by public health, social welfare, and mental health agencies in these peripheral jurisdictions.

A middle-income or transitional country with an entrepreneurial health system is the

Philippine Republic. There is a Ministry of Health in the central government, but its financial support in the early 1980s was modest—only 3.5 percent of the national government budget. There are 12 administrative regions and 76 provinces, with centrally appointed Provincial Health Officers. The scope of work of the provincial officers is limited largely to environmental and preventive services. Some 74 percent of hospitals and 55 percent of hospital beds were under private auspices in 1980, and their government regulation was quite limited. Public hospitals in the MoH are controlled by the central headquarters. About 72 percent of physicians, nurses, and midwives were in private practice or private employment. Private pharmacies are also abundant and their sale of drugs is essentially unrestricted. Even the great majority of medical and nursing schools are under private sponsorship—quite unusual in a developing country. When the Philippines enacted a social insurance program for hospital care and inpatient doctor's care in 1969, it was put under a separate Medical Care Commission, not the MoH. The Commission pays private doctors by fee-for-service. Family planning programs are numerous, but entirely under voluntary agencies. A 1980 survey found only 25 percent of all Philippine health expenditures to come from government and 75 percent from private sources.

Thailand is another transitional country, with an entrepreneurial health system, but a somewhat stronger Ministry of Health. Since 1918, a Division of Public Health had operated in the Ministry of Interior, concerned largely with police powers throughout the country. In 1942, this unit was removed from Interior and established as a cabinet-level Ministry of Health. Most of the government's health responsibilities are carried by the MoH, which has six major departments: (1) the Office of Under-Secretary of State for Health, which supervises all rural health service and personnel training; (2) the Department of Medical Services, supervising most of the nation's hospitals; (3) the Department of Health, responsible for major preventive campaigns, maternal and child health, nutrition, and environmental sanitation; (4) the Department of Communicable Disease Control; (5) the Department of

Medical Sciences, supervising a national network of laboratories; and (6) the Office of Food and Drug Committees, supervising drug production and distribution. At the level of Thailand's 71 provinces, there are Provincial Public Health Offices, headed by a Provincial Chief Medical Officer appointed by the Minister; each province has about 10 health districts, headed by a District Officer—usually a sanitarian or nurse.

Certain important health responsibilities in Thailand, however, are not within the MoH. A separate State University Office controls seven of the country's eight medical schools, along with their large teaching hospitals. Also, there remains in the Ministry of Interior a Department of Local Administration, which still carries certain preventive health responsibilities. Thailand also has many independent voluntary health agencies and an especially large market for private medical care. The private market consists of physicians (including private practice by government doctors), traditional healers, pharmacies, and even private hospitals; some 70 percent of all Thai health system expenditures come from the private sector. The Ministry of Health accounts for only 20 percent of the total.

Pakistan is a very low income developing country with an entrepreneurial type of health system. In the central government there is a Ministry of Health and Social Welfare, but substantial functions are performed also by other national public agencies. These include the Population Planning Division, the Science and Technology Division, the Labour Division, the Environmental and Urban Affairs Division, the States and Frontier Division, and the Kashmir Affairs Division—all of which are parts of other ministries. A Social Security program, providing health services to industrial workers and their dependents, is administered by three semiautonomous institutes, having no links with the MoH; services are delivered both by private practitioners (paid by the institute) and by salaried medical employees in institute facilities.

Below the top in Pakistan, there are four provincial Health Departments, with functions equivalent to those at the national level, but largely independent of national controls. Within each province are Health Districts,

headed by a District Health Officer, who reports to the Provincial Health Director-General. A major share of the health services received by the Pakistan population, however, is in the private market, quite outside the sphere of any level of the MoH. Out of 38,300 allopathic and Ayurvedic physicians in 1984, 56 percent were entirely in private practice. These practitioners absorb 46 percent of national health expenditures, and private pharmacies a further 25 percent. The Ministry of Health and Social Welfare and the corresponding Health Departments at provincial and district levels altogether accounted for only 17.2 percent of Pakistan health expenditures (excluding capital costs) in 1984.

Welfare-Oriented Health Systems. The *Federal Republic of Germany,* when it was in the western part of a divided Germany, illustrated an affluent industrialized country with a welfare-oriented health system. This was where the entire social security idea was born, and hundreds of semiautonomous sickness insurance funds still administer financial support for medical care. This far-reaching health insurance program is supervised by the Ministry of Labour and Social Affairs, rather than an MoH. In fact, at both federal and provincial levels, health comes under a Ministry of Youth, Family Affairs, and Health, and the services are limited essentially to preventive activities. Medical care is rendered principally by private practitioners, paid by fee-for-service. There is a large and highly productive pharmaceutical industry.

German physicians and other health personnel are trained in public universities and technical schools, coming under government educational authorities. In 1983, the German health system absorbed 8.2 percent of GDP; the largest share of this, 63 percent, came from social insurance; only 15 percent came from general revenues (for professional education as well as all public health). The national health insurance programs in other western European welfare-oriented systems is also under labor ministries, leaving the MoH with relatively modest responsibilities.

Mexico is a middle-income developing country, with a welfare-oriented health system, in which the Ministry of Health has a moderately broad range of functions. In the central government the MoH is known as the Secretariat of Health and Social Assistance, and in each of the 32 states there are equivalent health authorities. (In 1990 the Secretariat was renamed a ministry.) These come under the elected Governor of each state, and they are responsible for all preventive and certain curative health activities—delivered largely through a network of health centers—in the state. Until recently, governmental hospitals of the MoH came principally under the control of the central Ministry, but since 1987 in 12 of the 32 states, their management has been decentralized to the states.

A major framework of health services in Mexico, however, is the medical component of Social Security, which includes a large Mexican Institute for insurance of private employees and a separate institute for public employees. Altogether some 60 percent of the Mexican population is covered by the Social Security program, which delivers services through its own network of hospitals and polyclinics. In spite of this separate administration, the general budget and policies of the Social Security programs are subject to review and approval by the national Minister of Health. All drugs required by the Social Security and other public programmes, as well as the MoH, are purchased through a unified central mechanism. A national Center for Technological Development and Applications, within the MoH, does research and proposes standards for all agencies in the health system. Of all health expenditures in Mexico, only about 30 percent are made in the private market.

A very poor developing country, with a welfare-oriented health system is illustrated by *India,* where the Ministry of Health is a moderately strong governmental authority. Population growth in this large country became so explosive that in the early 1970s the name of the MoH was changed to the Ministry of Health and Family Welfare (MoHFW), and a major activity shifted to the promotion of contraception or family planning. At the national level the MoHFW formulates general health policy, operates research and training institutes, has certain regulatory powers, and directly oversees family planning activities. Most

personal and environmental health services are administered by the 31 state and union-territory MoHFWs, which derive two-thirds of their support from the state governments.

Within the states and territories of India, there are about 400 health districts (about 2,000,000 people each), in which a medical Officer of Health is responsible for the services of primary health centers as well as public hopsitals. There is also an extensive network of thousands of smaller subcenters staffed only by auxiliary health workers. Medical education is university based and supervised by the Ministry of Education, and occupational health in factories is controlled by the Ministry of Labor. There are also many voluntary health agencies—both religious and non-sectarian. The private market of both traditional (Ayurvedic) and modern medicine, however, is most extensive, and the majority of all doctors practice in it. Altogether the economic support of India's health system is drawn predominantly (about two-thirds) from private households.

Comprehensive Health Systems. Great Britain's health system illustrates the comprehensive type in a relatively affluent industrialized country; here the Ministry of Health performs a very wide range of functions. At the central level, the MoH operates essentially as the National Health Service (NHS) subdivision within the Department of Health and Social Security. At its beginning in 1948, the NHS was administered through four vertical pathways for: (1) general practitioner, pharmaceutical, and certain other ambulatory services, (2) specialist and hospital care, (3) local public health services, mainly preventive, and (4) teaching hospitals. At the top, however, all four of these pathways converged under one NHS headquarters. Then in 1974, the four separate lines of authority were brought together under the supervision of MoH staff in about 90 local Area Health Authorities; later the management was further decentralized to about 200 Health Districts.

General medical practitioners, dentists, pharmacists, and opticians remain in private practice, but their services are financed almost entirely by the British NHS, and they are subject to NHS regulations in most of their work. School health services, previously under educational authorities, are now within the NHS, but occupational safety and health remains separate under the Ministry of Labour. Pharmaceutical products and medical supplies are manufactured by private enterprises or imported from abroad, but the payment for and use of them are subject to public NHS regulation. In recent years, government policy in Great Britain has encouraged expansion of the private market for medical care, and this has occurred to some extent for specialist care and certain inpatient hospital services, with private health insurance to pay for these. The aggregate private market for health service, however, constitutes less than 10 percent of the total health system—whether measured by services or by expenditures—so that at least 90 percent of the British system is under the control of the MoH, as defined here.

Norway is another affluent industrialized country with a comprehensive health system and a moderately strong MoH. At the central level, it is responsible for the formulation of national health policies, and it does the planning of hospitals and other health facilities throughout the nation. At the next echelon (called *counties* rather than provinces), the County Health Officer is appointed by the central Ministry and carries responsibility for the maintenance of standards in all hospitals, as well as for the basic preventive services. The county governments own the vast majority of all general hospital beds, but their budgets are reviewed by the central MoH, and their specialist physicians are appointed from nominees of this Ministry. At the most local echelon, the Commune Health Officer is appointed by the local government, and he has a wide range of responsibility for local health affairs. He chairs an elected local Board of Health, which—within legal requirements—makes local public health policy. The social insurance program is controlled at the top by a National Institute of Health Insurance, also in the Ministry of Social Affairs. Payments of health care providers are made by a network of insurance offices in most of the communes; the Commune Health Officer often serves as a consultant to these offices. Medical schools come under a national Ministry of Church and Education, but they are all affiliated with large general hospitals in the MoH framework.

Costa Rica is a middle-income developing country with a comprehensive health system, but an MoH that is not very strong. This ministry has functioned since 1927, but after 1941 the great scope acquired by the Bureau of Social Security resulted in a reduction of responsibilities for the MoH. Social Security program coverage expanded quite rapidly, and in 1973 virtually all treatment services were transferred to the Social Security program; this included all hospitals and polyclinics for ambulatory care. The MoH was left to handle essentially the preventive services, especially in rural areas. Thus, government as a whole has major responsibility for Costa Rica's health system—accounting for about 75 percent of expenditures—but within it the MoH plays a relatively small part.

In *Sri Lanka*, a very poor developing country, the health system may also be considered comprehensive in type. The MoH is relatively strong. Within the central government almost all health activities are controlled by the MoH, except for the operation of medical schools in universities under the Ministry of Education and the largest hospitals under a Ministry of Teaching Hospitals. At the next lower level, there are 25 districts, each with a district hospital and a Director of Health Services. Each district has about 10 divisions, with divisional health centers. A fourth administrative level is served by subdivisional health centers, staffed by auxiliary but highly experienced health personnel; these subdivisions have an average population of about 20,000. Even a fifth level of health service consists of small clusters of villages with about 3,000 people, served by village health stations. With this exceptionally broad coverage of the country, almost the entire national population of 16,000,000 is within convenient reach of primary health care. At the same time there remains a significant private market for medical care (both modern and traditional) in Sri Lanka, and also for both modern and traditional drugs. As a percent of national health expenditures, private activities absorb about 45 percent of the total—much less, however, than the 70 percent reported for Thailand (World Bank data) or the 67 percent for India. The MoH is important enough to serve as the secretariat for an interministerial National Health Council, chaired by the Sri Lankan Prime Minister.

Socialist Health Systems. In the health systems of socialist and formerly socialist countries, the Ministries of Health all have exceptionally broad responsibilities, compared with such ministries in other types of system. The following account describes the health system before the break-up of the Soviet Union in 1991. The first such socialist health system was developed in the *Soviet Union* (USSR) after the Russian Revolution of 1917, and it is still the prototype of such systems in industrialized socialist countries. The MoH of the USSR oversees equivalent Ministries in each of the 15 republics, and these in turn supervise the work of 120 provinces (oblasts). The latter, in turn, supervise more than 3,100 districts (rayons). At all these levels the MoH responsibilities are congruent with almost all aspects of the national health system.

All hospitals, polyclinics, health centers, and other health-related facilities in the Soviet Union are owned and controlled by the MoH at some level. All health personnel, unlike policies in the United Kingdom, are salaried civil servants. The schools of medicine and institutions for training all categories of health workers are also under the control of the MoH, and not under separate educational authorities. Research in scores of subdivisions of the health sciences (e.g., cancer, cardiology, occupational diseases, child health, and nutrition) is conducted in special institutes controlled by the MoH. Pharmaceutical products are manufactured by the Ministry of Light Industry, but decisions on the drugs required are made by the MoH, and this Ministry distributes the drugs to all health facilities and MoH community pharmacies. Health services only for military personnel and a few other special groups come under the control of other ministries. Private medical practice has never been prohibited in the USSR, but until recently it was of very small proportions. The entire health system infrastructure is centrally planned by the MoH, in cooperation with a subdivision of the na-

tional agency for general economic and social planning (Gosplan).

In 1989, after great political upheavals in Eastern European socialist countries, major changes had to be expected in their national health systems. There were signs that health insurance programs, making payments to public and private physicians, would eventually replace the completely governmental control of the health system. The Ministry of Health would probably acquire a more limited role, but in 1991 its characteristics were not yet clear.

Cuba is the best example of a middle-income developing country with a socialist health system. At the central government level, the Ministry of Health is responsible for all aspects of health policy and planning. The country is divided into 14 *health provinces,* which in turn are subdivided into about 135 municipalities, urban or rural. MoH officials at the provincial level are appointed by the national Ministery, but at the municipal level, the Health Officers are chosen by elected People's Councils. At the most local community level there is a network of polyclinics for primary health care, each serving about 25,000 people, or 400 to cover the national population of 10,000,000. The polyclinics are staffed by teams of physicians, nurses, and allied health personnel, who provide both therapeutic and preventive services. A regionalized network of hospitals is also owned and supervised by the MoH and staffed by salaried specialists.

The Cuban medical schools, which were formerly in universities under the Ministry of Education, have been increased from one to four since the 1959 Revolution, and they have all been transferred to the MoH. The production of drugs is also a responsibility of the MoH. With its very large output of doctors, Cuba differs from other developing countries by making little use of *community health workers* or similar auxiliary personnel. In the mid-1980s, however, the Cuban MoH introduced a network of *family medical practitioners,* each serving only about 600 to 800 people for pirmary health care, in small units around a polyclinic. It is noteworthy that Cuba did not set out to recast its socialist economy with a free market, along the lines undertaken in Eastern Europe.

Finally, the implementation of a socialist health system in a very poor developing country is illustrated in *China*. Here the Ministry of Health is moderately strong, but not so all-embracing as in the more affluent socialist countries. At the top there is a Ministry of Health with seven principal divisions: (1) health and epidemic prevention, (2) medical care administration, (3) science and education, (4) maternal and child health, (5) pharmaceuticals, (6) traditional medicine, and (7) planning and finance. In each of the 21 large provinces and certain other areas, there is a comparable ministry with generally equivalent functions. Each province is subdivided into counties—some 2,300 in all—each headed by a Western-type physician. Within the county there are townships (formerly communes), with health centers staffed by auxiliary personnel. The network of hospitals and health centers covering this large country is almost entirely governmental in sponsorship (under the MoH), but services are not free. The services must be paid for, and in 1987 about 40 percent of the population had some type of insurance to help them pay and contributing 50 percent of the costs; about 18 percent of costs are borne by the MoH, and the remaining 32 percent must be paid by individuals. Since the late 1980s, China has been encouraging private practice by both traditional and modern doctors and by pharmacies, so that the scope of the MoH may be expected to decline.

These accounts of Ministries of Health in 14 national health systems should indicate their diversity in strength and scope, Everywhere that a national cabinet-level MoH exists, one can assume that the health of people has become a significant government responsibility and that substantial public expenditures are being made for its protection. Moving through four stages of health policy ideology—from entrepreneurial, to welfare oriented, comprehensive, and socialist—these ministries seem to grow generally stronger, but special political circumstances create several exceptions. Alternatives to Ministry of Health authority may be the result of a strong private health sector or to

substantial responsibilities vested in other branches of government. Some highlights of other government agency responsibilities in the national health system may now be explored.

OTHER PUBLIC AGENCIES WITH HEALTH FUNCTIONS

In virtually every national health system, there are governmental agencies, other than the Ministry of Health, with responsibility for certain functions. Only the highlights of these agencies can be considered.

Educational Authorities

The education of children in public schools is a responsibility of government in every country, usually under a Ministry of Education or its equivalent. One aspect of schooling, of course, is the maintenance of a clean and safe school environment, for which local school authorities are responsible. Another aspect is the education of children on elementary principles of hygiene, nutrition, and the requirements for maintaining good health. Such instruction is the task of teachers, while sometimes local public health nurses or doctors may be called on to help in the instruction. In most industrialized countries, such education is simply built into the regular curriculum, although in many developing countries this content may be quite meager.

In France, for example, a program of health service (examinations, immunizations, treatment of minor illness or injury, etc.) is a well-established part of local schooling. Medical and nursing personnel are engaged by the education authorities. In Great Britain, the local school agencies also had their own health personnel, until the reorganization of the National Health Service in 1974. In the United States, public education is also largely a local responsibility, and in most jurisdictions this includes health service and health education; in about one-third of the communities school health work has been assigned to the local public health agency.

Public education in developing countries is

more likely to be a central government function, through the Ministry of Education. Organized school health services and health education are typically weak. Socialist China is exceptional in putting high priority on school-based health education and on nutritious lunches for almost all school children.

The other aspect of education with an important place in national health systems is the preparation of professional personnel. In socialist countries and a few others the placement of medical and allied education under Ministries of Health is the exception. Almost everywhere else—both in industrialized and developing countries—university education, including medical and pharmacy schools, comes under the Ministry of Education or other special national agencies. Great Britain has its University Grants Committee, France has a separate Ministry of Universities, Sweden has a National Board of Universities and Colleges linked to the Ministry of Education, and Australia has a national Universities Commission also under the Ministry of Education.

In Brazil, the universities are under the supervision of the Ministry of Education, but the great proliferation of medical schools in the 1970s led to establishment of a national Committee on Medical Education within that ministry. In Egypt's Ministry of Education there is a Supreme Council of Universities, which has a Medical Education Board. Thailand has its State University Office, separate from the Ministry of Education. When medical schools control large teaching hospitals, as they do in Kenya, Malaysia, and Thailand, one or more important facilities in the health system are outside the control of the MoH.

Educational authorities, of course, can cooperate with Ministries of Health for the preparation of health personnel in the numbers and with the capabilities required in the health system. All too often, however, public health leaders decry the "high technology focus" of recent medical graduates and the limited appreciation of the primary health care needs of populations, especially in developing countries. When health leaders call for more generalists and fewer specialists, especially in surgery, they often encounter elitist and antagonistic responses.

Ministries of the Interior

It has been noted that government responsibilities for health were often lodged initially in Ministries of Interior, where a network of police usually operate to maintain law and order throughout a country. When most of these health functions are withdrawn and assigned to a Ministry of Health, however, certain health functions may remain under the mantle of local government. This has been true in countries such as Malaysia or Thailand, in which both preventive and hospital programs have stayed under the control of a Metropolitan Authority in the national capital—independent in many ways from the Ministry of Health.

Environmental sanitation in many countries is within the jurisdiction of local municipal governments, overseen by the Ministry of Interior. In the Federal Republic of Germany this Ministry has general responsibility for surveillance of most aspects of environmental sanitation. This field requires engineering and other skills not usually found in the MoH. Environmental protection functions in most U.S. states come under special agencies other than public health.

In Nicaragua and several other Latin American countries, the Ministry of Interior includes the national police, for whom a special health service is usually maintained. This is true also in Saudi Arabia. Ministries of Interior may encompass departments for construction of public works, which include hospitals and other health facilities; such construction is typically done in collaboration with the Ministry of Health. Sometimes these agencies are known as Ministries of Local Government.

Other Ministries with Health Functions

Several other types of ministry have selected health functions. Ministries of Agriculture carry out various social programs to benefit farm families and agricultural workers. These became prominent in the United States in the New Deal period of the 1930s and 1940s. The U.S. Department of Agriculture even organized hundreds of small health insurance plans for low-income farm families. In European countries with *agricultural extension services,* the education of rural people on nutrition, personal hygiene, and child-rearing is a frequent activity. Ministries of Agriculture in welfare-oriented developing countries, such as Brazil or Malaysia, may promote health as a part of *rural community development* schemes. This has been done also in the entrepreneurial health systems of Thailand and Kenya. In Burma, the Ministry of Agriculture has played a large role in the improvement of village water supplies. In countries with all types of health system, agricultural agencies are concerned with the control of animal diseases (zoonoses) transmissible to humans.

Ministries of Defense or of military affairs in virtually every country operate relatively well-developed health care programs for army, navy, and related personnel. Such programs also often serve high officials of government outside the military establishment. These will be discussed in Chapter 14.

In many countries veterans of military service are also entitled to health services for disabilities resulting from military action. In less developed countries, such care is usually given at the military health facilities, but in several industrialized countries there are special hospitals for veterans. In the United States and Canada there are special government agencies for Veterans Affairs, which operate V.A. hospitals; in the United States these serve veterans with *any* disability (not necessarily connected with military service), if private care would create a financial hardship. (On the average day two-thirds of V.A. hospital beds in the United States are occupied by veterans with conditions unrelated to military service.) These generous provisions were made for veterans after World War I—and expanded after World War II—probably because the United States lacked a national health insurance program such as operated in other countries.

Ministries of Justice or their equivalent often operate special health facilities for prison inmates. In federated countries, where certain prisons are operated by local units of government, prison health services also come under local control. The office of coroner or *medical examiner,* which investigates suspicious deaths, likewise includes a type of health service; this work is usually identified as *forensic medicine* or *forensic pathology.*

Ministries of Finance or Treasury or public agencies concerned with budgets typically have great power with respect to all functions of government, including health. There is often a subdivision for social services, inclusive of health matters. In the affairs of government, a decision on modified funding may be entrusted to the Ministry of Finance for implementation through the several other ministries involved. Similar across-the-board functions apply to Ministries of Planning

There are numerous other ministries that have health-related functions in selected countries. A Ministry of Cooperatives is important in Burma and India. There is a Ministry of Environment highly relevant to health in France. The Ministry of Land and Mines in Malaysia has health functions. Many countries have Ministries of Social Welfare—sometimes combined with Ministries of Health—providing health care to disabled or elderly persons. Ministries of Commerce may have significant roles in the distribution of pharmaceuticals. Government agencies responsible for railroads, airlines, or other means of transportation often operate special medical care programs for their personnel. This applies also in countries with quasipublic corporations operating telecommunications or public utilities. In most former socialist countries Ministries of Industry were concerned with the manufacture of drugs, medical supplies, and equipment.

To coordinate the heatlh activities of these several ministries, along with the Ministry of Health, some countries have established a *National Health Council* at the highest level. With or without such an agency, the MoH is usually expected to play the major coordinating role.

Perhaps the most significant government agency outside the Ministry of Health, especially in the most industrialized countries, is the Ministry of Labor. Two large health-related spheres are involved: occupational health services and social security programs. Because of the crucial place occupied by these activities in many health programs, they are the subject of the next chapter.

REFERENCES

Ackerknecht, Erwin H., *A Short History of Medicine*. Baltimore: Johns Hopkins University Press, 1982.

Brockington, C. Fraser, *Public Health in the Nineteenth Century*. Edinburgh: E. & S. Livingstone, 1965.

Chadwick, Edwin, *Report on an Inquiry into the Sanitary Condition of the Labouring Population of Great Britain, Poor Law Commissioners*. London: W. Clowes for the Majesty's Stationery Office, 1842.

Coleman, William, *Death is a Social Disease: Public Health and Political Economy in Early Industrialized France*. Madison, WI: University of Wisconsin Press, 1982.

Honigsbaum, Frank, *The Struggle for the Ministry of Health*. London: G. Rell and Sons, 1970.

Kramer, Howard D., "The Beginnings of the Public Health Movement in the United States." *Bulletin of the History of Medicine*, 21(3):352–376, May–June 1947.

Lidov, I. P., A. M. Stochik, and G. S. Tserkovny, *Soviet Public Health and the Organization of Primary Health Care for the Population of the USSR*. Moscow: MIR Publishers, 1978.

Marquez, Patricio V., and Daniel J. Joly, "An Historical Overview of the Ministries of Public Health and the Medical Programs of the Social Security Systems in Latin America." *Journal of Public Health Policy*. 378–394, Autumn, 1986.

Maxwell, Robert J., *Health and Wealth: An International Study of Health-care Spending*. Lexington, MA: Lexington Books, 1981.

Ministerio de Salud Publica, *Cuba: La Salud en la Revolucion*. La Habana: Ministerio, 1975.

Ministry of Health of Sri Lanka, *White Paper on the Reorganization of the Ministry of Health*. Colombo: The Ministry, 1980.

Mott, Frederick D., and Milton I. Roemer, *Rural Health and Medical Care*. New York: McGraw-Hill, 1948.

New Zealand Department of Health, *A Review of Health Serivces Administration in New Zealand 1872–1972*. Wellington, New Zealand, 1972.

Pater, John E., *The Making of the National Health Service*. London: King Edward's Hospital Fund, 1981.

Ringen, Knut, "Edwin Chadwick, the Market Ideology, and Sanitary Reform: On the Nature of the 19th Century Public Health Movement." *International Journal of Health Services*, 9(1):107–120, 1979.

Roemer, Milton I., *An Introduction to the U.S. Health Care System (Second Edition)*. New York: Springer, 1986.

Roemer, Ruth, C. Kramer, and J. E. Frink, *Planning Urban Health Services: From Jungle to System*. New Yorker: Springer, 1975.

Rosen, George, *A History of Public Health*. New York: MD Publications, 1958.

Sand, René, *The Advance to Social Medicine*. London: Staples Press, 1952.

Shattuck, Lemuel, *Report of the Sanitary Commission of Massachusetts, 1850*. Cambridge, MA: reprinted by Harvard University Press, 1948.

Sidel, Ruth, and Victor Sidel, *The Health of China*. Boston: Beacon Press, 1982.

Siem, Harold, *Choices of Health: An Introduction to the Health Services of Norway*. Oslo: Universitetsforlaget, 1986.

Soberon, Guillermo, J. Frenk, and J. Sepulveda, "The Health Care Reform in Mexico: Before and After the 1985 Earthquake." *American Journal of Public Health*, 76(6):673–680, June 1986.

Terris, Milton, "Epidemiology and the Public Health Movement." *Journal of Public Health Policy*, 8:315–329, Autumn 1987.

World Bank, *Pakistan Health Sector Report*. Washington, D.C.: (Report No. 4736-PAK), September 1983.

World Bank, *Population, Health, and Nutrition in the Philippines: A Sector Review*. Washington, D.C.: World Bank (Report No. 4650-PH), January 1984.

CHAPTER SIX

Social Security for Medical Care

Actions by government to support the costs of medical care for working people have a background very different from the background of public health preventive services. These developments evolved not from epidemics or environmental hazards, but from the conditions of life and work created by industrialization and early capitalism. They emerged from the organization of working people, for whom sickness meant a loss of economic livelihood.

BEGINNINGS OF SICKNESS INSURANCE IN EUROPE

Even before capitalism, in the Middle Ages of Europe, when manufacturing was principally by small independent craftsmen, there were guilds that made use of insurance. In the sixteenth and seventeenth centuries, guilds of carpenters, masons, and so on would collect from their members funds to help a colleague in distress—for example, from sickness and inability to work. The widow of a deceased guild member might also be helped.

Slowly in eighteenth century Europe, and more rapidly in the nineteenth century, workers lost their independence and were employed in factories. Here sickness caused even more hardship, because it meant the sudden termination of wages. In any individual, sickness could not be predicted, so that savings could not be relied on; in a group of workers, however, regular contributions could build up a fund to help the sick individual worker. This was called *sickness insurance,* and the idea spread rapidly through the working population of Europe. An especially large number of *krankenkassen* or sickness insurance societies developed in Germany, where industrialization was very robust. By 1850 there were hundreds of small autonomous sickness insurance funds, organized in various enterprises or communities.

In 1854, Prussia, one of the 30 German states, enacted a law that compelled workers with low wages to join a sickness fund; the employer was required to deduct a certain percentage of wages for this purpose and to contribute an equal amount from the enterprise. The workers affected, however, were relatively few and the idea of compulsory insurance did not spread. It planted a seed in German politics, nevertheless, that was to bear fruit 30 years later.

In 1871, Otto von Bismarck—a former Prime Minister of Prussia—became Chancellor of the German Empire, under Emperor William I. Bismarck is known as the statesman who unified the previously warring Germany states, but he also had another political objective—to destroy the rising socialist movement among workers. One strategy toward that end was to take over the sickness insurance movement, which was helping to build up labor unions and, with them, the Social Democratic (socialist) political party.

Accordingly in 1881, Bismarck introduced a bill in the *Reichstag* (parliament) that would have established a central national sickness insurance fund, which all low-paid workers would be required to join—along with substantial contributions from employers. The bill was opposed by the Social Democrats, who called it "beggar's insurance." It would merely prevent the worker from becoming a beggar, while making him pay for what he received; it did not attack the causes of working class misery, but only their results. Employer contributions, it was argued, would mean employer control of the insurance.

After extended debate, the idea of a large

central insurance fund was rejected, but in June 1883 a law was passed that marked the beginning of national social insurance for financing medical care. The law required that workers in listed occupations, earning below a certain monthly wage, must join one of the many existing sickness insurance funds or one to be created. Two-thirds of the premiums were to be contributed by workers and one-third by employers, with administrative responsibility shared proportionately. The benefits were (1) partial compensation for loss of wages (typically around 50 percent) after a waiting period, (2) the costs of medical care—principally general practitioners and drugs, (3) maternity benefits, and (4) funeral grants. Over the years other classes of worker were added, such as office workers, domestic servants, and higher paid manual workers. Dependents were finally added—for medical but not monetary benefits—in 1914–1918. Services were also extended to include hospitalization in semiprivate rooms, dental care, and optical appliances. It is noteworthy that physicians raised no objections to this legislation; it ensured payment for their services to low-income patients; more affluent middle class patients remained in the private market.

With these political origins, the social insurance idea soon spread to other European countries—first to the Austria-Hungarian Empire and eventually to every country on the continent. As the popularity of the programs with workers became apparent, the left-wing political parties changed their views and came to support the concept—calling for extension of both persons covered and benefits provided. The German pattern of mandating membership in local sickness insurance funds was emulated in every country. Sickness insurance societies everywhere became subject to government regulation, with respect to minimum benefits provided, investment policies, and annual reports. The government agency responsible for this surveillance in Germany and elsewhere was the Ministry of Labor, not the Ministry of Health.

In Germany insurance for general medical care costs and disability compensation came first; it was followed in 1884 by compensation and medical care for work injuries, financed solely by employers. Ths was managed in Germany by mutual trade associations for each industry, but in other countries by commercial insurance companies. Social insurance for old-age pensions and death benefits in Germany came still later—in 1889, with managment by regional government insurance agencies. Not until 1927 was social insurance added for unemployment compensation. Family allowances, to help meet the costs of raising children, came still later. A similar but slightly modified sequence of social insurance or social security benefits occurred in other European countries. Ministries of Labor were always at the helm in government.

The pattern of medical care delivery, associated with the pioneer German sickness insurance law, was simply an extension of the private practice model that had become firmly established by the 1880s. Since higher income patients were treated by individual doctors, rather than at crowded outpatient clinics of public hospitals, it was natural for insured workers to desire similar arrangements. Likewise medications would be obtained from private pharmacies. The sickness funds paid full physician charges, with no copayments by the patient. To ensure solvency, schedules of fees had to be negotiated in advance between the sickness funds and the doctors. To strengthen their bargaining power, many small sickness funds joined together in federations.

In response, German physicians also formed associations for negotiating with the federations of sickness funds. Eventually a pattern evolved in which the sickness fund paid the medical association a flat amount periodically (usually every 3 months) for each enrolled member. Then, the medical association paid fees for each service to the doctors, and since money is limited it had to exercise great care. This led to various techniques for identifying expensive abuses by doctors or patients. The whole process was complex, and if funds were insufficient to pay all fees in a quarter-year, doctors would have to accept less than full payment for services in that period. Eventually the mechanism was so well managed that reduced or prorated fees were rare.

The great complexities of German sickness insurance led to imposition of various constraints in the laws enacted by other countries. The Belgian law of 1894 did not mandate coverage of any workers, but simply regulated the operation of local sickness funds or *mutualities*. It subsidized the mutual societies to ensure their stability and help them enroll low-paid workers; not until 1944 was sickness fund enrollment made compulsory in Belgium for anyone. Although the funds were voluntary, utilization of medical care was constrained by requiring patients to pay a share (usually 25 percent) of all medical bills and prescriptions.

Legislation in Norway, enacted in 1909 and later in other Scandinavian countries, imposed copayment requirements on the patient from the outset. Eventually these payments were limited to the first two or three encounters in an episode of illness, on the grounds that subsequent services depended on the decision of the doctor rather than the patient. Copayments were waived for the indigent and pensioners, and were not required from anyone for hospitalization. In fact, Swedish and Norwegian general hospitals were financed mainly by provincial (also called county) revenues for every resident—not just for the poor—both before and after social insurance. This included the services of hospital doctors—specialists on full-time salaries from the hospitals. Initially coverage in the Scandinavian countries was through the enrollment of people in local sickness funds, as in Germany. Eventually, however (in Norway it was in 1930), the separate funds lost their autonomy and became branch offices of the National Insurance Institution.

The *national health insurance* law in Great Britain (departure from the *sickness insurance* term) was enacted in 1911, under Prime Minister Lloyd George of the Liberal Party. It mandated coverage of low-wage manual workers through membership in a "friendly society." The benefits were limited to general practitioner services and prescribed drugs. Hospital and specialist care had long been available to working class people without charge at local public general hospitals and some voluntary hospitals. Dependents of the insured workers were not covered by law, but they could involuntarily join the same friendly societies or purchase health insurance from a commercial company. Such companies also sold voluntary insurance for hospitalization, which would entitle the subscriber to a private or semiprivate hospital room and a personally chosen physician.

The special adjustment of the British health insurance program to the problem of cost control was to abandon the use of fee-for-service remuneration. British general practitioners themselves, in fact, favored this change, to avoid the policing of their performance to identify excessive servicing. Accordingly, all covered workers were required to choose a general practitioner from among these participating—virtually all GPs in an area. Then the local friendly society would pay a flat monthly amount for each worker on a doctor's list, regardless of the specific services rendered that month. Each practitioner would naturally try to attract as long a list of patients as possible to maximize monthly earnings. The doctor then had no financial incentive to render superfluous services, but still had to keep patients satisfied; they could sign up with another doctor at any time. Aside from its cost-control effects, this capitation payment pattern had the virtue of ensuring every insured worker a primary care provider at all times.

In 1912, prerevolutionary Russia enacted a sickness insurance law to cover its relatively small population of industrial workers. The same year Italy enacted social insurance, with benefits limited to maternity care. The first social insurance to be enacted in the United States was in 1908, when federal employees were covered by compensation for work-connected injuries, including the costs of medical care. By 1911, 10 U.S. states enacted similar work-injury compensation laws, but general medical care insurance at the federal level did not become law until 1965 (discussed later).

In 1928, France became the last major European country to enact social insurance for the medical care of industrial workers. As in the rest of Europe, hundreds of autonomous sickness funds or *caisses de maladie* had been operating for many years. The French medical profession was so individualistic and so strong, however, that it succeeded in having the insurance operate on an indemnity basis—that is, reimbursing workers only after they paid the doctor personally. Thus, doctors were initially free to charge patients whatever they wished, and patients could then seek reimbursement from their sickness fund only at a rate of 80 percent of an official "nomenclature" or fee schedule. In later years, especially when economic conditions worsened, French doctors agreed to follow the negotiated schedule of fees, but there have been recurrent controversies over this issue.

Finally, the "beginnings of sickness insurance in Europe" must recognize the effects of the Russian Revolution of 1917. Occurring at the end of World War I, this had an impact on every aspect of Russian life, including medical care—both its financing and delivery. An early action of the revolutionary Union of Soviet Socialist Republics (USSR) was to extend the limited health insurance for industrial workers to cover all employed persons in the cities, plus their families. With industry controlled by government, contributions became payable only by the enterprise. As this first socialist country became increasingly industrialized through the 1920s and 1930s, more workers became covered. Care was given in polyclinics and hospitals, staffed by salaried government doctors. Agricultural and other rural people, however, were not covered through the health insurance program, but through a separate network of health centers, staffed with salaried doctors and *feldshers* (medical assistants)—carried over from czarist times and paid entirely from general public revenues. Not until 1937, 20 years after the revolution, were these two subsystems unified into a national health service (see below).

INITIAL DEVELOPMENTS OUTSIDE EUROPE

After World War I (1914–1918), the idea of health insurance for industrial workers began to spread outside of Europe. The first such law was enacted by Japan in 1922. There was no background of worker's sickness funds in Japan, but managerial paternalism was the Japanese tradition and industrial enterprises became the framework for the insurance. Employees of large firms (300 workers or more) were insured through a fund established by the company; in firms of 5 to 300 workers, the insurance was administered by a department in the national Ministry of Health (not of Labor). The Japanese medical profession was strong, and there was free choice of doctor and fee-for-service remuneration, as in Europe. Dependents were partially covered with payment of 50 or 60 percent of private doctor fees. About half of the Japanese population was protected under this law; the other half was covered under a second health insurance law, enacted in 1938 but not fully implemented until after World War II. This latter insurance program, to cover employees of small firms (under 5 workers), the self-employed, and others, was administered by units of local government.

In 1924, Chile became the first developing country to enact statutory social insurance to cover its industrial workers for medical care costs. Since there were no local sickness funds, all workers were brought under one national scheme in the Ministry of Labor. Dependents were not included and the program reached only about 10 percent of the population. Unlike Europe, however, Chile did not use insurance money to pay fees to private doctors and pharmacies. Instead, the social insurance program established its own polyclinics and hired doctors (for 2, 4, or 6 hours per day) to serve the workers. Because the great majority of Chilean people were very poor, the market for private patients was small; doctors were glad to be offered steady salaries. Hospitalization was provided in the existing governmental or charitable *(beneficencia)* hospitals, with attendance also by salaried doctors. Since the workers were paying part of the costs, hospital amenities were somewhat better than those for the ordinary indigent person. Since dependents were not covered, a sick wife might be served in a large hospital ward, whereas her insured husband was in a semiprivate room.

Agricultural workers in Chile, despite being much more numerous than industrial workers, were not covered. White-collar employees, on the other hand, in banks, stores, government offices, and so on organized separate small health insurance societies. Later these were consolidated into a governmental National Medical Service for Employees (SERMENA).

A sweeping extension of Chilean national health insurance occurred after World War II and is discussed below.

Brazil started a national health insurance institute for industrial workers in 1931. Soon after, six other national institutes were established for transport workers, commercial employees, governmental civil servants, and so on. Each of these organizations had its own ambulatory care facilities with salaried personnel. Not until the 1970s—under a military government bent on efficiency and economy—were the seven separate health insurance institutes in Brazil unified into a national social insurance program (INPS).

Peru passed a law to cover industrial workers with health insurance in 1936. The charitable hospitals were especially deteriorated in Peru, and the social insurance program set out to improve hospital services. In 1939, it completed the construction of the first *hospital obrero* in Lima, exclusively for insured workers. This was an immediate success, and after 1940 several other Latin American countries followed the Peruvian model for insured hospital care. In 1948, a second health insurance program was launched in Peru for white-collar employees; this program also built its own hospitals—more spacious and better equipped than the workers' hospitals, commensurate with higher employee salaries and social status.

The separate *empleado* insurance programs in Peru and Brazil made other adjustments to higher social class conditions. A *dual choice* pattern of medical care delivery was arranged, under which the employee could either use an organized polyclinic or consult a private physician; if the latter option was chosen, a 50 percent copayment of the doctor's fee was required. Care in a private hospital could also be chosen, with 33 percent copayment.

The last major action in the health insurance saga before World War II occurred in 1939, when New Zealand became the first capitalist country to cover its *entire* population for medical care costs. Unlike Europe, this small South Pacific island-state had no local sickness insurance funds demanding an administrative role. From the beginning, the health insurance was managed by the national government—in the Ministry of Health, moreover, not the

Ministry of Labor. As in Europe, medical services in hospitals were provided mainly by salaried specialists, but ambulatory care was given by private general practitioners paid by fees; drugs were also purchased in private pharmacies on a fee-per-prescription basis.

DEVELOPMENTS AFTER WORLD WAR II

As in so many fields, World War II was a watershed event affecting medical care, both in its financing and organization, throughout the world. The health insurance concept, as an approach to improving the accessibility of medical care, spread to all the continents and changed its character in Europe as well.

The most dramatic action was taken by Great Britain, where the population had suffered through the bombings of the war, and where social planning had promised people a better future. During the war, the conservative government had issued the Beveridge Report, which called for a "national health service" to provide all residents with comprehensive medical and related services. Despite the wartime charisma of Winston Churchill, a postwar Labour Party was elected and promptly enacted the National Health Service (NHS) Act of 1946. Thirty-five years of limited health insurance for industrial workers (paying only for general practitioner care and drugs) and the wartime regionalization of hospitals had laid the groundwork. These provided two of the three pillars of the NSH, and local public health authorities provided the third. Every British resident became covered, and financial support was shifted mainly to general revenues.

The British NHS soon became a worldwide model for extending the coverage and benefits of national health insurance programs. The ambulatory service of general medical practitioners, dentists, pharmacists, opticians, and others was administered by *executive councils,* formerly linked to the friendly societies. Hospital and specialist services came under *regional hospital boards.* The local public health authorities handled not only community preventive services, but also ambulance and visiting nurse service. Everything was set in motion July 1948.

As noted previously, it took another 26 years before the three components of the British NHS were integrated, in 1974, under a network of 90 *area health authorities.* Later local administration was assigned to some 200 *health districts.* In each district there is a specialist in management, advised by a community medicine specialist (successor to the former Medical Officer of Health) and a community health council of local citizens. Private medical practice has never been forbidden in Great Britain, and by the late 1980s some 7 or 8 percent of the population had acquired voluntary health insurance to pay for private care—mainly elective surgery in private hospitals.

Other health insurance developments after World War II occurred in Asia and the Middle East. In 1945 Turkey started a statutory health insurance program for employed workers in its main cities—Istanbul and Ankara. Services were delivered through salaried medical personnel working in special Social Security polyclinics and hospitals. Soon other Middle East countries did the same—Iran in 1949, Iraq in 1956, Tunisia in 1960, and Lebanon in 1963. In Tunisia, however, the medical services were organized differently. As a former French colony on North Africa's Mediterranean coast, Tunisia was a poor country. Instead of building its own facilities and engaging its own personnel, the social insurance body contracted with the Ministry of Health to provide medical services for insured workers and their families; with the additional social insurance money, MoH resources could be expanded. Thus, the doctors and others serving insured people were part of the same corps of government personnel as those serving the general population. They did not have higher salaries and better working conditions—points of contention between Health Ministries and Social Security agencies in Latin America.

India started a social insurance program for certain industrial workers in 1948, implementing a medical care policy similar to that in Tunisia. Reflecting India's weak industrial development, the program was limited to (1) employees of private firms, (2) firms with 20 or more workers, (3) firms using electrical power,

and (4) workers earning under 500 rupees (about $100 at the time) per month. The Employees State Insurance Corporation (ESIC), which administered the program, covered about 15,000,000 workers initially (in 356 industrial locations), growing to about 25,000,000 in the mid-1980s. As a share of the large Indian population, this stayed at around 3 percent.

As in Tunisia, ESIC aimed to have its medical services integrated with those of the Ministry of Health. It contracted with the MoH in each Indian state to serve insured workers and their families through regular MoH resources. In some places, with large concentrations of covered workers, ESIC funds were used to support the construction of new MoH facilities. In large cities, workers could be served by private general practitioners paid on a capitation basis, as in Great Britain. This cooperation between social insurance and the MoH in India has clearly strengthened both programs.

The most far-reaching Asian development after World War II was undoubtedly the Chinese Revolution of 1949. In the first decade of the People's Republic of China, much guidance was offered by and accepted from the Soviet Union. In the cities, health insurance was extended for industrial workers, although large copayments were required for dependents. A separate subsystem was developed for the huge rural population, based essentially on the agricultural communes. Each commune of 25,000 to 60,000 people supported at least one health center, staffed by both modern and traditional Chinese doctors, along with other personnel. Several communes made up a country, of which there are 2,300, each having a hospital.

With the Great Proletarian Cultural Revolution in China (1965–1975), there was a dramatic shift of emphasis to improve health services for the rural population. Thousands of peasants received brief training as *barefoot doctors* to serve members of the *production brigades* (500 to 1,000 people), into which communes were divided. Cooperative insurance funds were organized in the production brigades to pay for services at a health center or hospital, on referral by the barefoot doctor. As a very poor socialist country, China decided to require payment for all personal treatment services.

With the death of Chairman Mao Tse-tung in 1976 and the formation of a new government, the People's Republic of China underwent further major changes. Much greater emphasis was put on modern scientific technology in all fields, including health care. The barefoot doctors received more thorough training, had to pass examinations, and became *village doctors.* The communes were converted to townships, as conventional units of government, and the health cooperatives were disbanded. On the other hand, social insurance for industrial and government workers and their families was expanded, reaching 40 percent of the population by the mid-1980s. Primary health care, with its great preventive emphasis, remained the central tenet òf Chinese health policy.

At the other end of the political spectrum in Asia, the Philippine Republic introduced a social insurance program for medical care in 1969. Reflecting its entrepreneurial character, the insurance was mandatory only for *higher* paid private employees and civil servants. Unlike what occurred in other developing countries, the Philippine Medical Care Commission did not develop its own resources, but made contracts to pay fees to private doctors and hospitals. Government health centers limited their services essentially to prevention.

In 1976, the Republic of South Korea also enacted social insurance for medical care, arranging for delivery of services through private doctors and hospitals. Enrollment, however, was mandatory along conventional lines for the lower paid workers. At first, only firms with 500 or more workers were covered, but this threshold was gradually reduced, the self-employed were added, and services for the indigent were provided in health centers. By 1989, nearly 100 percent of the Korean population were covered, although large copayments were required.

When Israel became an independent nation in 1948, a major sickness insurance fund was already well established; the *Kupat Holim* of the Jewish Federation of Labor had been in operation since 1912. Under the British mandate over Palestine after World War I, the

Kupat Holim grew rapidly, and by the time of statehood it covered at least half of the Israeli population. Although legally voluntary, this health insurance fund and several smaller funds protected about 85 percent of the population by the 1980s. Governmental social insurance in Israel was limited to maternity cash grants for working women or the wives of working men.

Unlike voluntary health insurance elsewhere, however, the Israeli program did not pay fees to private doctors. All health personnel were and are salaried employees of the insurance organization, providing service in health facilities owned by it. With its great political strength, the Labor Federation's sickness fund has been able to maintain its independence; numerous attempts of the government to absorb it into the MoH have been unsuccessful. The two agencies, of course, cooperate in many ways—especially through an integrated project in the Negev region.

Another Middle East country to develop social insurance after World War II was Egypt in 1964. The Egyptian Health Insurance Organization covered civil servants and employees in large private firms, with services provided through its own facilities and salaried personnel. By the 1980s, coverage was extended to workers in small plants, but still reached no more than 20 percent of the population. Libya, with its rich oil resources, enacted a social insurance program for medical care of workers and their families in 1957. By the 1980s, its coverage was extended to a substantial majority of the population. Health services were provided by salaried personnel in the special hospitals and health centers of the Ministry of Social Security or in the facilities of the Ministry of Health under contract.

In sub-Sahara Africa, Gabon, another oil-rich country, used its resources to develop a social insurance program for medical care. Started in 1963, it was gradually extended to cover private and then public employees, followed by the self-employed and the indigent in the 1980s. Eventually it reached a substantial majority of the Gabonese population, with services rendered mainly through medicosocial centers and special Social Security hospitals.

Kenya is one of the few other African countries to develop a social insurance program, although it is limited to payment for hospital services. It is also unusual in mandating enrollment, as in the Philippines, only for higher income employees. The explicit objective has been to increase the financial support and utilization of private hospitals.

South Africa is one of the few countries in the world to still mainly depend, like the United States, on voluntary insurance for employed workers. About 300 local voluntary insurance schemes have developed, mainly through employment groups, with premiums shared between employer and employees. In 1983 about 16 percent of the South African population were covered, but this consisted of 75 percent of the whites and only 6 percent of the other racial groups. As in United States, there is a small social insurance program for medical care, limited to elderly and totally disabled pensioners. The apartheid policy, of course, meant separate health facilities for the various races; this policy was significantly changed in 1990.

After World War II, action was finally taken in North America to develop social insurance for general medical care. The Canadian province of Saskatchewan took the first initiative. During the 1930s and the war years, this prairie province had suffered from both depression and drought—electing a semisocialist government (the Cooperative Commonwealth Federation or CCF) in 1944. By 1946, legislation was passed to cover the entire provincial population with insurance for complete general hospital care. Voluntary hospital insurance had been growing in Canadian cities at the time, but had little impact on the rural population. Soon the province of British Columbia followed suit. This experience proved so favorable that by 1957 the national government of Canada enacted legislation to share half the cost of any provincial hospital insurance program meeting federal standards. By 1961 all 10 Canadian provinces had social insurance for hospital care.

In 1962 Saskatchewan again pioneered a social insurance program for both ambulatory and inpatient physician's care. In spite of a "doctor strike" that delayed the start of the program for 23 days, it soon proved so suc-cessful that by 1966 the federal government again passed a law to share in the costs of any appropriate provincial program; all provinces joined the scheme by 1971. Thus the process of achieving social insurance for hospital and medical care in Canada, starting in 1946, took 25 years. Patterns of medical care delivery remained conventional (free choice of private doctors with fee-for-service payments) throughout Canada, except for negotiated fee schedules and construction of some community health centers. Hospitals, however, are paid on the basis of an annual prospective global budget (rather than by itemized billing or flat per diem), which promotes economical management and simplifies administration. Individual provinces are free to legislate additional benefits, such as drugs for the elderly or dental care for children. General long-term care became a benefit in all provinces, through Federal block grants, in 1977.

Statutory health insurance did not gain a foothold in the United States until 1965, beyond the worker's compensation laws for work-connected injuries, started in 1908. (These were not extended to all of the states until 1950.) In 1965, after a long period of political debate, the Social Security Act amendments for financing medical care of the aged were enacted. Voluntary health insurance plans, under both nonprofit and commercial sponsorship, had been expanding since the 1930s and increased their coverage greatly during and after World War II. Their coverage of elderly and retired people, however, was deficient, and the *Medicare* amendments filled this gap. It was noteworthy that the private health insurance plans had become so firmly established that they were used as agents or *fiscal intermediaries* in the administration of the Medicare Law. Attempts after 1970 to broaden the mandatory health insurance coverage to all employed workers and dependents were not successful at the U.S. federal level. A few states, however, passed laws in the 1970s and 1980s, to extend coverage.

Australia was still another country to develop health-related social insurance after World War II. Voluntary health insurance, sponsored by nonprofit agencies, had been growing for some time and in 1950 the first social insurance law was passed. The sole benefit was payment for costly and "life-saving" drugs—the only national health insurance program to start this way. Strictly speaking, this was not insurance, since it was financed by general revenues of the entire population. Gradually the pharmaceutical benefits were extended to virtually all prescribed drugs. Then in 1953 legislation was enacted to encourage greater enrollment in voluntary insurance, by governmental sharing in the costs of hospitalization for insured persons.

In 1972, after 20 years of relatively conservative government, the Australian Labour Party was elected to power, and in 1974 universal national health insurance with quite comprehensive benefits was enacted. A fiscal crisis developed in 1976, however, bringing to an end the Labour Party rule. The more conservative Liberal-Farmers Party coalition government then proceeded to dismantle the national health insurance or *Medibank* program step-by-step. By 1979, Australian health insurance had been returned essentially to its previous voluntary form. In 1983, however, the Labour Party was again elected to power and once more national health insurance (now called *Medicare*) was reinstated. Through all these financial gyrations, the pattern of private medical practice with fee payments for ambulatory care remained basically unchanged in Australia.

SPREAD OF NATIONAL HEALTH SERVICES

Latin American countries, although not deeply involved in World War II, made several major changes in health care financing after the war. In 1952 Chile—inspired by the British example—established a *Servicio Nacional de Salud* (SNS). The SNS covered about 70 percent of the population, and was financed mainly by general revenues. This was accomplished by (1) expanding Chile's 1924 health insurance to cover the dependents of industrial workers, (2) absorbing the national network of *beneficencia* and other hospitals, and (3) integrating all the programs together with the resources of the Ministry of Health. Chile was then divided

into 12 health zones, in which all three former health programs were brought under a single Zone Medical Director. Coverage was gradually extended further until, under President Salvador Allende (1970–1973), it reached more than 90 percent of the population.

In 1973 the Allende Popular Unity government was overthrown by a military coup, headed by General Augusto Pinochet. The military government immediately weakened the SNS by withdrawing the middle class families and requiring them to obtain private health insurance; the SNS, with severely reduced resources, then served only the poor. After 17 years in 1990, the Pinochet government was defeated in a national election, and steps were taken to reconstruct the SNS. With private insurance still viable for higher income families, in late 1990 Chile was left with a two-class health system, and the future was unclear.

Another crucial event in Latin America was the Cuban Revolution of 1959. Unlike most Latin American countries, Cuba had not developed a general statutory health insurance program for industrial workers, but only maternity benefits for their wives and for working women. About 7 percent of the population—mainly middle income people in the cities—were members of voluntary prepaid medical care plans or *mutualistas.* These were usually organized by groups of doctors who owned a clinic and small hospital. After the revolution, these mutual aid societies continued to operate as a division of the Ministry of Public Health (MINSAP) until around 1970, when they were absorbed into the national public system.

Based on advice principally from Czechoslovakia, socialist Cuba developed a health system largely on the Soviet model. It did not train feldshar-type medical assistants, however, but greatly increased the output of doctors—needed with special urgency because of the flight of half the country's previous doctors. Several hundred polyclinics, staffed by teams of doctors and allied personnel, were built as the basic framework of the system. Each unit serves about 25,000 people for complete ambulatory care, with priority for rural areas. All health services are financed from general revenues, except out-of-hospital drugs, for which small charges are personally payable at government pharmacies. In later years, much authority was delegated to about 150 locally elected Municipal Health Officers. Also, small health stations, staffed by a family doctor and nurse, were set up around the polyclinics to serve some 600–800 people for primary health care.

Several other Latin American countries developed Social Security programs for medical care after World War II. In 1946 Colombia enacted such legislation, establishing one central fund for all classes of worker. Unlike the multiclass patterns in Peru and Brazil, this unified and more democratic pattern may have been influenced by the wartime victory of democracy over fascism. Bolivia developed another unified Social Security program in 1949, followed by several Central American countries. In 1958, Uruguay became the last of the Latin American countries to cover its industrial workers with socially insured medical care.

Progress was also made elsewhere in Latin America. Coverage was extended to beyond 50 percent of the population in Mexico and Brazil. In Argentina, the enrollment of hundreds of *obras sociales* was increased beyond 75 percent of the people, and services were coordinated through a National Institute of Social Programs (INOS). With special constitutional goals in Costa Rica, coverage was extended to practically 100 percent of the population.

Europe, where national social insurance for health care was already well advanced, did not stand still after World War II. In addition to Great Britain with its NHS, several other countries took important actions. Germany and France greatly extended their national health insurance coverage by mandating enrollment for additional classes of agricultural and self-employed persons. Since the relatively small number of higher income people not covered by law has nearly always purchased private insurance protection, these countries came to claim universal coverage. The same applied also to Belgium and the Netherlands, although the latter country counted most of its coverage as voluntary.

The most sweeping postwar changes after the British NHS occurred in the Scandinavian countries. By 1956, Norway had some 90 percent of its population statutorily enrolled and,

therefore, questioned why it needed an elaborate bureaucracy to exclude 9 or 10 percent. It decided simply to cover 100 percent of Norwegian residents. Similar action was taken by Sweden in 1962 and by Denmark in 1971. Finland's initial social insurance legislation was enacted only in 1963, but from the outset it covered 100 percent of its population for medical care. In all four of these Scandinavian countries, furthermore, the delivery of services became much more highly organized. Health centers were widely constructed to house teams of general practitioners and nurses for primary health care. This pattern became especially widespread in Sweden and Finland, where the great majority of GPs became publicly employed. Employment of hospital specialists on salary had long been the policy in all these countries.

The Eastern European countries, under fascist regimes during World War II, became socialist under Soviet influence after the war. Poland, Hungary, East Germany, Czechoslovakia, and the others all transformed their halfway social insurance programs for wage earners into tax-supported national health services for the total population. Networks of polyclinics and hospitals were established, all staffed by salaried government physicians and allied personnel. Resources were greatly expanded, preventive and treatment services were integrated, and central planning replaced the private market for medical care. Socialist health policy dominated the entire Eastern European scene for some 40 years until the late 1980s, when it was explicitly rejected. As in the Soviet Union or earlier, health leaders throughout Eastern Europe looked to social insurance, with private and public medical practice, as the preferred alternative for health system design.

In the 1970s and 1980s, a further chapter was written in national health insurance developments when major new laws were enacted in the Southern European countries. For many years Italy, like other European countries, had numerous sickness insurance funds, first with voluntary and then mandatory enrollment. After World War II, with the fall of fascism, the mutual societies were converted into local branches of a national health insurance program. By the 1970s, coverage reached 90 percent, although the range of benefits differed among local funds. In 1977 Italy's several left-wing political parties, especially the communists, gained substantial strength in the parliament. In 1978 a National Health Service, under which 100 percent of the Italian population became eligible for complete medical care, was legislated. Financial support was shifted gradually from the insurance funds to general revenues.

Italian physicians were free to remain in private practice or to be publicly employed—in hospitals on salaries and in health centers on a capitation basis. The whole program is administered by a strengthened Ministry of Health, through a network of 20 political regions and hundreds of local health units of 50,000 to 200,000 population each. By 1988 the Italian NHS had been properly implemented in only 8 of the 20 regions, but progress was gradually being made.

In Greece, the population had been protected by similar sickness insurance funds for many years, until by 1980 coverage had reached 95 percent. Two large funds operated their own polyclinics, and numerous smaller funds paid fees to private doctors. In 1983 a national health system was legislated, and support was shifted to general revenues. A network of health centers was built to make services more available in rural areas. All doctors staffing health centers and hospitals were paid by salary, and this organized delivery pattern was gradually replacing private medical practice.

Spain was under a fascist dictatorship from 1939 to 1975, when General Franco died. The new democratic government promptly extended Social Security (under the Ministry of Labor) and brought its health service aspects under the control of a greatly strengthened Ministry of Health. Within this ministry the National Institute of Health (INSALUD) extended coverage to 93 percent of the population, financed three-fourths by employer and one-fourth by worker contributions. The INSALUD program operates a large network of its own hospitals and clinics, but much service is also purchased from private doctors and hospitals under contract. In 1990 the Spanish

health system was still rapidly changing, with an increasing share of support being derived from general revenues.

National Ministries of Labor, it has been noted, have been the principal government agencies responsible for supervising social insurance programs—especially in Western European countries, where the idea originated. This has been true also in most of Latin America, but in countries undergoing social revolutions and in countries without a strong labor movement Ministries of Health have had greater responsibilities. Whichever government agency may play the major supervisory role over social insurance, however, in one other health field Ministries of Labor are clearly the main actors—occupational safety and hygiene. The inspection of factories and mines to detect accident hazards and mandate their correction has been a Ministry of Labor responsibility in almost all countries. This large subject is discussed in Chapter 14.

OVERALL HEALTH INSURANCE COVERAGE AND COMMENTARY

As of 1990, some 70 countries, with a majority of the world's population, provided Social Security or equivalent health care protection for all or some portion of their national populations. The coverage is universal or nearly so in 34 countries, all but a few of which are industrialized. Coverage is only partial in 36 countries, all of which are economically developing, except the United States. In these countries coverage is gradually broadening, although in many it still constitutes only a small fraction of the population.

In Table 6.1, the 70 countries are listed in three sets, according to the percentage of national population with Social Security coverage and indicating the national GNP per capita. If we take $4,000 for GNP per capita as the dividing line between industrialized and developing countries (as of 1986), it may be noted that all but 5 of the 34 countries in the set with 90–100 percent coverage are industrialized. Among the 15 countries with 25–89 percent coverage, only 2 are industrialized, the

Table 6.1. Countries Listed According to Social Insurance Coverage (as Percent of National Population) for Medical Care and GNP per capita, 1986

Country	GNP per cap.
Coverage 90–100 percent	
Switzerland	$17,808
Iceland	16,444
Luxembourg	15,740
Norway	15,109
Canada	14,124
Sweden	13,734
Denmark	12,907
Japan	12,809
Australia	12,454
Finland	12,343
West Germany	12,049
France	10,986
Austria	10,159
Netherlands	9,861
Italy	9,330
Belgium	9,298
Great Britain	9,009
East Germany	8,808
Soviet Union	8,442
New Zealand	7,115
Czechoslovakia	6,688
Hungary	6,212
Israel	6,181
Spain	5,248
Ireland	5,198
Poland	5,034
Bulgaria	4,955
Greece	4,617
Romania	4,024
Yugoslavia	3,659
Portugal	2,628
Cuba	1,999
Costa Rica	1,458
Nicaragua	845
Coverage 25–89 percent	
Libya	$5,290
Cyprus	4,195
Taiwan	3,611
Venezuela	2,922
Mexico	2,678
Korea, South	2,418
Argentina	2,373
Panama	2,150
Uruguay	1,900
Brazil	1,809
Turkey	1,409
Chile	1,309
Philippines	590
Bolivia	541
China	299
Coverage under 25 percent	
United States	$17,148
Algeria	2,654

Country	GNP per cap.
Iraq	2,308
South Africa	2,077
Iran	1,637
Guatemala	1,292
Colombia	1,290
Peru	1,153
Tunisia	1,121
Ecuador	1,097
Paraguay	921
El Salvador	821
Dominican Republic	816
Honduras	752
Egypt	749
Indonesia	491
Pakistan	331
Guinea	305
India	272
Burma	191
Lebanon	

Source: Ruth Leger Sivard, *World Military and Social Expenditures 1989.* Washington: World Priorities, 1989.

rest being developing. And among the 21 countries with less than 25 percent coverage, only one, the United States, is in the industrialized category.

As we have seen in this chapter, coverage of 90–100 percent of national populations has usually come after a long historical process, although sometimes after a social revolution. Coverage of less than 90 percent has several possible meanings. Most often it means that coverage is limited to industrial and commercial workers in a country that is mainly agricultural; sometimes families may not be covered. Often there are separate social insurance programs for public and private employees. The self-employed may or may not be covered, although if not statutorily they often can purchase private insurance. In both the United States and South Africa, the low percentage covered means the limitation of social insurance to the elderly and (in the United States) the severely disabled.

Health service benefits may differ for dependents and primary workers, and for private employees compared with public. In some developing countries a major distinction is made in services for blue-collar and white-collar workers. In general, primary beneficiaries are entitled to the complete services of physicians (generalists and specialists), hospitalization, most prescribed drugs, diagnostic tests, rehabilitative therapy, and maternity care. In addition, many of the higher income countries support the costs of dental care, eyeglasses and other appliances, transportation, and home nursing. The emphasis of all these programs has been on treatment of the sick and injured, but in recent years they have come to recognize the value of providing health promotion and disease prevention.

With respect to the method of payment for health services under social insurance, there are several variations. In several countries, the patient must pay doctor and other provider bills first and then seek reimbursement from an insurance office. Usually the refund is 75 or 80 percent of an official fee, so that the patient ends up paying the balance personally. (Copayments may apply only to the first few services in an illness.) The U.S. Medicare program for the elderly is the only one in the world in which there are no officially negotiated fees and patients may be charged any amount (although reimbursed for only 80 percent of a government maximum). The U.S. program is also the only one with an annual *deductible* expenditure, before the insurance takes effect.

The realities of Social Security coverage and benefits for health care in countries are often not as good as the letter of the law. Legal entitlement does not necessarily mean accessible care. The law may be very broad, but the resources in doctors, hospitals, drugs, and so on may be quite inadequate. There may be waiting lists for certain nonurgent services or long distances to reach a doctor or hospital bed. This has, in fact, been a problem in countries with such diverse health systems as Canada, Great Britain, and the Soviet Union. Even within one country, the needed resources may be abundant in one region and deficient in another. Many political factors—most commonly the competing military budget—determine whether entitlements to health care are translated into reality.

Regarding patterns of health care delivery, as explained in this chapter, there are other basic variations. Of the 70 countries with statutory health insurance, 22 (31 percent) depend essentially on private physicians and other providers in private settings. This pattern is used mostly in the older industrialized countries,

where the private market for medical care has been strong; in these countries, social insurance is largely a mechanism for paying conventional medical bills. Many of the inefficiencies and "perverse incentives" of private medical practice, paid for by fees for each unit of service, are tolerated to gain political acceptability and to get legislation.

In the developing countries, where the income level is much lower and the private market for medical care is relatively small, the strategy for delivering services under social insurance has usually differed. Public employment of health care providers and public ownership of health facilities have, on the whole, proved to be more cost-effective than the private alternative. Quality control, greater efficiency, and lower costs can be better achieved by organizing doctors and others in governmental polyclinics and hospitals, paying all personnel by salary (full time or part time), and establishing needed resources under a regional plan. (A few exceptions to such public control are seen in certain very entrepreneurial developing countries, such as South Korea, the Philippines, and South Africa.)

Organized patterns of health care delivery have come to prevail also in countries where the major type of financing has changed from social insurance to general revenues—either by evolution or by revolution. This has been the sequence in Great Britain, the Scandinavian countries, Italy, Greece, and Spain. It has, of course, also been conspicuous in the Soviet Union and all the socialist countries influenced by it. Except for the United States and Canada, furthermore, in all countries with any form of health insurance, virtually every physician in a hospital works on salary, full time or part time.

The form of social financing of health care—whether by social insurance or general revenues—has a bearing on the distribution of services. When social insurance is the method, entitlement to care is limited to individuals (with or without dependents), who have paid premiums. Even if 95 percent of people are covered, 5 percent are excluded. Unfortunately in the 36 countries with less than 90 percent coverage, the form of financing is almost always by social insurance. In these countries, health care protection may be lost by unemployment or even by employment in a type of work not covered under the law.

In spite of this inequity, history suggests that health care financing through social insurance has many practical advantages. First, being based on a special levy on earnings (usually with employer contributions), it raises money without touching general revenues; this has made it politically attractive. Second, taking a fixed percentage of earnings may be only slightly "progressive," but giving health services irrespective of monetary input is very progressive. Third, the insurance mechanism is organized self-help, and is psychologically associated with health service as a right, not a charity; this has important implications for patient–doctor relationships. Fourth, the development of social insurance for health care in countries has shown that, in time, both the population coverage and the scope of services tend to expand.

This overview of worldwide experience with social insurance for health care, and the previous accounts of specific country experiences, shows how closely this movement is linked to economic and political developments. The emergence of the insurance mechanism to handle medical care costs was basically an outgrowth of the Industrial Revolution, the emergence of a large working class dependent on wages for survival, and recognition of the value of cooperation to cope with the risks of sickness. Beyond this, one may identify several notable features in the development of health insurance programs.

1. The growth of voluntary insurance leads eventually to statutory insurance, under government, because of both the strengths and weaknesses of voluntary programs. On the one hand, voluntary health insurance demonstrates the feasibility and value of the idea; on the other hand, its operation leaves various inadequacies and inequities that can be corrected only by governmental action.
2. Voluntary organizations that have acquired a social role are usually incorporated in some way in the operation of a statutory social insurance program.
3. In affluent industrialized countries, health

insurance starts typically as a mechanism for paying charges under medical care delivery patterns that previously existed. In time, the rise in expenditures—the result of both increasing rates of utilization and advanced technology—leads to increased measures of regulation or public control and generally increased health care organization.

4. In economically less developed countries, where the past market for private medical care has been relatively small, health insurance usually starts with an organized pattern of health care delivery, in the interests of both economy and quality.
5. Social insurance of private health care costs may be abruptly transformed into completely socialized systems of health service, as a result of social revolutions. Under such circumstances, financing becomes shifted mainly to general revenues, all resources become governmental, and all people become legally entitled to health care.
6. In the absence of social revolutions, *national health services,* through which all people become entitled to comprehensive health care as a right of national residence, are achieved only after many years of experience with more limited social insurance and political developments conducive to change.
7. Even without development of full-scale national health services, national health insurance programs tend to evolve toward wider population coverage and broader scopes of health services. This is true under both private practice and organized frameworks of medical care delivery.
8. Mounting pressures for efficiency and effectiveness in the use of public funds have led everywhere to increased rationalization of health care delivery. This has encouraged strategies that promote prevention, maximize the use of auxiliary health personnel, and stress ambulatory care rather than costly hospitalization.

Beyond these general features of the health insurance movement, there are many other trends in national health systems to which health insurance contributes. These include such processes as health planning, regionalization, quality control and evaluation, and the whole social dynamics in back of the global movement for achieving health care equity. These subjects are explored further in later chapters.

REFERENCES

Benatar, S. R., "Medicine and Health Care in South Africa." *New England Journal of Medicine,* 315(8):527–532, 21 August 1986.

Beveridge, William, *Social Insurance and Allied Services* (American Edition). New York: Macmillan, 1942.

Bloom, G., M. Segall, and C. Thube, *Expenditure and Financing of the Health Sector in Kenya.* Nairobi: Kenya Ministry of Health, 1986.

Carney, Kim, "Health in Egypt." *Journal of Public Health Policy,* 5(1):131–142, March 1984.

Deeble, J. S., "Health Care under Universal Insurance: The First Three Years of Medicare." Canberra (Australia): Department of Community Services and Health, 1987 (processed).

Emery, George M., "New Zealand Medical Care." *Medical Care,* 159–170, July–September 1966.

Field, Mark G., *Soviet Socialized Medicine—An Introduction.* New York: The Free Press, 1967.

Fulcher, Derick, *Medical Care Systems: Public and Private Health Care Coverage in Selected Industrial Countries.* Geneva: International Labour Office, 1974.

Glaser, William, *Health Insurance Bargaining: Foreign Lessons for Americans.* New York: Gardner Press, 1978.

Gruat, J. V., "The Social Guarantee in the Gabonese Republic: A New Kind of Social Protection in Africa." *International Social Security Review,* 2:157–171, 1985.

Levitt, Ruth, *The Reorganized National Health Service.* London: Croom Helm, 1976.

"Libya" in *The Europa Yearbook 1987: A World Survey,* Vol. I. London: Europa Publications, pp. 1747–1760.

Marmor, Theodore R., *The Politics of Medicare.* Chicago: Aldine, 1973.

McGreevey, William, *Brazilian Health Care Financing and Health Policy: An International Perspective.* Washington, D.C.: World Bank, November 1982.

Mera, Jorge Alberto, *Politica de Salud en Argentina: La Construccion del Seguro Nacional de Salud.* Buenos Aires: Libreria Hachette, 1988.

Mesa Lago, Carmelo, *Social Security in Latin America.* Pittsburgh: University of Pittsburgh Press, 1978.

Moon, Ok-Ryun, *The National Health Insurance Policy in Korea.* Seoul: Seoul National University, School of Public Health, 1987.

Reinhardt, Uwe E., "Health Insurance and Health Policy in the Federal Republic of Germany." *Health Care Financing Review,* 3(2):1–14, December 1981.

Robb, J. Wesley, "The British Choice in Health Care: A Report from London." *The Pharos,* 33–37, Winter 1985.

Rodwin, Victor G., "The Marriage of National Health Insurance and 'La Mèdecine Libèral' in France: A Costly Union." *Milbank Memorial Fund Quarterly,* 59(1):16–43, 1981.

Roemer, Milton I., *Medical Care in Latin America.* Washington, D.C.: Organization of American States, 1963.

Roemer, Milton I., *The Organization of Medical Care under Social Security: A Study Based on the Experience of Eight Countries.* Geneva: International Labour Office, 1969.

Roemer, Milton I., "Health Development and Political Policy: The Lesson of Cuba." *Journal of Health Politics, Policy and Law,* 4(4):570–580, Winter 1980.

Scarpaci, Joseph L., *Primary Medical Care in Chile: Accessibility under Military Rule.* Pittsburgh: University of Pittsburgh Press, 1988.

Sen, Pedro, "Financing of Medical Care Insurance in the Philippines." *International Social Security Association Bulletin,* No. (2):139–150, 1975.

Siem, Harold, *Choices for Health: An Introduction to the Health Services in Norway.* Oslo: Universitetsforlaget AS, 1986.

Sigerist, Henry E., *Man and Medicine.* New York: Norton, 1932.

Sigerist, Henry E., "From Bismarck to Beveridge: Developments and Trends in Social Security Legislation." *Bulletin of the History of Medicine,* 8:365–388, April 1943.

Steslicke, William E., "Development of Health Insurance Policy in Japan." *Journal of Health Politics, Policy and Law,* 7(1):197–226, Spring 1982.

Taylor, Malcolm G., *Health Insurance and Canadian Public Policy: The Seven Decisions That Created the Canadian Health Insurance System.* Montreal: McGill-Queen's University Press, 1978.

U.S. Social Security Administration, *Social Security Throughout the World—1987.* Washington, D.C.: Government Printing Office, 1988.

World Bank, *The Health Sector in China.* Washington, D.C. (Report No. 4664-CHA), 13 April 1984.

World Bank, *Turkey: Health Sector Review.* Washington, D.C. (Report No. 6089-TU), September 1986.

World Health Organization, "India" in *Health Care in South-East Asia.* New Delhi: Regional Office for South-East Asia, 1985, pp. 91–110.

Zschock, Dieter K. (Editor), *Health Care in Peru: Resources and Policy.* Boulder, CO: Westview Press, 1988.

CHAPTER SEVEN

Voluntary Health Agencies

Organized activities outside of government for a health objective are another part of the national health system in virtually every country. The health objectives may be very different and the strategies employed quite diverse, but health services are influenced in some way.

HISTORIC DEVELOPMENT

If we regard any organized activity outside of government but not in the private commercial market as *voluntary,* then the earliest such activities were undertaken by religious groups. In Chapter 3, we saw how in the third and fourth centuries the Christian church under Constantine established merciful institutions for the care of the poor, the aged, and the sick in and around Constantinople. These hostels or hospitals became better developed in western Europe in the eleventh and twelfth centuries. St. John's, the first English hospital, was built by the church at York in 1084, and the Hospital of the Holy Ghost was built in Berlin in 1070. Not until the late twelfth and thirteenth centuries were local government funds put into church hospitals, enabling them to provide more than simple custodial care. With the crusades from western Europe to the east, hospitals were built for pilgrims in Jerusalem.

Much later, in the eighteenth and nineteenth centuries, Christian sects from Europe sent missions to Asia and Africa to spread Christianity. Medical care in hospitals and clinics has been a major strategy in spreading the gospel, and thousands of hospitals have been established for this reason. In many developing countries, mission hospitals have pioneered the techniques of Western medicine, especially in rural areas. Sometimes these hospitals trained nurses and other local personnel, but they did not engage in community health programs. Church supported hospitals in Africa and Asia have usually retained their sovereignty, but they could not survive without additional financial support. This has usually been obtained by substantial charges for patient care and also some subsidy from government.

In Latin America, the *beneficencia* (charity) hospitals, organized originally by Catholic Church groups coming with the conquerors from Spain and Portugal, continued to serve the poor long after national independence was achieved (1820–1830). Eventually these hospitals were subsidized by government and, after the mid-twentieth century, most were taken over by Ministries of Health.

Philanthropic foundations carried out other forms of health-related functions outside the domain of government. The earliest major gifts to charity were entrusted also to the Christian church, but as guilds arose in the cities they were given royal charters and also entrusted with large donations. After the French Revolution, separate philanthropic bodies required governmental approval and they did not grow extensively. In the Anglo-Saxon countries, private philanthropic charities were encouraged. As early as 1612, an English philanthropist, Thomas Sutton, gave money for the establishment of a hospital and a free grammar school. In 1724, Sir Thomas Guy used his wealth to build Guy's Hospital in London (criticized for the egoism and the use of "tainted money").

In the laissez-faire economy and permissive culture of the United States, philanthropic foundations have multiplied rapidly. In the early twentieth century millionaires such as Andrew Carnegie and John D. Rockefeller established foundations (Carnegie in 1911 and

Rockefeller in 1913) that served as models for many others. By 1980 there were 26,000 foundations in the United States, a large proportion of which carried out health-related programs. To a lesser degree, there were philanthropic foundations in 45 other countries. In several Latin American countries, foundations were set up—even linked to government—to carry out public health work unrestricted by official bureaucratic procedures.

Still other nongovernmental bodies within national health systems have been the professional associations in medical and related disciplines. The antecedents of modern medical associations were the Royal College of Physicians of London, granted a charter by the king in 1518, and the Royal College of Surgeons, chartered in 1800. These royally sanctioned bodies became an elite group, but medical associations for all physicians were organized in Great Britain in 1832, in the United States in 1847, and eventually in almost every country. The same applies to associations of nurses, pharmacists, and numerous other health professions.

Following the development of nongovernmental organizations with health-related objectives, voluntary health agencies, organizations of people devoted to a health objective through numerous donations of work and money outside of government, arose. The health objective may be of three principal types: (1) to fight (through treatment, prevention, or other means) certain diseases, (2) to help certain types of people, or (3) to provide certain types of health service. Sometimes two or all three of these purposes may be embodied in a voluntary health agency. It is with voluntary health agencies that this chapter is mainly concerned.

The earliest of such voluntary health activities—for certain types of person—were carried out in France, in connection with childbirth. In 1786, the French *Societé de Chartre Maternelle* was organized to provide relief for poor women during confinement. In 1784, the *Institut des Mères Nourrices* was organized by humanitarian doctors and others in Lyons. In the nineteenth century, wealthy benefactors in France and Germany established nurseries,

milk stations, and consultation clinics for mothers and babies. Infant welfare stations, to promote the health of well babies, rather than to treat sick ones, were organized outside of government in Nancy and Paris in the 1890s. These voluntary initiatives spread to England and the United States at the turn of the twentieth century, years before they were undertaken by official public health departments.

The earliest organized voluntary effort directed against a certain type of disease appeared in London in 1879. The value of silver nitrate drops in preventing eye infections in newborns had just been demonstrated, and in 1879 the London Society for the Prevention of Blindness and the Improvement of the Physique of the Blind was founded. The work of this society was primarily educational. After the initial leadership of physicians, the wives of many middle class businessmen became involved in these agencies.

Another relatively early voluntary agency for a disease-specific objective was devoted to the fight against tuberculosis. In 1882, Robert Koch in Germany had discovered the tubercle bacillus, but the significance of this for disease control was not immediately appreciated. In 1891, a French League Against Tuberculosis was founded at Bordeaux. The next year, in 1892, a Philadelphia physician and associates organized the Pennsylvania Society for the Prevention of Tuberculosis—one of the few health system innovations to originate in the United States and then spread to Europe. In 1904, the U.S. National Association for the Study and Prevention of Tuberculosis was organized, mainly to promote popular education and medical research. In 1907, the agency began selling "Christmas seals" for fund-raising—a technique continuing to the present time. In 1918, the U.S. organization changed its name to the National Tuberculosis Association, with hundreds of local chapters throughout the country. Although started by a physician, it was soon made up of thousands of men and women from every walk of life.

Voluntary agencies, concerned mainly with certain types of health service, were devoted to the extension of visiting nurses to help poor families. The first such Visiting Nurse Association (VNA) was organized in Liverpool,

England in 1959, from the efforts of a wealthy humanitarian, William Rathbone. The nurses provided bedside care in homes to spare the low-income patient from the discomfort and danger of hospitalization. In 1874 a National Nursing Association was formed in England to provide voluntary trained nurses for the poor. An especially dedicated group of English women organized the Victorian Order of Nurses (V.O.N.) around 1890 for hospital work, and then after World War I for public health nursing. V.O.N. nurses were very active in Canada.

CONTEMPORARY VOLUNTARY HEALTH AGENCIES

The flowering of medical knowledge at the end of the nineteenth century, along with the great extension of general education, led to the rapid growth of voluntary health agencies. Almost every major health need generated a nongovernmental group of citizens to tackle it. This was especially true in the United States, where government's role in the health system was relatively weak, but in different forms it was evident also in Europe. Extension of voluntary health agencies to the less developed countries of the other continents came somewhat later. In all types of country, the voluntary health agency that mobilizes the efforts of large numbers of people depends on a socioeconomic setting in which a significant portion of the population have incomes beyond their immediate needs.

The most numerous types of voluntary health agency almost everywhere are those concerned with particular diseases or disorders.

Disease-Specific Agencies

Voluntary health agencies to fight against blindness and tuberculosis had arisen after important technical discoveries in the nineteenth century, but voluntary campaigns against *venereal disease* grew from other roots. In 1876, a Committee for the Prevention of the State Regulation of Vice was organized in New York City (where prostitution was tolerated and reg-

ulated). The concern was clearly morality, not disease control. In 1895 the name was changed to the American Purity Alliance. Somewhat more health consciousness was shown in France, where the *Societé Francaise de Prophylaxie Sanitaire et Morale* was formed in 1901. Then in 1905, the American Society for Sanitary and Moral Prophylaxis was founded—rather more specifically to fight both prostitution and venereal disease. This was the time when syphilis became better understood, with the discovery of the spirochete by Schaudinn in 1905 and of the drug salvarsan by Ehrlich in 1910.

In 1910 the American Federation of Sex Hygiene was formed, becoming the American Social Hygiene Association in 1914. Its program was largely to educate parents, teachers, and adolescents about sexual behavior; it also became deeply concerned about "cleaning up the U.S. Army." This meant a political role for a voluntary health association—to promote legislation; in 1918 the U.S. Congress (during the World War I) passed the Chamberlin–Kahn Act to provide federal grants to the states for venereal disease control, especially near military bases. The VD-control objective of the voluntary social hygiene movement was soon fully adopted by government public health agencies, so that the volunteers could direct their efforts elsewhere. In the 1980s, another sexually transmitted disease, AIDS, became the center of attention for a new generation of disease-specific voluntary health agencies.

A very different type of challenge for voluntary action was presented by *cancer*. This was a disease shrouded in mystery and demanding a vast range of medical research. In 1892 a League Against Cancer was formed in France, and in 1900 a National Cancer Commission was set up by the Royal Colleges of Physicians and of Surgeons in Great Britain. These bodies were composed primarily of physicians, and their objective was to attract money, from both private and public sources, to support cancer-related research.

The most vigorous voluntary movement to fight cancer arose in the United States some years later. In 1912 the American College of Surgeons set up a committee for cancer education, and in 1913 the American Gynecological Society did the same. Soon these two professional groups got together and formed the American Society for the Control of Cancer. Their goal was "to disseminate knowledge concerning the symptoms, diagnosis, treatment and prevention of cancer, to investigate the conditions under which cancer is found, and to compile statistics in regard thereto." In 1927 they offered a $50,000 prize to anyone finding a cure for cancer, but after 5,000 entries no one won. The society's work focused on education about early detection of cancer, and it mobilized the General Federation of Women's Clubs toward this end. In 1936, over one million women were estimated to be doing this educational work.

A National Advisory Cancer Council was organized in the United States in 1937 to promote research. This body influenced the law establishing the National Cancer Institute within the U.S. Public Health Service that year. In 1944 the American Society for the Control of Cancer became the American Cancer Society and embarked on a program for cancer research, education, prevention, and early detection. Local chapters helped cancer patients with the personal aspects of the disease, but not with specific medical treatment. They publicized the "seven warning signs of cancer" and broadcast the message that "every doctor's office is a cancer detection center."

As human longevity increased, cancer became a conspicuous disease in more and more countries. By 1980, there was a national association in 31 countries, and in 1982 they formed a World Federation for Cancer Care. The countries included six in Asia, six in Africa, seven in Europe, and seven in the Americas. The cancer societies, in conjunction with voluntary agencies for heart and lung diseases, have undertaken a worldwide campaign to combat the global tobacco epidemic.

Early in the twentieth century, *heart disease* became the first cause of death in the industrialized countries. Voluntary actions were first launched in the United States. In 1915 the Association for the Prevention and Relief of Heart Disease was formed by a number of physicians, but disbanded during World War I. It resumed activities in 1919 and began to include nonmedical members. In 1947 it became

the American Heart Association (AHA) and undertook major fund-raising efforts, with much success. Its program has stressed education of the general population and of doctors and grants for medical research. The AHA helped to secure passage of the 1948 law setting up the National Heart Institute in the U.S. Public Health Service.

Heart disease, despite its great prevalence, has not had the popular appeal of other diseases spawning voluntary health agencies. There are some small heart associations in Western Europe, but very few in developing countries. The name of the international body in this field—the *International Society and Federation of Cardiology*—reflects its quite technical orientation.

Mental disease, although much less lethal than heart disease, has given rise to voluntary health agencies in many countries. Inspiration for the idea is usually attributed to Clifford Beers, who reported his own grim experience in an American mental hospital in a book, *A Mind That Found Itself,* published in 1907. This led to the organization of the Connecticut Society for Mental Hygiene the same year, followed soon by the U.S. National Committee for Mental Hygiene in 1909. The goals were to broaden general understanding of mental illness—stigmatized for centuries—prevent mental disorders by early treatment, reform the conditions in state mental hospitals, and protect the legal rights of mental patients. By 1945, there were mental hygiene societies in 29 countries, beside the United States.

In the years 1970–1972, a major international survey of voluntary health organizations was launched by the American Public Health Association. Organizations devoted to mental health were found to be active in 17 industrialized and 15 developing countries. More than most voluntary health organizations, those in the mental health field have been concerned with improving the quality of patient care in governmental facilities.

Still another disease-specific voluntary health agency to originate in the United States was the National Foundation for Infantile Paralysis. The disablement from this disease of President Franklin D. Roosevelt, as an adult, surely contributed to the birth of the organization in 1938. The cause and mode of spread of *poliomyelitis* were unknown at the time, and most of the money raised went to support research. Most notable was the foundation's support for Jonas Salk's work, leading to an effective immunization; since Salk's ideas were contrary to conventional thinking, his applications for government research support had been rejected. This was a great triumph for voluntary health agencies, and subsequent campaigns against polio throughout the world have been undertaken by governments. Few other countries have established voluntary agencies for this disease. (In the United States, after immunization reduced cases of polio nearly to zero, the National Foundation directed its efforts to fighting against birth defects.)

The origin of a society for the prevention of *blindness* in England in 1879 has been noted. Blindness from infection in countries of the Middle East and from degenerative disease (cataracts and glaucoma) in European countries became conspicuous problems in the early twentieth century. Many countries organized national associations of blind persons to promote instruction in Braille reading, the use of "seeing eye" dogs, and other measures of rehabilitation. The American Association for the Conservation of Vision was formed in 1911, and it joined with other groups in 1928 to form the National Society for the Prevention of Blindness. A World Union of the Blind was organized in 1984, with scores of national member associations. Similar voluntary agencies have been formed to respond to the needs of the deaf.

Pregnancy, of course, is not a disease, but childbirth is a specific health problem that has led to voluntary social movements for centuries. Since the writings of the British economist Thomas Malthus in 1798 about the hazard of overpopulation in relation to the earth's resources, *birth control* has become a major political issue throughout the world. In nineteenth-century Europe there were Malthusian Leagues, devoted to population control, but in the twentieth century the birth control issue became formulated much more in terms of family welfare and the emancipation of women.

In 1878, the first birth control clinic was organized in Amsterdam, amid great controversy. In 1921, the British Malthusian League organized such a clinic in London. In the United States, a public health nurse, Margaret Sanger, concerned about poor women with many children, did the pioneering. In 1916, she opened a birth control clinic in Brooklyn, New York, and she was promptly arrested. After serving a jail sentence, she helped to organize the American Birth Control League, which in 1942 became the Planned Parenthood Federation of America. After World War II, as the population problem became prominent in many developing countries, this organization became the International Planned Parenthood Federation (1952) and then Planned Parenthood-World Population (1961). By 1973 there were 79 countries with such organizations.

In the 1970s the many strategies for contraception became formulated as *family planning,* with extensive support by governmental Ministries of Health. A major objective of U.S. foreign aid programs was the promotion of family planning in developing countries; India even changed the name of its governmental health agency to *Ministry of Health and Family Welfare.*

Objections to contraception by major religious groups (especially Catholics), however, made many governments wary about direct operation of family planning (FP) programs. Education and dissemination of FP techniques had an obvious place in the well-established maternal and child services of the public health agencies, except for the political sensitivity. The solution almost everywhere was for government to use voluntary health agencies to do FP work. Family planning agencies were created by government where they did not already exist. In the 1970–1972 international survey of voluntary health organizations, noted earlier, family planning agencies were reported in 20 industrialized countries and 35 developing countries. In nearly all of these the necessary funding came mainly from government.

Numerous other specific diseases or disorders have given rise to voluntary health agencies. The *crippled child* and later the disabled adult have been objects of social concern since the early twentieth century. An Association for the Aid of Crippled Children was founded in New York City in 1900, and Rotary Clubs of businessmen supported similar agencies elsewhere in America and other countries. Cerebral palsy became a more specific object of voluntary agency work later in the century. In 1969 an International Cerebral Palsy Society was formed, with headquarters in London and representatives from 60 countries. Special agencies have also arisen to tackle the problems of epilepsy, multiple sclerosis, and other crippling disorders.

Since 1950, few major diseases are without a voluntary health agency in the United States and many other countries. Diabetes, arthritis, hemophilia, cystic fibrosis—disorders common or rare—have generated voluntary health agencies. These groups attract their members and support largely from victims of these diseases and their families. Their objectives usually stress the promotion of research and the greater mobilization of public funds to fight the selected disorder.

A special type of disease-specific health agency is that devoted to self-help—the self-treatment of persons with a certain health problem. Most highly developed is Alcoholics Anonymous, founded in the United States in 1935 and spread to many other countries. Persons suffering from alcoholism join together in these clubs and influence each other psychologically to overcome their addiction. Similar self-help groups have been organized to help drug addicts, women following mastectomies, parents of retarded children, and others.

Voluntary Agencies for Certain Persons

Throughout the World, children have been the objects of social concern, especially children's health. Almost every country of Latin America has a national society for the *health care of children,* whose president is typically the wife of the highest elected official in government. These agencies typically sponsor clinics for malnourished children, assist in immunization campaigns, and help to operate well-baby sessions. Most of the financial support usually comes from governmental grants. So strong is the appeal of children that in the United Nations family of agencies, the one for children, UNICEF, is based on the voluntary contributions of countries.

In certain countries, preventive health services for children have been so extensively developed by voluntary agencies that this entire field of work is turned over by government to the voluntary body. This is true in New Zealand, where the Plunket Society was organized by women in 1907. The well-baby counseling clinics were so well managed that the Ministry of Health simply supported them, in place of MoH clinics. In 1970 there were more than 600 Plunket Society branches in New Zealand employing their own nurses to run the clinics and make home visits.

In Belgium the voluntary *Oeuvre National de l'Enfance* or ONE plays a similar role. It carries out and directly provides a broad range of preventive services for children and expectant mothers. In 1980, ONE operated 1,141 infant welfare clinics, 665 clinics for preschool children, and 224 antenatal clinics; it also provided home nursing to families with newborn babies. Unlike practices in other European countries, most of the clinics are attended by both a physician and a nurse. The costs of these services are met mainly by government grants to ONE.

The health and welfare of *elderly people* have given rise to voluntary agencies in several industrialized countries. Senior citizen activity programs have been organized by these groups. The Social Security Act 1965 amendments in the United States, supporting medical care of the aged, were promoted in large part by voluntary groups of senior citizens.

Military veterans have also formed organizations to advance their personal welfare. In spite of large government programs to help veterans in the United States and a few other countries, disabled veterans in several countries have organized to mobilize greater support.

Most organizations for farmers, industrial workers, women, and youth cannot be considered voluntary health agencies in the sense of this chapter. Yet in socialist and some other countries these organizations provide volunteer support for various personal and environmental health programs of government. In labor unions and farm organizations, committees are often devoted to legislative issues on health care. *Fringe benefits,* including medical care insurance, figure prominently in labor–management negotiations.

Voluntary Agencies for Certain Services

The nineteenth century origin of *visiting nurse services* in England has been noted. In 1877 the idea of district nurses, engaged by voluntary agencies to visit the sick poor in their homes spread to the United States. Starting in New York City, the idea was taken up also in Buffalo, Philadelphia, and Boston, where the agencies were called *instructive district nursing associations.* In addition to bedside nursing, the nurses were expected to educate families on how to take care of their sick relatives. Eventually they all changed their names to *visiting nurse associations* (VNAs). The VNAs were started typically by middle-class women's groups and funded by private donations.

As public health nursing has developed in the programs of official public health agencies, its role has become quite distinguishable from that of the VNAs. Public health nurses follow up cases of communicable disease in the home and visit mothers with newborn babies. By contrast, VNA nurses give bedside care in the homes for surgical patients recently discharged from a hospital or for chronically ill patients. When the British National Health Service reorganized the entire British health system in 1948, these two forms of community nursing were administratively integrated at the local level, but in the United States, they still usually remain separate. American VNA services, however, are no longer dependent on voluntary donations for support, but are typically paid for by public (e.g., Medicare) or private health insurance programs. VNA services have come to include physical therapy, nutritional counselling, and nursing.

In the Netherlands a unique type of voluntary health agency has been operating since the late nineteenth century to provide a variety of preventive services—primarily through home nursing. These are the "Cross Associations" (the White Cross, the Yellow and Green Cross, etc.), organized in local communities to help families with newborn babies, tuberculosis cases, patients with cancer, rheumatism, and so on. In 1980, there were 1,670 branches of the Cross Associations in the Netherlands, with 3,000,000 members and a staff of 3,720 nurses. Members pay an annual subscription, and substantial subsidies are received from central and local governments.

The *Red Cross Societies* are probably the most internationally widespread voluntary health agencies of any type. Their mission everywhere is to help people confronted with natural or man-made disasters. In 1859, Henri Dunant, a Swiss businessman, saw the tragic bloodshed at the battlefield of Solferino, Italy. He convinced an international conference in Geneva in 1864 to organize volunteer national societies to help the wounded on any side of a battle. Because of the emblem worn on the sleeves of volunteers, these groups became the Red Cross Societies.

National Red Cross Societies were gradually organized throughout Europe and America. The first societies were in Germany, Belgium, Denmark, France, Italy, and Spain, and were oriented to military battles. Their functions were soon extended to general relief in any type of disaster. The American Red Cross, established in 1881, was incorporated by Act of Congress in 1900. Its charter states that its purpose is "to furnish volunteer aid to the sick and wounded of armies in time of war, in accordance with the spirit and conditions of the Geneva Convention, to continue in time of peace . . . to mitigate suffering caused by pestilence, famine, fire, floods, and other natural calamities." By 1965, the American Red Cross had more than 3,700 local chapters, with 2,000,000 volunteer members; its funds came from the donations of over 44,000,000 people.

By 1990, there were national Red Cross Societies in 149 countries on every continent. In developing countries, the Red Cross has become identified with services needed in natural disasters, but also in many other circumstances. Almost everywhere they operate ambulances and maintain blood banks. In all developing countries, the Red Cross is heavily subsidized by government, and it functions in close relationship to the facilities of the Ministry of Health. In countries where Islam is the dominant religion, the agencies are known as the Red Crescent Societies.

Unrelated to the Red Cross is another voluntary agency providing ambulance services. In England, the St. John Ambulance Association was organized by volunteers in 1878. In 1888, it was formally sanctioned by Queen Victoria and became the St. John Ambulance Brigade, with volunteer men and women in uniforms. The Brigade stands by to help whenever crowds gather at large public meetings. This agency has also been established in other British Commonwealth countries, such as Australia and Canada.

Another type of voluntary health agency providing many types of service is illustrated by the Norwegian Women's Public Health Association (NKS is the Norwegian acronym). In 1975, NKS had 1,300 local branches and operated 670 health facilities. Its program included the operation of nursing homes and schools for the mentally retarded, provision of home care for the chronically ill, rehabilitation of the disabled, supplemental feeding of children, and training of nurses. Some 90 percent of the NKS costs are met by grants from the Norwegian government, but thousands of volunteer women contribute their time and effort.

Religious missions, originating in the industrialized countries and operating in the developing countries, constitute another special type of nongovernmental health organization. Their principal role has been to establish and run hospitals, especially in rural regions, where governmental facilities are scarce. After they are set up, at the expense of the foreign donor church, mission health facilities charge patients for the care provided, and they are also usually supported by government grants.

Mission health facilities under Protestant and Catholic sponsorships are organized quite separately in each country. To coordinate the medical work of these churches around the world, in 1968 the Christian Medical Commission was established. This is independent of the World Council of Churches, which is es-

sentially Protestant, and the equivalent Catholic organization. The commission estimates that the worldwide count of all Christian health care programs is about 5,000 (in 1975). They are located mainly in Asia and Africa, and to a lesser extent in Latin America.

The quality of medical care in mission hospitals is generally regarded as very good, and somewhat better than in government hospitals of the same size. With payments from patients and overseas support, their resources—especially the supply of drugs and laboratory supplies—are usually greater. In recent years, mission health programs have been extending outside the hospitals into the community to provide primary health care. In African countries, governments often regard mission hospitals as part of the national network of public facilities for medical care. Larger mission hospitals often provide training for nurses, technicians, and other health personnel.

Finally, the various *professional associations* in medicine, nursing, pharmacy, dentistry, and other health fields must be considered voluntary agencies oriented to a certain type of service. Their purpose is generally to advance the position and the role of the members of each discipline, and therefore the type of service that each group offers. The early antecedents of professional associations in the British Royal Colleges were noted previously.

By 1990, virtually every country in the world had its national medical association, carrying on educational work among its members, maintaining relationships with government, and explaining to the population the scope of physician services. About as many associations exist in dentistry and the other fields. A 1970–1972 world survey of the American Public Health Assoction found medical associations in 19 industrialized and 33 developing countries, dental associations in 21 industrialized (more than medical) and 29 developing countries (fewer than medical), and nursing associations in 22 industrialized and 35 developing countries. In recent years many of these professional associations have become involved in insuring their members against legal malpractice actions by patients. In some countries they also play a role in upholding standards of ethical behavior, although this is often done by separate professional bodies set up by government statute or regulation.

A striking reflection of the scope of voluntary health organizations throughout the world is given by the numerous international nongovernmental organizations in various fields. These are reported in the *Encyclopedia of Associations* for 1988. Selecting only examples from the several hundred "health and medical organizations" listed, they may be classified under the categories used in this chapter:

In addition to these three categories of international nongovernmental organization (NGO), there are several others that span the entire scope of health systems. These NGOs typically have a membership of specialized organizations, rather than national representatives. They are illustrated by the chart at the top of page 115.

Finally, the professional associations of nations have joined together in several international organizations. These are illustrated by the chart at the bottom of page 115.

Agencies	Year of Founding	Countries Represented
Disease-Specific		
International Union Against Tuberculosis and Lung Disease	1920	116
International Diabetes Federation	1949	88
World Psychiatric Association	1961	72
International Federation of Anti-Leprosy Associations	1966	22
International Cerebral Palsy Society	1969	60
World Federation for Cancer Cure	1982	75
World Federation for the Deaf	1951	83
World Blind Union	1984	7
For Certain Persons		
International Union of School and University Health and Medicine	1959	34
International Union of Railway Medical Services	1948	37
International Council of Prison Medical Services	1976	—
International Committee of Military Medicine and Pharmacy	1921	—
International Association of Agricultural Medicine and Rural Health	1961	—
International Commission on Occupational Health	1906	24
Maternal and Child Health Programs	1920	100+
For Certain Services		
International Union for Health Education	1951	29
International Society of Blood Transfusion	1937	79
International Council of Home-help Services	1959	11
International Society for Disaster Medicine	1975	8
International Federation of Health Records Organization	1968	17

Association	Year of Founding	Organizations Represented
Council for International Organizations on Medical Science	1949	89
International Federation for Hygiene, Preventive and Social Medicine	1948	39
International Academy of Legal and Social Medicine	1938	—
International Association for the Study of Living Conditions and Health	1953	25
International Federation of Voluntary Health Service Funds	1968	165

Each of these sets of international NGOs contains many more associations than indicated above. Those selected are intended to reflect the numerous types of voluntary health agency within countries with the vitality to establish international associations. These associations generally promote the formation of equivalent voluntary agencies in countries that lack them, and they help to strengthen the national agencies that exist. They contribute to the development of national health policy standards in their respective fields.

National and international NGOs are concerned mainly with strengthening services in well-established health programs, such as are reviewed above. In addition, the NGO is a natural vehicle for promoting nonconventional or *alternative* types of healing. Thus there are associations to advance homeopathy, naturopathy, acupuncture, herbal medicine, and so on. These are found mainly in several nations of Europe—often linked to *green* political parties—and also in the developing countries of Asia.

GENERAL COMMENTARY

The underlying purpose of voluntary health agencies has invited several sociological generalizations. It is said that voluntary health agencies respond to a social need before government is prepared to do so. It is also said, on the contrary, that voluntary groups take action to forestall government intervention in a particular field. Many voluntary agencies are actually set up by government to undertake tasks that would be politically sensitive for the public authority. Depending on which of these reasons is valid for a particular agency, the relationships between government and the agency would be friendly or hostile.

Association	Year of Founding	Countries Represented
World Medical Association	1947	42
International Dental Federation	1900	80
International Pharmaceutical Federation	1912	—
International Council of Nurses	1899	99
International Confederation of Midwives	1919	51
Medical Women's International Association	1919	38
International Association of Medical Laboratory Technologists	1954	32
International Society of General Practice	1959	—

In fact, all three of the above rationales are true at different times and places. Certainly services for maternal and child health promotion were provided by voluntary groups before government was ready, and then many of these groups dissolved when government undertook the work. Yet in certain countries the voluntary agencies performed so well that even when government was ready, it asked the voluntary agencies to continue and used public funds to subsidize them. In tuberculosis control, pioneered by voluntary agencies, government took over the treatment task in sanatoria; the voluntary TB associations usually did case-finding and general education.

Aggressive voluntary efforts to forestall government action is best illustrated by a type of health agency not discussed in this chapter. Voluntary sickness insurance (later health insurance) agencies in the late nineteenth and early twentieth centuries sought vigorously to maintain their role, when government action was taken to mandate such insurance by law. In certain countries (United States, Australia, South Africa) voluntary health insurance agencies have pursued policies deliberately to forestall government measures in the same field. To a lesser extent, this has sometimes applied to services for crippled children.

The delegation to voluntary agencies of services that would be politically embarrassing for government is well illustrated in the field of family planning. Almost everywhere, this has been the strategy. Sometimes official public health agencies will conduct a modest FP program, whereas extensive services are offered by the nongovernmental groups. In the early 1970s, such voluntary FP agencies were funded almost wholly by governments in at least 20 industrialized countries and at least 35 developing countries. In the latter, financial support came principally from international (bilateral) public sources.

Aside from their relationships with government, voluntary health agencies differ in several other ways. They vary greatly in size (both membership and budget) and in age. Those in industrialized countries tend to be much larger and older. Of the voluntary agencies found in developing countries in the 1970–1972 survey, only one-third had been founded earlier than 1940. The typical voluntary health agency in an industrialized country has numerous branches in the major cities; in the developing countries, there is usually a major office in the capital city and relatively few branches.

Most significant are the variations in the source of funding of voluntary health agencies. In spite of their usual origin from the donations of private citizens, once they are operating, government support becomes a major source of funding. In the United States this is seldom seen, but for all industrialized countries in 1971, according to the APHA international survey, government subsidy accounted for 14 percent of the funding. Voluntary donations made up 61 percent of the funding, and 23 percent came from income from charges for services rendered by the agency. In developing countries the contributions of government were much greater. Subsidy from domestic government sources accounted for 18 percent of funding, and international government support for an additional 29 percent—47 percent in all. Income from service charges contributed 22 percent of funding and only 31 percent came from voluntary donations.

The breakdown of expenditures by voluntary health agencies is often guarded from public view, but the 1970–1972 international survey was able to collect this information on many agencies. It was found that considering funds from all sources, 57 percent of all expenditures went for overhead—to manage the agency's affairs; only 43 percent went for health activities to which the agency was ostensibly devoted. This distribution was essentially the same in developing and industrialized countries. (One can understand why government authorities are often skeptical about voluntary agencies.) One of the incentives for voluntary donations in most countries is their tax-exempt status, but in many developing countries this feature is not relevant.

Taking a world overview of voluntary health agencies, it is clear that they operate in nearly all countries, but there are great differences in their numbers and strength. In general, where the national government is strong and quite centralized, voluntary health agencies are relatively weak. This is most evident in the socialist countries, with their centrally planned health systems, but it is observable also in welfare-oriented health systems such as those of France or Japan. In the more pluralistic and permissive health systems, such as those of the United States, Australia, the Philippine Republic, or India, voluntary health agencies are more numerous and stronger. In the United States it has been estimated that, counting all branches of national bodies, there were as many as 6,000,000 local voluntary health agencies in the 1980s. Although voluntarism plays a more modest role in most other countries, it is nevertheless an important stimulus and supplement to governmental action.

REFERENCES

Akerele, O., I. Tabibzadeh, and J. McGilvray, "A New Role for Medical Missionaries in Africa." *WHO Chronicle*, 30:175–180, 1976.

American Public Health Association, *The Role of National Voluntary Health Organizations in Support of National Health Objectives: Phase II Report*. Washington, D.C.: American Public Health Association, October 1974.

Bader, Michael B., "The International Transfer of Medical Technology." *International Journal of Health Services*, 7(3):443–458, 1977.

Breslow, Lester, *A History of Cancer Control in the United States, 1946–1971*. Washington, D.C.: U.S. Public Health Service, 1977.

Carter, Richard, *Breakthrough: The Saga of Jonas Salk*. New York: Trident Press, 1966.

Cavins, H. M., *National Health Agencies*. Washington, D.C.: Public Affairs Press, 1945.

Committee of the Christian Medical Association, *The Ministry of Healing in India: Handbook of the Christian Medical Association*. Mysore, India: Wesleyan Mission Press, 1932.

Dayton, Edward R., *Medicine and Missions: A Survey of Medical Missions*. Wheaton, IL: Medical Assistance Programs, 1969.

Draper, Elizabeth, *Birth Control in the Modern World*. London: Allen & Unwin, 1965.

Garrison, Fielding H., *An Introduction to the History of Medicine*, 4th ed. Philadelphia: W. B. Saunders, 1929.

Govan, E.S.L., *Voluntary Health Organizations in Canada*. Ottawa: Commission on Health Services, Queen's Printer, 1966.

Gunn, Selskar M., and Philip S. Platt, *Voluntary Health Agencies: An Interpretive Study*. New York: Ronald Press, 1945.

Hampton, I. A., *Nursing of the Sick 1893*. New York: McGraw-Hill, 1949.

Hodson, H. V. (Editor), *The International Foundation Directory*. Detroit, MI: Gale Research, 1979.

Huber, M., *The Red Cross Principles and Problems*. Geneva: A. Kundig Press, 1950.

Kanagaratnam, Kandiah, "The Concern and Contribution of the World Bank in Population Planning." *International Journal of Health Services*, 3(4):709–718, 1973.

Katz, Alfred, *Helping One Another: Self-Help Groups in a Changing World*. Oakland, CA: Third-Party Publishers, 1990.

Leake, Inger R., "The Norwegian Women's Public Health Association." *World Health Forum*, 11:332–335, 1990.

Obermann, C. E., "The Red Cross." In *A History of Vocational Rehabilitation in America*. Minneapolis, MN: T. S. Denison, 1965.

Puddy, E., *A Short History of the Hospital of St. John of Jerusalem in Norfolk*. Norfolk: G. M. Starling, 1961.

Ravenholt, Reimert T., "United States Agency for International Development (USAID) Contributions to International Population Programs." *International Journal of Health Services*, 3(4):641–660, 1973.

Robertson, B. D., *Voluntary Associations: A Study of Groups in Free Societies*. Richmond, VA: John Knox Press, 1966.

Roemer, Milton I., "Resistance to Innovation: The Case of the Community Health Center." *American Journal of Public Health*, 78(9):1234–1239, September 1988.

Rosen, George, *A History of Public Health*. New York: MD Publications, 1958.

Sigerist, Henry E., "Medical Societies, Past and Present." *Yale Journal of Biology and Medicine*, 6:351–362, 1934.

Thompson, Helen M., "The Red Cross Takes up the Challenge." *World Health Forum*, 7:402–405, 1986.

Weaver, W., *U.S. Philanthropic Foundations: Their History, Structure, Management, and Record*. New York: Harper & Row, 1967.

World Health Organization, "Netherlands." In *Health Services in Europe*, 3rd ed. Copenhagen: WHO Regional Office for Europe, 1981, Vol. 2, pp. 133–140.

CHAPTER EIGHT

Private Sector Health Care

When all the organized health programs discussed in Chapters 5, 6, and 7 have been accounted for, there remains a private sector of health care in every health system. It varies enormously among countries in size and character, but everywhere it is a residual part of the health system structure. It is not organized deliberately in the usual sense, but is governed by economic forces of supply and demand, competition and price, and various aberrations of these forces, found in every market.

PRIVATE SECTOR MEANINGS

The private sector in health care has several possible meanings. The provider of health service may be a private agent, as distinguished from an agent of government, or the source of money paying for the health service may be private, as distinguished from public. Various combinations of these two dimensions of private and governmental health activities may be involved, as shown in the simple matrix of Figure 8.1.

In Figure 8.1 the four cells refer to possible health care policies in a national health system. Several illustrative situations may be cited. Cell number 1 refers to both the source of money and the provider of service as being pri-

vate; this applies to the majority of personal health services rendered in the United States. Both the buying and selling of service are private. This also applies to most of the personal health services in India, where private medical or Ayurvedic practitioners are paid for by private individuals. To some extent this pattern is found in virtually all countries.

In cell number 2 health services are provided by public entities, such as personnel in government health centers and hospitals, for which private payments are made. Such a policy is followed in the Philippines and Thailand, where public support for the health system is relatively weak, so that charges are made for service provided in governmental health facilities. The very poorest people are not required to pay, although some small payment may be made as a matter of pride. This applies particularly to payment for drugs dispensed at a government health center or health post.

In cell number 3 health services are rendered by private physicians, pharmacists, and others, for which payments are made from funds in a governmental financing program. In fact, the governmental program often makes use of private entities (such as sickness insurance societies) for the actual transmission of money. The latter arrangement prevails in Germany, France, Belgium, and other countries in which social insurance was enacted after a long history of voluntary insurance paying private providers. Government then regulates the intermediary private agencies in ways that affect the ultimate payments received by doctors and others. In other countries, such as Canada, Japan, and South Korea, governmental agencies pay private providers of service directly.

In cell number 4 health services are provided by governmental personnel and facilities that are financed also by governmental funds. This

Source of Money	Provider of Services	
	Private	Public
Private	1	2
Public	3	4

Figure 8.1. Matrix of the source of money and provider of services in a health system, classified by private and public sectors.

is the pattern in the Soviet Union, Cuba, and other socialist countries that developed a general public system of health services. (Many changes were occurring in these systems in the early 1990s, but the conventional socialist pattern continues to varying extents.) The pattern also applies to almost all hospital services in the Scandinavian countries and to public sector hospital services in many other countries. Cell number 4, therefore, has no relevance to the private sector.

The partially public sector role in cells number 2 and 3 has conventionally been regarded as influencing the character of services in these cells. When, as in cell number 2, the services are provided by public agencies, private payments may restrain the rate of utilization, but little more; in any event, such payments typically cover only a fraction of the costs. When, as in cell number 3, the payments come from public programs (with or without private intermediaries), public authorities tend to have substantial influence on the character of the services. Various public regulations affect the performance of private providers of services, financed from the public sector.

Thus, it is only in cell number 1 that one finds the unfettered operation of a free market of health service. Only when both payment for and provision of services are private are the classical profit incentives experienced by providers, and the classical constraints of price felt by consumers. Profits, of course, may encourage hard work, but they also can encourage unnecessary services. Price may encourage high or low demand, with little relation to the extent of true health need. The full implications of private sector health care, therefore, appear only in cell number 1. Hence, this chapter will be devoted primarily to health services defined by cell number 1, as they exist throughout the world.

Within the boundaries of cell number 1, the greatest volume of activity almost everywhere is by wholly private consumers and wholly private providers. Two variants within cell number 1, however, are found in most health systems. In the first the consumer side has been organized by the management of a private enterprise; here typically an employer organizes personal health services for his employees. In the second the financial side has been organized by a private enterprise; here typically a commercial insurance company organizes the payment for health services. The operation of these two variants of the wholly private market of health care will be examined separately.

WHOLLY PRIVATE HEALTH CARE MARKETS

The wholly private market, in which health care is both financed and provided privately, has several subdivisions. It may apply to (1) the services of traditional healers and birth attendants, (2) the services of modern medical practitioners, (3) drugs and pharmacies, (4) hospitals and nursing homes, and (5) other health services and appliances.

Traditional Healers

As discussed in Chapter 1, traditional healers function within the health systems of all developing countries. They are much more formally trained in Asia (especially in India and China) than in Africa and Latin America, but their services are always rendered primarily in the private sector. Payment is based on a fee for each treatment, although this is sometimes paid in the form of barter—typically food. The fees are usually much lower than those charged by modern physicians, but there are exceptions. Occasionally a traditional healer acquires a great reputation, attracting patients from a large region and charging high fees.

The market for traditional healing is usually larger in populations with limited education. It is also greater in areas in which modern personnel—either in private practice or in public facilities—are scarce. For both of these reasons, healers play especially large roles in rural areas. In a household survey made in Colombia in 1967, it was found that only 3 percent of all ambulatory care encounters in cities were with *curanderos,* but in the rural areas such encounters were 17 percent of the total. In Indonesia in 1985, traditional healing was found to absorb 6 percent of household health expenditures, but this percentage was lower in the cities and higher in rural areas. A survey in Tanzania in 1971 found that 25 percent of urban families consulted traditional healers at a rate of 1.0 visit per family per year; among rural families, 40 percent consulted healers at a rate of 1.8 visits per family per year.

Traditional healers are usually consulted in their own homes, but when the sickness is severe the healer comes to the patient's home. The great majority of healers in the late twentieth century make use of traditional drugs, even if magical incantations or other procedures are also used. Charges to the patient are then made for the drugs but not for the other services.

Traditional birth attendants (TBAs) render childbirth services in the patient's home. Their fees are very low, not only because of the poverty of the families they serve but also because of the nature of the competition. The alternative childbirth service available in many developing countries is a government midwife, whose attention is free. The outcome of this competition in Thailand in 1974 was strongly in favor of the TBA—63 percent of childbirths, compared with 14 percent by the government midwife and the balance by others. In Malaysia, on the other hand, government midwife services were highly developed, so that by 1982 they handled 76 percent of all deliveries, compared with less than 24 percent by TBAs.

Modern Physicians

The services of modern physicians in the wholly private sector are found in virtually every country in the world. In Tanzania in the 1980s and also in Somalia, laws were passed to prohibit private medical practice, but their complete enforcement was questionable. In all other countries, private practice along with payment from private sources is found, ranging in extent from a small share to an overwhelming proportion of all medical services.

Private physician services in the entrepreneurial health system of the United States play a dominating role. Over several recent decades, the proportion of U.S. personal health expenditures derived from purely private sources has declined substantially, but in 1987 it was still 60 percent. More than half of this

Table 8.1. Personal Health Expenditures by Source of Funds: Percentage Distribution, United States, 1950–1987

Sources of Funds	Percentage		
	1950	1970	1987
Personal payment	65.5	40.5	27.8
Voluntary insurance	9.1	23.4	31.4
Philanthropy and industry	2.9	1.7	1.2
Government, federal	10.4	22.2	29.6
Government, state and local	12.0	12.1	10.0
All sources	100.0	100.0	100.0

Source: U.S. Public Health Service, *Health United States 1989.* Washington, D.C.: Government Printing Office, 1990, p. 236.

percentage was cushioned by voluntary health insurance, but this was still in the private sector. The details for all sources of U.S. personal health expenditures are shown in Table 8.1. It is evident that over three decades the contribution of federal government spending and voluntary insurance increased about three times. These figures are heavily influenced by spending for hospital care, and it is known that both government support and voluntary health insurance are less developed for physician services.

Other data for the United States indicate that patient contacts with physicians in 1988 occurred at the rate of 5.3 per person per year. Of these 59.3 percent took place in the physician's private office, another 13.7 percent by telephone, and 1.4 percent by home calls—a total of 74.4 percent in private sector settings. Physician contacts in all organized settings—hospital outpatient departments, health centers, special clinics, and so on—accounted for 25.6 percent of the total. In the U.S. health system, personal payments to private physicians may be made also for inpatient care, since medical staffs in hospitals are open generally to private physicians.

Equivalent data on sources of personal health expenditures are available on six other industrialized countries, as well as the United States, for 1974–1975. These are shown in Table 8.2, in which it is evident that the sum of personal payments and voluntary insurance in all the countries is much lower than that in the United States. This sum varies from 34.9 percent in Australia to 7.0 percent (5.8 plus 1.2 percent) in Great Britain. In all the countries

Table 8.2. Personal Health Expenditures by Source of Funds: Percentage Distribution, Selected Industrialized Countries, 1974–1975

Country	Percentage					
	Personal Payment	Voluntary Insurance	Social Insurance	General Taxation	Other	Total
United States	27.1	25.6	11.7	31.0	4.6	100
Australia	21.1	13.8	1.7	62.7	0.7	100
France	19.6	3.0	69.0	7.0	1.4	100
Canada	19.5	2.5	9.1	66.3	2.6	100
Germany, West	12.5	5.3	62.5	14.6	5.1	100
Sweden	8.4	—	13.1	78.5	—	100
Great Britain	5.8	1.2	5.0	87.3	0.4	100

Source: Maxwell, Robert J., *Health and Wealth—An International Study of Health-Care Spending.* Lexington, MA: Lexington Books, 1981.

except the United States and Australia, voluntary insurance accounted for a very small percentage of personal health expenditures in 1974–1975. (After 1985 voluntary insurance became less important in Australia but more important in Great Britain.)

Such refined data are not available for many other industrialized nations, but for several countries one can report the percentage of expenditures for ambulatory medical care derived from public and private sources. These countries are listed in Table 8.3, ranked according to the share of ambulatory care billings

Table 8.3. Ambulatory Care Billings to Private or Public Sources: Percentage Distribution, Selected Industrialized Countries, 1987

Country	Percent from	
	Private Sources	Public Sources
Germany, West	8.0	92.0
Sweden	10.0	90.0
Great Britain	12.0	88.0
Japan	15.0	85.0
Switzerland	15.0	85.0
Greece	15.0	85.0
Austria	20.0	80.0
Iceland	20.0	80.0
Italy	20.4	79.6
Denmark	24.0	76.0
Canada	27.9	72.1
Finland	30.0	70.0
France	37.9	62.1
Australia	38.8	61.2
United States	44.0	56.0
Belgium	50.0	50.0
Ireland	53.0	47.0
New Zealand	53.0	47.0
Netherlands	56.0	44.0

Source: Organization for Economic Cooperation and Development, *Health Care Systems in Transition.* Paris: OECD, 1990, p. 147.

derived from private sector sources in 1987. These private sources in some countries (e.g., the United States, Australia, or the Netherlands) supported wholly private payments for private ambulatory service. In most countries, however (e.g., New Zealand, Belgium, France, Austria, or Switzerland), they supported the substantial copayments required for ambulatory care, even under social insurance. In other countries in which copayments are not required and purely personal spending is rare—such as Great Britain, Italy, or Ireland—private sources are accounted for mainly by voluntary health insurance that has developed along with the public medical care program.

In all these industrialized countries, private sector physician services are usually characterized by elegant conditions. In contrast to public sector services even in very affluent countries, they are provided in office settings in which the patient receives extremely gracious and courteous attention. Most private physicians have nursing and clerical assistants who help with the interview and examination. Patients are seen mainly by appointment, so that waiting times are short. The patient disrobes for a physical examination, which is done with thoroughness and sensitivity.

The setting of private medical practice in the developing countries is quite different. In Asia, Africa, or Latin America, the typical private practitioner has two simple rooms—one for patients to wait in and the other for medical examinations. In the main cities, where several doctors may share the same quarters at different times, there may be a few more amenities—examining tables, medical instruments, and so on. In the small towns serving rural populations, office facilities are small and drab.

From the strict viewpoint of efficiency, private solo medical practice in any type of country is likely to be less efficient than service delivery by an organized team of health personnel. Efficiency becomes important when financial support is derived from public or other social programs. Economies become important when the expenditure of public funds is at stake.

Private medical practice in developing countries is of two general types: by doctors who are exclusively in such practice and by doctors who work part of each day for a government agency and spend the rest of their time in private work. Exclusive private practice is more common in the very poor countries, where public programs are relatively weaker. In the entrepreneurial health system of Pakistan, about 50 percent of all physicians were in full-time private practice in 1984. In the similar type of health system of Kenya, 70 percent of all physicians in 1982 were exclusively in private practice. Even in the welfare-oriented health system of India (also of very poor economic level) only 41 percent of scientifically trained physicians worked for government agencies in 1987, another 12 percent worked mainly in nongovernmental organizations, and 47 percent were entirely in private practice. Furthermore, almost 100 percent of the large stock of Ayurvedic practitioners in India were wholly in private practice.

In the transitional developing countries, where resources are generally greater, private practice is also very extensive, but it is not so exclusive. In Thailand, only 10 percent of physicians are exclusively in private practice, but the 90 percent working in government or other organized programs spend a large part of each day in private practice. In the Philippines— like Thailand, entrepreneurial in its health system—59 percent of physicians in 1981 were entirely in private practice and most of the 41 percent in public employment practiced privately part-time. Egypt is a transitional level developing country with a welfare-oriented health system, and only 9 percent of its physicians are exclusively in private practice; most

of the employed physicians, however, spend substantial time each day in private work.

Analyzed in terms of health expenditures, a World Bank report shows the proportions of private and public expenditures in very poor and transitional-level developing countries, to be as indicated in Table 8.4. It may be noted that among the five countries with over 60 percent of health expenditures coming from private sources, all but one (Uganda was not studied) were considered in Volume I to have entrepreneurial-type health systems. Among all 21 other developing countries, with less than 60 percent (mostly under 50 percent) of expenditures being private, none was considered to have an entrepreneurial health system. These private health expenditures, of course, were only partially for physicians and tradi-

Table 8.4. National Health Expenditures from Private and Public Sources: Percentage Distribution, Selected Developing Countries, 1980–1984

| Country | Private Public | Percent from | |
		Private Sources	Public Sources
Uganda	4.09	80.4	19.6
Philippines	2.77	73.5	26.5
Pakistan	2.46	71.1	28.9
Thailand (1979)	2.34	69.9	30.1
Indonesia	1.64	62.1	37.9
Swaziland	1.50	59.9	40.1
Egypt (1977)	1.37	57.8	42.2
Morocco	1.22	54.9	45.1
Somalia	1.03	50.7	49.3
Zambia	0.98	49.5	50.5
Peru	0.90	47.4	52.6
Ethiopia	0.85	45.9	54.1
Botswana (1978)	0.77	43.5	56.5
Jordan	0.73	42.2	57.8
Sri Lanka	0.67	40.2	59.8
Zimbabwe	0.66	39.7	60.3
Ecuador	0.63	38.6	61.4
Senegal	0.60	37.5	62.5
Colombia (1978)	0.50	33.3	66.7
Jamaica	0.49	32.9	67.1
China	0.47	31.9	68.1
Burkina Faso	0.46	31.5	68.5
Rwanda	0.37	27.0	73.0
Niger	0.35	25.9	74.1
Burundi	0.20	16.7	83.3
Lesotho	0.13	11.5	88.5

Source: Derived from World Bank, *Financing Health Services in Developing Countries.* Washington, D.C.: World Bank, 1987.

tional healers. A large part of them were for self-prescribed drugs purchased from drug sellers or private pharmacies, as discussed below.

Drugs and Pharmacies

As a part of the wholly private health care market, the purchase of drugs is even more extensive than consultation with physicians. In industrialized countries, where social insurance or general revenue support covers all or the great majority of people, physician's care is always a benefit, but drugs may not be. Drugs are not a nationwide benefit in Canada, nor even for the socially insured elderly population of the United States. In the national medical care programs of most industrialized countries, drugs require substantial copayments, and in the socialist countries they have conventionally (with various exceptions) required full payment by the patient.

In countries, both industrialized and developing, where hospitals and other health facilities are predominantly governmental, pharmacies are typically private. If prescribed drugs are partially financed by a statutory program, patients still purchase nonprescribed drugs at their personal expense. Both prescribed and nonprescribed drugs are sold by pharmacies (with and without trained pharmacists), and nonprescribed drugs may also be sold by stores that are mainly selling food.

Private pharmacies are of two general types—those devoted entirely to selling drugs and some medical supplies, and those selling many types of merchandise along with drugs. In the United States and Canada, for example, the latter type predominate and might best be called drugstores. Around 1980, there were 51,000 drugstores in the United States and about 5,100 in Canada; this meant about one drugstore to 4,500 people in both these countries. In the Scandinavian countries, on the other hand, pharmacies, restricting their sales to drugs, predominate, so that each one can serve more people. In 1975, there were 555 pharmacies in Finland, for a ratio to population of 1:8,320, and in Denmark there were 335 pharmacies, for a ratio of 1:15,300.

In Australia, with its Pharmaceutical Benefits Scheme enacted in 1950, the supply of private drugstores is especially large—5,000 in the mid-1960s; this was a ratio of one drugstore to 2,300 residents or double that in the United States and Canada. Likewise in New Zealand, with its universal health insurance coverage (including drugs) since 1939, drugstores existed at a ratio of 1:2,045 residents. In Japan, even though most physicians dispense many of their own prescriptions, there were 21,000 drugstores in the mid-1960s, for a ratio of 1:4,790 people.

In developing countries, private drugstores are found in the main cities, but in rural regions most drugs are sold by food stores or untrained and unlicensed drug sellers. In the mid-1960s Indonesia had so few drugstores that its ratio was 1:206,000 population; in Nepal it was 1:204,000. Thailand, with many traditional Chinese medicine shops, had 1,100 drugstores and pharmacies, for a ratio of 1:27,000. In India, where both western and Ayurvedic drugs are sold, the pharmacies and drugstores in the mid-1960s numbered 40,000, for a ratio of 1:15,000 population. The Philippines health system was so strongly entrepreneurial that its 5,025 pharmacies (many selling traditional Chinese drugs) meant a ratio of 1:5,400. Egypt also has a large stock of pharmacists, as well as doctors, so that in 1980 it had over 5,000 registered pharmacies, for a ratio of 1:8,000 population. Nigeria, on the other hand, had only 1,200 private pharmacies for its large population in 1980, for a ratio of only 1:71,000 people; in addition there were some 20,000 small shops selling *patent medicines.*

In developing countries and in low-income areas of more affluent countries, the private pharmacy or drugstore is regarded by many people as a resource for inexpensive medical care. Poor people with illness that does not seem alarming will go to the drug shop, explain their symptoms to the pharmacist or sales clerk, and ask for a suitable medicine; this is much less expensive and faster than consulting a physician. A 1979 study in Botswana (in southern Africa) found that of all household health expenditures, 21 percent went for drugs. A similar household survey in Afghanistan

(1976) found this proportion to be 38 percent. In Bolivia (1977) a rural population was found to use as much as 76 percent of household health expenditures for purchasing drugs. In South Korea, before its 1976 health insurance law, some 75 percent of patients with acute illness were found to take medication recommended by druggists or friends before visiting a health facility.

When the patient seeks help in a drugstore to alleviate a symptom, the advice most likely comes from an untrained sales clerk rather than a qualified pharmacist. This is especially true, of course, in developing countries. Whatever limited knowledge the clerk may have, he or she is more likely to recommend drugs that are in ample supply and that yield a good profit. Private shops in developing countries are a major resource for both advice and medication on family planning. Sometimes a druggist will give injections, which are usually highly valued by patients.

The private drugstore, both in affluent and developing countries, is typically open for long hours each day—a special convenience to many patients. The druggist and drug clerks are, more likely than physicians, to be culturally compatible with clients—from the same social class and speaking the same language; for this reason, many patients feel more comfortable visiting the drugstore than entering a doctor's office. There is no proper substitute for knowledge, however, and especially in developing countries, this may be seriously deficient. A study in Egypt in the 1980s arranged for women to visit 20 different pharmacies, inquiring about the treatment for a case of childhood diarrhea; not one of the pharmacists questioned recommended ORT (oral rehydration therapy). Many private drugstores, on the other hand, encourage the sale of infant formula products, to the detriment of breast-feeding. Also antibiotics may be copiously dispensed, both with and without prescriptions, so that drug resistance develops in the population.

Private Hospitals and Nursing Homes

In many countries, hospitals and nursing homes have been established by private indi-

viduals and groups, and operated for profit. This practice in the United States, with its entrepreneurial health system, has attracted a great deal of attention, even though the extent of proprietary ownership of hospitals is actually greater in several welfare-oriented health systems of Europe and elsewhere (see Table 8.5). The overall supply of U.S. hospital beds in the 1980s was about 5.9 per 1000 population, and in 1980 some 7.75 percent of these beds were in proprietary facilities. With extension of chains of proprietary hospitals, this proportion rose to 10.11 percent in 1987, but 90 percent of the beds were still in voluntary nonprofit or public hospitals. American proprietary hospital chains were active in establishing hospitals in Great Britain and elsewhere, with the intention of enlarging the private health care sector in those countries.

The large percentages of proprietary hospital beds in several European countries—Sweden, Switzerland, Germany, France, Spain, and Greece—are referable largely to beds in long-term care facilities for the elderly, chronically ill, and mental patients; in other countries, these facilities might be classified as nursing homes, rather than hospitals. Insofar as general hospitals are included, these are typically small facilities with generous amenities, serving maternity and simple surgical cases. (The high proportions of proprietary beds in Australia,

Table 8.5. Proprietary Hospitals in Welfare-Oriented and Comprehensive Health Systems: Industrialized Countries, 1978–1981

| Country | Hospital Beds | |
	Per 1,000 Population	Percent Proprietary
Canada	9.80	1.73
Sweden	14.71	5.08
Switzerland	11.24	7.39
Ireland	9.71	8.08
Germany	11.49	12.47
Australia[a]	12.05	12.79
France	7.19	16.63
Spain	5.15	18.61
New Zealand[a]	10.20	23.55
Greece	6.25	41.02
Japan[a]	11.63	59.10

[a]General hospital beds only.
Source: Derived from World Health Organization, *World Health Statistics 1983.* Geneva: WHO, 1983.

New Zealand, and Japan, however, apply solely to general hospitals.)

The extent of proprietary hospital beds in entrepreneurial health systems of Africa and Asia is shown in Table 8.6. The extraordinarily high percentages in five such countries reflect health system policy and are not explained by long-term beds, as in Europe. They apply mainly to beds in small general hospitals, built by private physicians to serve affluent patients in the main cities. Such proprietary hospitals are found also in the countries of Latin America and the Middle East, even with welfare-oriented health systems shown in Table 8.7. The construction of these hospitals has actually been encouraged by government to enlarge the usually small supplies of general hospital beds. Private investment in hospitals clearly enlarges resources, although the beds are available only to upper-income families.

In both industrialized and developing countries, proprietary general hospitals serve predominantly higher-than-average income groups for relatively noncomplicated diagnoses. Maternity care and simple elective surgery (hernias, appendicitis, tonsillectomies, etc.) are the most frequent causes for admission. These hospitals do little in the way of research, personnel training, or outpatient or emergency service. Nursing care is usually better developed than in public or voluntary nonprofit hospitals, rooms are private and tastefully dec-

Table 8.7. Proprietary Hospitals in Welfare-Oriented Health Systems of Latin America and Middle East, 1979–1981

Country	Hospital Beds	
	Per 1,000 Population	Percent Proprietary
Latin America		
Costa Rica[a]	3.37	1.86
Haiti	0.7	4.14
Guyana	4.69	4.30
Guatemala	2.19	6.60
Chile	3.42	6.94
El Salvador	1.94	9.00
Peru	2.11	12.30
Honduras	1.28	17.63
Middle East		
Iraq	1.88	1.33
Algeria	2.92	1.51
Israel[a]	5.10	2.67
Turkey	2.11	4.09
Egypt	2.00	5.75
Iran	1.56	13.41
Saudi Arabia	1.55	17.18
Syria	1.11	20.21
Malaysia (Peninsular)[b]	2.70	8.36

[a]These countries have comprehensive, rather than welfare-oriented, health systems.
[b]Located in Southeast Asia.
Source: Derived from World Health Organization, *World Health Statistics 1983.* Geneva: WHO, 1983.

Table 8.6. Proprietary Hospitals in Entrepreneurial Health Systems of Developing Countries, 1979–1981

Country	Hospital Beds	
	Per 1,000 Population	Percent Proprietary
Ghana	1.32	1.64
Rwanda	1.56	1.85
Thailand	1.52	4.47
Sierre Leone	1.13	5.37
Zambia	3.17	8.91
Mauritius	3.14	9.71
Pakistan	0.57	16.46
Zaire	3.13	17.94
Indonesia	0.68	26.03
Jordan	0.81	28.26
Philippines[a]	1.93	54.58

[a]General hospital beds only.
Source: Derived from World Health Organization, *World Health Statistics 1983.* Geneva: WHO, 1983.

orated, and meals allow a choice of menus. Yet if an affluent person needs complex surgery or management of a serious chronic illness, she or he is more likely to seek care in a public hospital with the most qualified physicians on staff.

Nursing homes for the elderly and chronic sick, as distinguished from hospitals, are dominated by private ownership in the United States. A unique feature of U.S. Social Security legislation contributed importantly to this development. The initial act of 1935 provided that no old-age pensions were payable to any person in a public residential facility (with the objective of closing down many inferior public almshouses). As a result, a large proprietary nursing home industry arose and continued to thrive even after the 1950s, when this legislation was changed. As of 1980, of all nursing homes in the United States (accommodating more patients than all general hospitals), 81 percent of the structures with 68 percent of the total beds were in proprietary units. This was true even though 56 percent of their financial support came from governmental programs.

This large a proportion of proprietary nursing homes is not found in any other country, although in Western European countries such nursing homes have recently been growing. The great majority of beds for the elderly and chronic sick in industrialized countries, outside the United States, are in public facilities, sponsored mainly by units of local government. In the developing countries, where nursing homes are very rare, they are typically sponsored by voluntary nonprofit or religious groups. Many elderly patients with chronic illness, lacking a family to take care of them, are simply kept for long periods in public general hospitals. This is true also in Japan and South Korea, where elderly people are rapidly increasing. The entire issue of long-term care of all sorts is discussed more fully in Chapter 13.

Other Health Services and Appliances

Beyond these major services in private health care markets, there are other services and appliances in many national health systems. Dental care is needed in every population and yet, except for children, may be only meagerly supported or provided by public programs; it often occupies a large place, therefore, in the private sector. In developing countries there are *denturists,* dental technicians, and others who cater to private patients of low income. In all countries, dentists in exclusive private practice tend to be a greater share of the total than are physicians.

In most industrialized countries, there are nonmedical optometrists or opticians who analyze defects of vision and prepare corrective eyeglasses. In many, there are podiatrists who treat superficial disorders of the feet. Audiologists may test hearing and sell hearing aids. Such personnel are mainly in private practice. Physical therapists are employed mainly in organized rehabilitation services, but some may be in private practice, which applies also to clinical psychologists and some psychiatric social workers. Orthopedic braces, prosthetic limbs, trusses, surgical corsets, and other such appliances are made and sold predominantly by small private shops in the cities. Even when public programs pay for these services and appliances, their provision comes mainly from private resources.

In developing countries, the range of these specialized but nonmedical services is much smaller. Optical shops may be found in the main cities, but little more. As a result, the general medical practitioner or the surgical specialist sometimes fills the need. The fitting of a prosthetic appliance or a hearing aid in many developing countries is a luxury that only the wealthy patient may enjoy by traveling abroad.

PRIVATE HEALTH CARE WITH PUBLIC FINANCING

The previous section has focused on private health care with private financing, as conceptualized by cell number 1 of Figure 8.1. But much private care throughout the world is defined by cell number 3 in this table—that is, health care given by private providers although financed by public or statutory funds. Also a much smaller amount of health care is privately financed but provided by public resources, as defined by cell number 2 in Figure 8-1.

Medical care given by private physicians and financed by public programs abounds in the welfare-oriented health systems of Western Europe, Canada, Japan, Australia, and New Zealand. This is predominantly care by general medical practitioners, since most specialists are employed by public or voluntary hospitals on salary. In the health system of the United States, as well as Canada, where hospital staffs are generally open to all qualified private physicians, this mixed pattern applies to specialists also. The two largest publicly financed medical care programs in the United States, Medicare and Medicaid, pay fees to private providers for services to eligible persons.

Because of the potential abuses of private medical practice, with fee-for-service payments, all of the public financing programs use various procedures to identify overservicing. Statistical techniques are applied to identify deviance from averages or norms. Exceptionally numerous visits or procedures for a given diagnosis can be readily identified. Prior authorizations are required before performance of certain elective procedures. Doctors seeking reimbursement for unusually large numbers of prescriptions, injections, or certain diagnostic procedures may be professionally investigated. A great deal of bureaucratic paperwork is one of the prices paid for this retention of private practice with public medical care financing.

One strategy for overcoming the abuses of fee-for-service remuneration has been to change to a capitation method. The effects of this are shown in physician utilization data of several European countries. In Great Britain, and to a significant extent in the Netherlands and Denmark, general practitioners are periodically paid by flat capitation amounts for each person selecting a doctor. In Canada, France, Germany, and Japan, fee-for-service remuneration is still the only method of payment. The number of contacts with a physician in a year is strikingly greater in the latter countries. The rate of contacts for one year in the period 1981–1986 was as follows:

Capitation Payments		Fee-for-Service	
Great Britain	5.2	Canada	7.1
Denmark	5.2	France	7.8
Netherlands	5.4	Germany	10.8
		Japan	12.8

Public payment for drugs dispensed by private pharmacies or drugstores does not require as much surveillance. Where drug prices are regulated, some oversight may be necessary, and the dispensing of narcotics is subject to control in almost all countries. Prescribing practices, in general, call for surveillance of the physician.

Public payment for care in private hospitals entails greater complexities. In most countries, remuneration of public hospitals has become based increasingly on negotiated and approved global budgets (that is, budgets for all hospital operating expenses: personnel, supplies, etc.); after these are finalized, the hospital is paid a fixed amount very month or more often. (Germany, however, uses per diem payments for both its public and private hospitals.) With nonpublic hospitals—both nonprofit and proprietary—payment must usually be based on calculation of per diem costs. This entails cost accounting according to various commercial conventions. In Canada, where both public and private hospitals depend entirely on public financing, global budgeting is applied to both types of facility.

In developing countries, public hospitals—including those sponsored by Social Security programs—are typically supported by periodic payments based on annual global budgets. Nonpublic hospitals, both nonprofit and proprietary, must usually be paid on a per diem or even a per item basis. The enactment of social insurance for medical care in the Philippines and Indonesia was motivated, in large part, by the objective of increasing the occupancy of these private hospital beds. The same applies to the special hospital insurance for higher income employees in Kenya.

A major strategy for cost containment in many industrialized countries, furthermore, has been government regulation of the construction of nonpublic hospitals. Since, in the presence of social financing, available hospital beds tend to be used, planning authorities limit new construction or expansion of beds to those for which health need can be well demonstrated. This is done in France and Germany, and was done extensively in the United States in the 1970s.

COMMERCIAL HEALTH INSURANCE

Another aspect of the private market for health care is the sale of private insurance by commercial companies to pay for such care. This type of insurance is extensive in the United States, where it covers more people—55 percent of all persons insured for hospital care—than any other type of health insurance. The role of private commercial insurance for private health care in other industrialized countries is not as great, but it has been growing in Great Britain, Germany, France, New Zealand, and elsewhere to enable an affluent 5 or 10 percent of the population to opt out of the public program for largely private medical services. Even though the proportion of people covered by private insurance is small, it contributes strongly to the development of a two-tier health system—a public one for the great majority of the population and a private one for the economically elite.

In some developing countries, private commercial health insurance has also come to play a role. South Africa is a developing country of transitional economic level, with an entrepreneurial type of health system. (In 1983 only 16 percent of the national population had voluntary health insurance, but this was 75 percent of the white residents and under 6 percent of the other racial groups.) Voluntary insurance was sponsored by both nonprofit and for-profit commercial entities, and this provided the insured people much greater access to private health care resources. The same disparity existed in the welfare-oriented health system of Zimbabwe (formerly Southern Rhodesia), where only 3 percent of the population had the advantage of private insurance coverage. In Malaysia, about 100,000 people (less than 1 percent of the national population) have purchased private health insurance from eight commercial companies, to facilitate their access to private medical care. Private insurance companies are prominent also in Jamaica, Trinidad, Botswana, Malawi, and Thailand. Voluntary commercial health insurance was promoted in 1990 by the government of Indonesia.

Commercial insurance companies sell health care policies also in Latin America, especially in Brazil and Argentina. Such insurance is sold at group insurance rates to large enterprises, for providing access of employees to private resources, and at higher individual rates to affluent consumers. This is done also in Chile, Venezuela, Peru, and Guyana. Sometimes private physicians are organized in group practice clinics, as in U.S. private health maintenance organizations.

Private commercial insurance, both in industrialized and developing countries, usually means indemnification of the patient rather than reimbursement for the provider. Indemnification is ordinarily intended to be at 80 percent of a "reasonable fee," so that the patient still must make a copayment of 20 percent or more. Sometimes there are also "deductibles" of the first $100 or more in a year, before the insurance takes effect. Thus, commercial health insurance involves a contract between the company and the patient, without relation to the health care provider.

With respect to compensation for medical care costs from work-connected injuries, commercial insurance companies play a large role in every region of the world. National legislation in all types of health system usually requires such insurance coverage to be purchased by employers. With respect to first-aid and emergency care, legislation also requires large firms (with 100 or more workers) to maintain minimal medical or nursing services at the workplace.

EMPLOYER-SUPPORTED HEALTH CARE

A final type of health care wholly in the private sector—both for financing and provision of services—is that organized by employers to serve their employees. In addition to services for work-connected injuries, the managements of certain large private enterprises throughout the world have organized general medical care programs to serve their workers and often their dependents.

In the United States, where national health insurance protection has been lacking, certain large enterprises have organized comprehensive medical care programs, staffed by salaried personnel in special facilities, to serve employees and often their families. The earliest such programs (around 1913) were financed mainly by periodic deductions from wages, with a partial contribution from the employer. In a few large firms—such as the Endicott-Johnson Shoe Company or the Consolidated Edison (electrical utility) Corporation—management took full financial responsibility. The enactment in the U.S. of compensation laws for work-connected injuries after 1910 led many large companies to provide limited first-aid medical services at the worksite, if only to reduce compensation insurance costs. The most extensive organized services at the worksite for *general* medical care, however, were established in isolated industries, such as mines, lumbering, and railroads. Only a few employer-sponsored general health service programs were organized in the main cities.

Since 1940, as voluntary health insurance, organized through places of employment, has grown in the United States, these in-plant medical services have declined. Most workers and their families prefer to have access to all doctors in an area, rather than only those at the worksite. Where such community doctors are few, as at very isolated mines and railroad junctions, organized worksite clinics and medical personnel have survived the longest.

In other industrialized countries, where national health insurance or national health services have been enacted, the impetus to establish comprehensive health care programs at worksites has not been as great. A few large corporations have done so, nevertheless, either for reasons of paternalism or sound personnel policy. These are illustrated by the Philips Company in the Netherlands, Nuffield in Great Britain, or the large automobile firms in France (Renault) and Italy (Fiat). The major emphasis of these programs, however, is health promotion, first aid, occupational safety and hygiene, and rehabilitation services that are not as readily available in the community.

In the developing countries, where the quality of health service for the general population is seriously deficient, employer-supported medical care programs have been established extensively. The greatest development has been by oil extraction and mining companies, but several other types of industry have also organized programs. Good medical care not only helps attract and hold high quality skilled workers, but can also reduce absenteeism and heighten loyalty to the company.

In Latin America, on-site medical services have often preceded the enactment of Social Security for medical care, so that these statutory employer contributions are waived, as long as the company-sponsored service continues. Brazil has several mining companies, and also large automotive manufacturers, with strong management-operated programs. Oil exploration firms and coffee plantations also support such services in Colombia. Smaller countries, such as Guatemala, the Dominican Republic, Guyana, and Honduras, have large agricultural enterprises with employer-supported health programs. The U.S.-based United Fruit Company has been important in these countries. In Venezuela, Peru, and Trinidad, oil extraction is the main such industry. The Creole Corporation (linked to U.S. Standard Oil Company) in Venezuela had (1980)

70,000 employees plus dependents served by two company-owned hospitals and 15 ambulatory care clinics.

General health services in Africa are especially weak, so that numerous multinational corporations have organized health programs. In Angola, two large petroleum companies have done so, as have two such companies in Nigeria. In Botswana, several foreign mining companies operate small hospitals for their own employees, as do mining companies in Ghana. Sudan, Kenya, and Somalia also have management-sponsored health services provided by foreign petroleum companies. The U.S. Firestone Company in Liberia operates a large comprehensive medical care program with its own 2 hospitals, 7 clinics, and 46 first-aid stations. In Zaire, the Unilever Company does vegetable oil extraction, with employees served by 9 small hospitals and 4 clinics.

Middle East countries also have several multinational oil corporations, as well as other enterprises with worksite medical services. In Saudi Arabia, ARAMCO (Arab-American Corporation) has had 127,000 employees and dependents, served by 10 of its own clinics and a large 360-bed hospital, with a medical and allied health personnel staff of 1,600 persons. Comprehensive health services are also provided by large oil companies operating in Jordan, Libya, Egypt, Oman, Tunisia, Morocco, and the Yemen Arab Republic. In these countries, large textile manufacturing firms, chemical corporations, construction companies, and in Lebanon the American University at Beirut operate organized medical care programs for employees through their own resources.

In Asia, Indonesia is host to several large multinational corporations, that operate worksite medical care programs; these include oil extraction, metal mining, and construction enterprises. The Cal-tex Oil Corporation there covers 30,000 employees plus dependents and operates two hospitals. Malaysia and the Philippines also have oil companies with their own programs. Several large tea and rubber estates in Malaysia formerly provided limited hospital care for their workers, until these were replaced by stronger governmental services. In India, Hindustan Lever, Ltd. is unusual in providing health services in 35 villages where it acquires dairy products. Tata Industries in and around Bombay is a large complex of domestic textile, vegetable oil, hydroelectric and other production units, which have for many years provided comprehensive preventive and curative series for many thousands of employees. In Pakistan, the once private Railway Corporation became a parastatal agency, which operates 18 small hospitals and 52 clinics to serve 150,000 employees and dependents.

In all these developing countries, especially in the isolated regions, the company-supported medical services usually become a prominent feature of the health system in their local areas. Most of them, therefore, are willing to give some care to the surrounding population, when it is paid for privately. In a few countries, labor unions may take the initiative to provide health services to workers, either by themselves or in collaboration with employers. This has been done to develop a *Mokpo Labor Hospital* in South Korea, and to support four maternal and child health clinics in Zaire. In agricultural enterprises, where there is no formal employer, farming people may sometimes organize health cooperatives (a type of health insurance) to pay for medical care; this is discussed in Chapter 14.

COMMENTARY

These several types of private sector health care throughout the world call for general comments. In all but a few of the industrialized countries, health services that are privately financed and also privately provided constitute only a small percentage of the total. Yet such private care usually makes claims on a disproportionately large share of available national resources. The question of when such inequity should generate corrective political action in an industrialized country is not easy to answer. If 5 percent of a national population coopts 10 percent of health resources, the inequity may be small enough to tolerate, in the interest of harmonious political relationships. If, however, 5 or 10 percent of a population absorbs the attention of 30 percent of the health resources, it may be time for societal correction of the inequities.

In developing countries, where the overall supply of doctors and other health resources is usually inadequate, the inequities of private health services are usually more serious. When the national stock of physicians, dentists, and hospital beds is deficient, and a small elite class of people in the national capital claims the attention of one-fourth or one-third or even one-half of these resources, the remaining personnel and facilities for the mass of the population are seriously inadequate. These are the realities in most very poor developing countries and many at a transitional economic level.

Among the several types of private health care reviewed previously—by traditional healers, modern physicians, pharmacies, hospitals and others—that given by private physicians has overriding importance. For most people, the physician is the port of entry into the modern health system. He or she influences the use of hospitals, the purchase of drugs, and numerous diagnostic and therapeutic procedures. Most analysis of the private sector in health systems, therefore, has focused on the private physician.

The effects of private medical practice have been discussed and debated throughout the world for many decades. When medical service is wholly private—both in provision and financing—social constraints beyond market dynamics are few. But even when financing is public, regulatory influences to protect populations have limited impact. Nevertheless, certain advantages of private practice, with payments of a fee for each service, are real and must be recognized:

1. Private medical practice with fee payments encourages hard work and diligent attention to each patient.
2. In a competitive market, private practice induces the physician to give service of a high quality, both technically and personally, so as to attract and retain patients. Competition leads to innovation.
3. Private practice ensures the doctor freedom in exercising his or her professional judgment to help patients in every possible way.
4. Market forces theoretically encourage doctors to go to areas where other doctors are scarce and competition is minimal.
5. The sovereignty of private practice tends to

ensure high professional morale in day-to-day work.

6. Private practice allows the patient to make choices among doctors, selecting the one with whom he or she feels compatible. If dissatisfied, the patient may change to another doctor.

7. The patient is free to consult different private doctors before deciding on a course of therapy.

8. The offices or clinics of private doctors are open after normal working hours (evenings and weekends), for the convenience of many patients.

On the other hand, private medical practice causes problems for patients and for the operation of health systems, that are widely recognized:

1. Private medical practice, with fee payments for each service, may and often does lead to excessive services—beyond the health needs of the patient, to maximize the doctor's income.

2. Excessive services may and sometimes do include elective surgical procedures, cesarian operations for childbirth, and other services that may be harmful and even fatal.

3. Private fee payments may lead the doctor to "hold on" to patients who should properly be referred to another medical specialist.

4. Market forces lead the private doctor to set up practice in areas where the prospects of income are good, and to avoid localities where such prospects are poor. This usually results in severe shortages of doctors in rural areas and urban slums, where health needs are great.

5. The education of doctors in most countries is at public expense, but private practice yields private profits, earned from this social investment.

6. To impress patients, the private doctor may use the most complex and expensive technology, when simpler methods of diagnosis and treatment would be quite adequate.

7. Private practice stresses therapy of many types, but seldom includes prevention or health promotion.

8. The choices of private doctors mady by many patients may be based on faulty criteria that are not in the best interests of the patient.

This catalogue of advantages and defects of private medical practice is probably not complete. Various adjustments made in medical care programs, however, reflect the occurrence of both types of effect. As for advantages, in those organized settings where physicians are publicly employed on salaries, additional rewards are sometimes given to encourage diligent work. Free choice is also sometimes introduced even in public medical care programs, where several doctors are available.

The adjustments to correct or compensate for the problems in private practice are more numerous. When the financing is organized, bills submitted by private doctors are reviewed in various ways. In addition to prior authorizations for elective surgical operations, "second opinions" may be solicited. To compensate for the concentration of doctors in attractive cities, laws are enacted to require new medical graduates to serve for periods of time in rural areas or to prohibit settlement in "overdoctored" localities. To encourage preventive services, doctors are educated continually and special fees are offered.

The difficulties of private practice with fee-for-service remuneration are evident in all types of country, but in the developing countries they are more serious. A 1982 study on Cesarian sections in Brazil showed the effects dramatically. On indigent patients, served by salaried public doctors, the rate of C-sections was 25 percent; on insured patients, served by both salaried and private doctors, it was 40 percent; and on wholly private patients, served by private fee-for-service doctors, the rate of C-sections was 75 percent.

Geographic maldistribution can be horrendous. In Thailand, 75 percent of the doctors are in Bangkok serving 9 percent of the population; the remaining 91 percent of the people must get along with 25 percent of the doctors. In Peru, the capital city, Lima, has 16 percent of the national population but 65 percent of all doctors in private practice (Lima also has the great majority of doctors in public employment). Countries in every world region (e.g., Mexico, Nigeria, Iran, Thailand) have mandated periods of public service for new medical graduates to counteract this problem. Without such mandatory rural service, the situation would be still worse. These physician shortages in rural areas have been the major reason that so many developing countries have trained various types of auxiliary medical assistants and community health workers. Yet medical associations in some world regions, especially in Latin America, have opposed such training and delayed its development (claiming it would reduce the quality of care when, in fact, they fear competition).

Defenders of private practice in both developing and industrialized countries often claim that private doctors improve the operations of a national health system by "reducing the load" on the public services. This argument, however, overlooks the finite quantity of doctors in any health system. If 30 percent of the doctors, let us say, are withdrawn into the private sector to serve an affluent 5 percent of the population, then the remaining 70 percent of doctors face a *heavier* load to serve the remaining 95 percent of the population. The greater time spent per patient in private practice means inevitably less medical time per patient in public programs. The disparities between private and public services in most developing countries are typically much greater than these percentages suggest.

The inequities in medical services for public and for private patients in developing countries are seldom so neatly quantifiable. In most developing countries, private practice is not mainly exclusive and full-time, but predominantly carried on part of the time each day, after public duties are finished. In a 1-hour period the doctor typically earns much more money in private practice than in a salaried government post. As a result, doctors are naturally tempted to maximize the time spent in private practice, at the expense of their time in public practice; 4 hours of public duty is completed in 3, and 3 hours in 2. Such shortcuts in public medical service are observable in developing countries in all regions of the world. Yet, doctors' public medical posts legitimate them to the local population and even help them recruit private patients. Sometimes, as in Egypt or Kenya, doctors may even use public facilities to see private patients.

In Pakistan, physician unemployment in the cities has led the government to offer loans to encourage private doctors to set up practices in rural areas. Several Ministries of Health in developing countries actively encourage their doctors in rural posts to engage in private practice, to supplement their very low MoH salaries; in Egypt such private earnings are even nontaxable. In this way, private payments compensate for meager public salaries.

A few developing countries, on the other hand, have prohibited government physicians from engaging in private practice; a supplemental *nonpracticing allowance* is even added to the official salary. This has been the policy in India for many years, but it has not been rigorously enforced. Still, it has resulted in more than 50 percent of Indian doctors engaging in full-time private work, and also in a great deal of emigration, while many vacancies remain in rural government posts. Even where private practice is permitted and encouraged for government doctors, of course, as in Kenya or Ghana, there are still numerous vacancies in MoH rural posts.

It may not be obvious, but in all countries there is a reciprocal relationship between the private health care market and all organized health programs (predominantly public). If public programs are well developed and meet the needs of people, there will not be much demand for private medical care. If public programs are weak or unsatisfactory, patients who can afford the price will seek care privately. If a health problem is distressing enough, even poor people will seek private care.

In summary, private medical practice favors the more affluent families over the poor (contrary to health needs), the urban over the rural, and elaborate therapy over simple treatment and prevention. Yet these tendencies are not absolute, and poor people even in rural areas are sometimes helped by private practitioners. A household survey in Java, Indonesia in 1978 quantified these relationships remarkably well, and portrayed a situation that doubtless applies to most developing countries. The findings are presented in Table 8.8. Some of the use of modern physicians shown in this table may refer to doctors in government health facilities, but most refers to private practitioners.

Table 8.8. Illness Treatment by Provider and Household Income
Level Percentage Distribution, Indonesia (Java), 1978

| | Household Income | | |
Provider of Care	Lowest 40 percent	Middle 40 percent	Highest 20 percent
Urban Java			
Healer, auxiliary, self-care	87	50	28
Modern physician	13	50	72
Rural Java			
Healer, auxiliary, self-care	84	79	59
Modern physician	16	21	41

*Source:*Derived from Chernichovsky, Dov, and Oey Astra Meesook, *Poverty in Indonesia: A Profile.* Washington, D.C.: World Bank (Staff Working Papers No. 671), 1984.

Although consultation with private doctors is markedly greater in the higher income groups, it occurs to a small extent even among the very poor. Many private doctors charge poor patients lower fees.

Private medical practice and other private sector health care will doubtless continue throughout the world for many years to come. In the 1980s, political trends in many countries led to a *privatization movement,* on the alleged grounds, by no means proven, that the private sector was more efficient (or certainly more "attractive") than the public sector. Even the most effective and efficient health system under government, however, will not satisfy everyone, and private money will be used to make a stronger claim on available health resources. In the interest of humanity, we may hope that health resources everywhere will be great enough to make any resultant inequity very small.

REFERENCES

American Public Health Association, "Issue Paper on Nongovernmental Resources for Primary Health Care." Washington, D.C.: APHA, March 1986 (processed document).

Bannerman, R. H., John Burton, and Ch'en Wen-Chieh, (Editors), *Traditional Medicine and Health Care Coverage.* Geneva: World Health Organization, 1983.

Berliner H. S., and C. Regan, "Multinational Operations of U.S. For-Profit Hospital Chains." *American Journal of Public Health,* 77:1280–1284, 1987.

Dunlop, David W., "Health Care Financing: Recent Experience in Africa." *Social Science and Medicine,* 17(24):2017–2025, 1983.

Federation of Asian Pharmaceutical Associations, *Aspects of Asian and Pacific Pharmacy.* Tokyo: Federation of Asian Pharmaceutical Associations, 1966.

Gray, Bradford (Editor), *For-Profit Enterprise in Health Care.* Washington, D.C.: Institute of Medicine, 1986.

Health Insurance Association of America, *1986–1987 Source Book of Health Insurance Data.* Washington, D.C., 1987.

Heggenhougen, H. K., "Bomohs, Doctors and Sinsehs—Medical Pluralism in Malaysia." *Social Science and Medicine,* 14B:235–244, 1980.

Janowitz, B., et al., "Caesarian Section in Brazil." *Social Science and Medicine,* 16:19–25, 1982.

Lee, Kenneth and Anne Mills (Editors), *The Economics of Health in Developing Countries.* Oxford: Oxford University Press, 1983.

Management Sciences for Health, *Managing Drug Supply: The Selection, Procurement, Distribution and Use of Pharmaceuticals in Primary Health Care.* Boston, March 1982.

Mangay-Maglacas, A., and H. Pizurki (Editors), *The Traditional Birth Attendant in Seven Countries.* Geneva: World Health Organization (Public Health Papers 75), 1981.

Nortman, Dorothy L., Joanne Fisher, *Population and Family Planning Programs: A Compendium of Data through 1981.* New York: The Population Council, 1982.

Organization for Economic Cooperation and Development, *Health Care Systems in Transition.* Paris: OECD, 1990.

Roemer, Milton I., "On Paying the Doctor and the Implications of Different Methods." *Journal of Health and Human Behavior,* 3:4–14, Spring 1962.

Roemer, Milton I., "Private Medical Practice: Obstacle to Health for All." *World Health Forum,* 5:195–210, 1984.

Scarpaci, Joseph L. (Editor), *Health Services Privatization in Industrial Societies.* New Brunswick, NJ: Rutgers University Press, 1989.

Segall, Malcolm, "Planning and Politics of Resource Allocation for Primary Health Care: Promotion of Meaningful National Policy." *Social Science and Medicine,* 17(24): 1947–1960, 1983.

Silver, George A., *A Spy in the House of Medicine.* Germantown, MD: Aspen Systems, 1976.

Southby, Richard M., and Warren Greenberg, *The For-Profit Hospital.* Columbus, OH: Battelle Press, 1986.

Starr, Paul, "Escape from the Corporation 1900–1930." In *The Social Transformation of American Medicine.* New York: Basic Books, 1982, pp. 198–232.

Stern, Bernhard J., *Medicine in Industry.* New York: Commonwealth Fund, 1946.

Stinson, Wayne, *Community Financing of Primary Health Care.* Washington, D.C.: American Public Health Association, 1982.

Telecky, Ludwig, *History of Factory and Mine Hygiene.* New York: Columbia University Press, 1948.

U.S. Public Health Service, *Health United States 1989.* Washington, D.C.: Government Printing Office, 1990.

World Health Organization, *World Health Statistics 1983:* Geneva: WHO, 1983.

PART THREE

ECONOMIC SUPPORT AND MANAGEMENT

CHAPTER NINE

Economic Support of Health Systems

Of all the features of a country that influence its health system, none is more important than the economic level. Beyond its basic influence on people's health, the country's economic level determines the size of expenditures in the national health system. In 1987, according to the World Bank, health system expenditures in all industrialized countries amounted to $670 per person per year, in developing countries of middle income, it came to $31 per capita, and in very low income developing countries it was $9 per capita. These enormously different per person expenditures obviously paid for very different amounts and quality of health resources and health services.

Understanding the economic aspects of a national health system is important because money obviously sets limits on all health resources and services. Furthermore, monetary units provide a practical method of quantifying the mixture of diverse activities in a health system. They permit one to add together the value, for example, of medical consultations, clean drinking water, and drugs, for comparison with hospitalization or scientific research.

TOTAL HEALTH SYSTEM EXPENDITURES

More meaningful than the per capita health expenditures of a country, in U.S. dollars, is the percentage of national wealth in each country devoted to its national health system. In the 1980s, this varied from less than 2.0 percent in several countries of Africa to more than 11.0 percent in the United States. As a general rule, the industrialized and more affluent countries spend greater proportions of their wealth—typically more than 6.0 percent of gross domestic product (GDP)—on health

than the developing countries. The latter have lesser GDPs per capita, and they spend a lower percentage of them on health—typically much less than 6.0 percent.

The most complete and accurate information on national health expenditures is available for the industrialized countries belonging to the Organization for Economic Cooperation and Development (OECD). These are predominantly Western European countries and a few others with similar economic systems. (Eastern European and socialist industrialized countries are discussed later.) Data for 1960 and 1987 from 24 OECD countries are presented in Table 9.1.

Table 9.1. Total Health Expenditures as a Percent of Gross Domestic Product: Industrialized Countries, 1960 and 1987

Country	1960	1987
Greece	2.9	5.3
Spain	—	6.0
Denmark	3.6	6.0
Great Britain	3.9	6.1
Portugal	—	6.4
Japan	3.0	6.8
Italy	3.9	6.9
New Zealand	4.4	6.9
Australia	5.1	7.1
Belgium	3.4	7.2
Finland	4.2	7.4
Ireland	5.9	7.4
Luxembourg	—	7.5
Norway	3.3	7.5
Switzerland	3.3	7.7
Iceland	5.9	7.8
Germany, West	4.8	8.2
Austria	4.4	8.4
Netherlands	3.9	8.5
Canada	5.5	8.6
France	4.3	8.6
Sweden	4.7	9.0
United States	5.3	11.2

Source: Organization for Economic Cooperation and Development, *Health Care Systems in Transition.* Paris, 1990.

These health expenditure data are based on defining *health activities* as any activity whose *primary* purpose is advancement of health—through either treatment or prevention. For ordinary personal health services, this definition is easy to apply, but there are borderline functions. Thus, an old people's residential facility would not be included, but a nursing home for the aged and chronically ill would be. Likewise a school lunch program for all children would not be counted, but a feeding unit for malnourished babies would be. Professional education of doctors in most countries is considered a health expenditure, although in the United States it is counted under "education."

It is evident from Table 9.1 that in every industrialized country the share of GDP devoted to health has risen substantially between 1960 and 1987. In several countries—Japan, Belgium, Norway, Switzerland, Netherlands, and the United States—the share has more than doubled. Numerous factors contribute to this growth of health expenditures. To cite only the most important, they are (1) advances in the health sciences, many (though not all) of which are costly; (2) changing age composition of the population, with larger proportions of the elderly in whom serious illness is more common; (3) greater education of people leading to heightened demand for services; (4) urbanization of populations, so that health care can be more readily provided; (5) the vast extension of health insurance (both public and private) and other methods of mobilizing funds to facilitate support of health services; (6) expansion of the health professions that create demand, as well as responding to it; (7) the occurrence of new diseases, such as AIDS, to replace old diseases, such as smallpox, that have been eradicated; and (8) the very extension of the human life span, so that people live on with many disorders that require medical care.

Equivalent information on health expenditures in the developing countries is not so readily available. A World Bank report, appearing in 1985, assembled previously published data on developing countries that were considered relatively reliable. These figures on

Table 9.2. Total Health Expenditures as a Percent of Gross National Product: Developing Countries for Stated Years in the 1970s and 1980s

Country	Year	Percent of GNP
Burundi	1982	1.5
Lesotho	1979	1.6
Bolivia	1974	2.0
Philippines	1976	2.2
Syria	1975	2.3
Indonesia	1980	2.8
Tanzania	1977	3.0
Upper Volta	1981	3.2
India	1976	3.3
Sudan	1976	3.4
Rwanda	1982	3.5
Turkey	1987	3.5
Kenya	1975	3.7
Colombia	1978	4.0
Malawi	1980	4.0
Zimbabwe	1980	4.2
Ghana	1976	4.2
Thailand	1975	4.2
Peru	1981	4.5
Jamaica	1980	5.0
Sri Lanka	1982	5.1
Zambia	1981	5.6
Honduras	1976	6.0

Sources: de Ferranti, David, *Paying for Health Services in Developing Countries—An Overview.* Washington, D.C.: World Bank (Staff Working Papers No. 721), 1985. For Turkey the source is the OECD citation in Table 9.1.

health expenditures as a share of gross national product (GNP), which is very close to GDP, are shown in Table 9.2. It is clear that all but one of these 23 developing countries spent less than 6.0 percent of GNP for health; in Table 9.1 only 1 of the 23 industrialized countries spent under 6.0 percent of GDP on health.

Time trends for developing country health expenditures as percentages of GNP can be reported for only a few countries. Data on six countries from 1970 and 1976 permit the following estimates along a 6-year time span:

Country	1970	1976
Philippines	1.9	2.2
India	2.5	3.3
Sudan	3.7	3.4
Ghana	4.0	4.2
Sri Lanka	3.0	5.1 (1982)
Honduras	5.1	6.0

Among these six developing countries, the health expenditure trend was upward except in Sudan.

The generally lower percentage of lesser national wealth in the developing countries suggests that in those countries health care is a "luxury good." Of the total income available to a family, so much must be spent for food and shelter that little is left for medical care. Within government, so much is allocated for military purposes, transportation, education, and building the basic infrastructure for economic development that little is left for health purposes. Despite these handicaps, the trend of health expenditures in developing countries—at least in the 1970s—has been generally upward.

Overall health system expenditures in the socialist countries of various economic levels are especially difficult to determine. Marxist theory counts only physical products, not services, in the output of an economic system. Even if adjustments are made for this, the necessary data are not readily available. Nevertheless, in the Soviet Union all health expenditures in 1970 were estimated to be equivalent to 3.3 percent of GNP, rising to about 4.0 percent in 1986. According to the declared intent of *perestroika,* these expenditure rates were to be doubled by the year 2000. In Hungary, national health expenditures were reported to come to 3.52 percent of "national income" in 1965, rising to 3.87 percent in 1980. (Translating "national income" into GNP would reduce these percentages slightly.)

World Bank reports on China, a very poor socialist country, indicated health expenditures as 2.3 percent of GDP in 1957, 3.3 percent in 1981, and 4.0 percent in 1987. Only in Cuba, a socialist developing country of middle income level, were health expenditures relatively high. Because of heavy subsidies from the Soviet Union, Cuba has been able to promote education and health with exceptional economic support. Based on United Nations data, it may be estimated that in the 1980s, Cuba was spending some 4 or 5 percent of its GNP on health.

The generally low health expenditures of the socialist countries call for some comment.

Most of any country's health spending is for personnel, and we know that the salaries paid to physicians and other health workers in these countries are especially low. For many political reasons, skilled industrial workers receive the highest salaries, and those who give services, as opposed to those who produce commodities, are meagerly rewarded. There have also been special reasons to downgrade the medical profession, with its customary opposition to revolutions. Frugality has likewise been the rule in health facility equipment. Administrative costs, furthermore, are low in a regimented health system. Finally the widespread "gifts" to personnel in socialist health systems may add significantly to costs, but are difficult to estimate.

Viewing the entire world, the share of almost every country's wealth devoted to its health system has been significantly rising. The reasons for greater demand have been noted, and the general expansion of national economies (albeit at very different rates) have enabled countries to devote somewhat lesser shares to food and shelter and greater shares to health. The exact source of these health expenditures must now be examined.

SOURCES OF HEALTH EXPENDITURES

In every country the funds for supporting the health system are derived from several different sources. The very oldest source is the family or private individual, who makes payments to a healer or doctor for personal medical care. In primitive societies, such payments were mainly in the form of barter, such as food or tools, but the principle of paying a fee for each service was established. Sometimes, when treatment was given by a tribal chief or spiritual leader, the service was regarded as a gift.

In the city-states of classical Greece, physicians were paid by monetary fees. For treating slaves, whatever payment the doctor received came from the slave owner. For treating impoverished freemen, however, a city-doctor was sometimes employed on salary. The money for this was raised by local government taxation—a source quite different from the private individual. Taxation in the ancient world was based mainly on the ownership of land, but over the centuries local governments have derived revenues in other ways.

In Medieval Europe, the Christian church acquired wealth from the donations of the common people and the bequests of the rich. Religious charity therefore became another source of economic support for the health system, and subsequently charitable donations of many types have arisen. Donations from very rich individuals or from their estates became known as *philanthropy*. Local tax revenues also contributed to the maintenance of hospitals and the care of the poor.

As industrialization grew in central Europe, a working class took shape, dependent on factory wages for survival. Sickness could mean disaster, so that workers developed sickness insurance societies to help a worker disabled by illness. Sometimes employers contributed to the sickness fund. This was the birth of voluntary health insurance in the early nineteenth century.

Under Germany's powerful leader, Otto von Bismarck, a law was passed in 1883 requiring low-income workers in selected occupations to enroll in a sickness fund, and these funds became subject to various government regulations. The mandatory aspect made this "social insurance" for medical care.

In the early twentieth century, some large industrial enterprises in Europe and America took action to provide their workers with general medical care at the worksite; dependents might also be served. The enactment of worker's compensation laws for work-connected injuries stimulated the organization of some limited medical services in most large plants. In colonies and also developing countries, the owners of isolated enterprises organized general medical care programs for their workers and dependents.

As the importance of health services, for both prevention and treatment, became more widely appreciated in the nineteenth and twentieth centuries, central governments began to contribute to, and then increased their support of, national health systems. National governments could draw revenues from many types of taxation—such as personal incomes, exports, imports, general sales, corporate profits, inheritances, entertainment, and luxuries—beyond the power of local government. These national revenues were used to support health services directly and indirectly, through grants to provincial or local units of government.

Although newer sources of health money developed, the older sources did not die out. As in biological evolution, they all continued side by side, often in changing proportions. Thus in the modern world, in virtually every country, the national health system is supported by funds from a mixture of sources. The exact proportion derived from each source is often difficult to determine. In almost every country there is one, or sometimes two, sources that account for the majority of health expenditures; the other sources account for a minor fraction. The identities of these sources exert a large influence on the general characteristics of the national health system.

In the United States, the proportions of the various sources of health expenditures are known in some detail for 1988, as shown in Table 9.3. It may be noted that more than half of the federal funds (16.6 of 29.2 or 57 percent) is derived from social insurance. The largest single source of U.S. health system funding is from voluntary insurance, and the second largest source is from private individuals and families. Private sector funding accounts for well over half of the total—a situation not found in any other industrialized country in the world.

Table 9.3. Health Expenditures by Source of Money: Amount in Billions of U.S. Dollars and Percentage Distribution, United States, 1988

Source	$ Billion	Percent
General taxation		
Federal government	68.1	12.6
State and local governments	59.1	10.9
Social insurance		
Federal government	89.7	16.6
State governments	10.5	1.9
All public sources	(227.4)	(42.1)
Voluntary insurance	174.9	32.4
Philanthropy and industry	24.3	4.5
Individuals and families	113.2	21.0
All private sources	(312.4)	(57.9)
All sources	539.9	100.0

Source: U.S. Department of Health and Human Services, *Health Care Financing Review,* 11(4):1–41, Summer 1990.

Table 9.4. Overall Health Expenditures by Source of Funds: Percentage Distribution in Welfare-Oriented Health Systems of Six Industrialized Countries, 1974–1975

Source of Funds	Country					
	Australia	Switzerland	Netherlands	France	Canada	West Germany
General taxation	62.7	41.7	15.1	7.0	66.3	14.6
Social insurance	1.7	24.8	56.0	69.0	9.1	62.5
All public	(64.4)	(66.5)	(71.1)	(76.0)	(75.4)	(77.1)
Private insurance	13.8	} 33.5	} 27.3	3.0	2.5	5.3
Individuals and families	21.1			19.6	19.5	17.8
Charity and industry	0.7	—	1.6	1.4	2.6	5.1
All private	(35.6)	(33.5)	(28.9)	(24.0)	(24.6)	(22.9)
Total (all sources)	100.0	100.0	100.0	100.0	100.0	100.0

Source: Maxwell, Robert J., *Health and Wealth—An International Study of Health-Care Spending.* Lexington, MA: Lexington Books, 1981.

In 1989 total U.S. health spending came to $604 billion or $2,400 per capita.

For other industrialized countries, somewhat equivalent breakdowns of overall health expenditures are shown in Tables 9.4 and 9.5. Table 9.4 gives the health expenditures in six countries with welfare-oriented health systems; in these, funds came from government sources in 1974–1975 at rates between 64 and 77 percent. In three of the six welfare-oriented health systems, the public funds came mainly from general taxation, and in the other three mainly from social insurance. Private sources in these countries were contributing 22.9 to 35.6 percent of the funding in 1974–1975.

In Table 9.5, the health expenditures in three countries with comprehensive health systems are shown, and their share from public sources is seen to exceed 90 percent. (It is note-

worthy that Italy gave this overwhelmingly public support to its health system even before 1978, when it legislated a *national health service*.) Thus in 1974–1975 private funds accounted for less than 10 percent of health expenditures in these countries. If we regard private sector expenditures as measuring potential inequities, we may conclude that in the three industrialized countries with comprehensive health systems, these would be of very small proportions.

Regarding industrialized countries with socialist health systems (at least before 1989), very little information is available on the sources of funding. Data on the Soviet Union, published in 1976, apply to 1968, and show the following distribution:

Source of Funds	Percent
Government revenues	77.1
Government enterprises (agricultural and industrial)	13.7
Social insurance (rest homes only)	5.5
Personal households	3.7
All sources	100.0

The economic effects of the major movements of Eastern European countries toward market economies after 1989 have not yet been quantified.

Among the many developing countries, the several sources of health system funding can be identified in a small number. In almost all developing countries, the Ministry of Health, op-

Table 9.5. Overall Health Expenditures by Source of Funds: Percentage Distribution in Comprehensive Health Systems of Three Industrialized Countries, 1974–1975

Source of Funds	Country		
	Great Britain	Sweden	Italy
General taxation	87.3	78.5	23.8
Social insurance	5.0	13.1	67.5
All public	(92.3)	(91.6)	(91.3)
Private insurance	1.2	—	} 8.7
Individuals and families	5.8	8.4	
Charity and industry	0.4	—	—
All private	(7.4)	(8.4)	(8.7)
Total (all sources)	100.0	100.0	100.0

Source: Maxwell, Robert J., *Health and Wealth—An International Study of Health-Care Spending.* Lexington, MA: Lexington Books, 1981.

Table 9.6. Overall Health Expenditures by Source of Funding: Percentage Distribution in Four Developing Countries with Entrepreneurial Health Systems, 1975–1984

	Country			
Source of Funds	Thailand (1983)	South Korea (1975)	Pakistan[a] (1982)	Kenya[a] (1984)
Ministry of Health	19.6	6.2	1.8	42.1
Other local government agencies	7.5	7.2	15.8	6.8
Social insurance	—	—	1.4	—
Foreign aid	1.5	—	—	—
Public sector	(28.7)	(13.4)	(19.0)	(48.9)
Charity and industry	1.0	2.6	9.9	7.5
Individuals and families	70.3	84.0	71.1	43.6
Private sector	(71.3)	(86.6)	(81.0)	(51.1)
All sources	100.0	100.0	100.0	100.0

[a]Recurrent expenditures only (representing over 90 percent).
Sources: Derived from tables in Volume I, pp. 289, 304, 482, and 498.

erating at different jurisdictional levels, is especially important, so that this is usually identified as a source of funds (even though it is also a major provider of services). For four developing countries with entrepreneurial types of health systems, the sources of funding are indicated in Table 9.6. The first two countries, Thailand and South Korea, are of a middle (transitional) economic level, and the last two, Pakistan and Kenya, are of a very poor economic level.

Limited data are also available from South Africa, a middle-income developing country with an entrepreneurial health system, where the sources of health expenditures in 1982 were as follows:

Source	Percent
Government (all levels)	49.0
Voluntary insurance schemes	24.0
Enterprise programs	1.3
Individuals and families	25.7

Very limited data are also available from a very poor country with an entepreneurial health system, Indonesia; in that country for 1986–1987, the sources of health expenditures were distributed as follows:

Source	Percent
Government	30.7
Quasigovernmental agencies	5.7
Private sources	63.7

Including South Africa and Indonesia, these six developing countries with entrepreneurial health systems all derived more than 50 percent (five of them over 60 percent) of their health expenditures from the private sector. Even in South Korea, which enacted a large social insurance program in the 1980s (after the data shown were collected), personal copayments required were so high that in 1985 the private sector was still the source of 64 percent of health expenditures.

In Table 9.7, the sources of health expenditures are shown for the welfare-oriented health systems of six developing countries, three of middle (transitional) economic level and three of very poor economic level. For a seventh developing country with a welfare-oriented health system, Malaysia, the general public sector accounted for 74.3 percent of the funding and the private sector for 25.7. Thus for seven developing countries with welfare-oriented health systems, the private sector accounted for less than 60 percent of funding, in contrast to the countries with entrepreneurial health systems in which four of five derived more than 60 percent from the private sector. (In fact, as noted in Volume I, Liberia's system might no longer belong in the welfare-oriented category.)

The missing values for *foreign aid* call for comment. In the several countries where these data are lacking, foreign aid has probably been included within the funds of the Ministry of Health or other government agencies to which this aid was given. The small percentages re-

Table 9.7. Overall Health Expenditures by Source of Funding: Percentage Distribution in Six Developing Countries with Welfare-Oriented Health Systems, 1976–1984.

	Country					
Source of Funds	Peru (1984)	Guatemala (1976)	Turkey (1983)	Burma (1984)	Zimbabwe (1981)	Liberia (1984)
Ministry of Health	27.3	23.1	17.2	29.3	51.2	36.4
Social insurance	32.9	20.9	12.6	—	—	—
Other government agencies	6.3	3.5	12.2	4.4	8.5	5.4
Foreign aid	—	—	—	11.6	0.4	—
Public sector	(66.5)	(47.5)	(42.0)	(45.3)	(60.1)	(41.8)
Charity and industry	8.2	3.6	—	1.9	4.3	28.7
Individuals and families	25.2	48.8	58.0	52.7	35.6	29.5
Private sector	(33.4)	(52.4)	(58.0)	(54.6)	(39.9)	(58.2)
All sources	100.0	100.0	100.0	100.0	100.0	100.0

Sources: Derived from tables in Volume I, pp. 342, 361, 392, 517, 544, and 550.

ported for Thailand and Zimbabwe are probably accurate; the relatively high percentage for Burma in 1984 is probably referable to major bilateral assistance that year, after many years of Burma's isolation. The missing values for social insurance in Burma and in Kenya (Table 9.6) are caused by the inclusion of these small amounts in the Ministry of Health figures; in South Korea social insurance was started after 1975. In Peru, Guatemala, and Turkey, social insurance obviously plays a large economic role.

The sources of health expenditures may be reported in three other countries—two (Nicaragua and Israel) considered to have comprehensive health systems and one (China) with a much modified socialist system. Israel, although located in the developing region of the Middle East, is actually no longer a developing country by customary definition. China, with its broadly socialist ideology, does not claim to have a socialist health system. Despite these qualifications, the data in Table 9.8 may be of interest. The most unusual figure in this table is the high proportion of Israeli health funds derived from voluntary insurance, charity, and industry. Outside of the United States (and possibly South Africa), Israel is the only country of any economic level with such large funding from these private sources.

Data on charity and industry as sources of health funding are particularly unreliable in the developing countries. In Latin America, lotteries are a favorite method of raising funds for charitable *beneficencia* hospitals, but only

Table 9.8. Overall Health Expenditures by Source of Funding: Percentage Distribution in Three Developing Countries with Comprehensive or Socialist Health Systems, 1980–1986.

	Country		
Source of Funds	Nicaragua (1986)	Israel (1980)	China (1981)
Ministry of Health	40.4	60.0	30.0
Other government agencies	9.1	3.0	
Social insurance	—	—	31.0
Public sector	(49.5)	(63.0)	(61.0)
Voluntary insurance	—	21.0	7.0
Charity and industry	4.2		—
Individuals and families	46.2	16.0	32.0
Private sector	(50.4)	(37.0)	(39.0)
All sources	100.0	100.0	100.0

Sources: Derived from tables in Volume I, pp. 426, 441, and 598.

a small fraction of the money goes to the hospital. Such lotteries started in Ireland in 1746. The equivalent of "charity" is often given in the form of donated labor for constructing health facilities or sanitary pipelines in the villages. Management support for direct health services may be included in contributions to social insurance. In Nicaragua, social insurance premiums are paid, but are integrated into government general revenues.

Data on time trends of the several sources of health system expenditures in industrialized countries are available only for the broad categories of public and private sectors. Such data are given in Table 9.9 for the 27-year period from 1960 to 1987. Countries are listed in the rank order of the proportions of their national

Table 9.9. Public Sources as Percentage of National Health Expenditures in 23 Industrialized Countries, 1960–1987

Country	Year			
	1960	1975	1980	1987
United States	24.5	42.9	42.4	41.1
Netherlands	33.3	76.6	79.3	77.6
Iceland	40.7	89.8	89.1	88.5
Canada	43.6	76.7	75.7	75.6
Australia	47.1	63.2	61.5	71.8
Finland	54.8	79.4	78.5	78.4
France	58.1	76.5	81.6	77.9
Greece	58.6	61.0	81.4	75.5
Portugal	—	59.4	71.2	60.9
Japan	60.0	72.7	70.3	73.5
Belgium	61.8	79.3	81.8	76.4
Austria	65.9	69.9	69.6	67.9
Germany, West	66.7	79.5	78.5	76.8
Switzerland	—	68.6	68.5	67.6
Spain	—	70.6	74.6	71.7
Sweden	72.3	90.0	91.6	91.1
Ireland	75.0	83.1	91.8	86.5
New Zealand	75.0	84.4	83.3	82.6
Norway	78.8	95.5	98.5	98.7
Italy	82.1	86.2	82.4	78.3
Great Britain	87.2	90.9	89.7	86.9
Denmark	88.9	92.3	85.3	86.7
Luxembourg	—	91.2	92.6	92.0

Source: Derived from Organization for Economic Cooperation and Development, *Health Care Systems in Transition.* Paris, 1990.

health expenditures derived from public sources in 1960. Several observations may be made from these OECD data.

Between 1960 and 1975, in all 19 countries for which data are available, the proportion of health spending derived from public sources increased substantially; private sources, therefore, declined relatively. Between 1975 and 1980, in 10 of the 23 countries the rise in public sources continued, but in 13 of these countries the trend reversed, and public sources declined as a share of the total. Between 1980 and 1987, the upward trend in public spending was resumed in only 4 countries, but in the other 19 it continued downward. Only in Norway, among the 23 countries, was the upward trend in public spending uninterrupted during the 27-year period.

These data indicate that in almost all industrialized countries of the world, an upward trend in public support of national health systems was evident from 1960 to 1975; this trend undoubtedly began many years before 1960.

In 1980, national health policies changed, and in nearly half the industrialized countries public funding was relatively reduced, so that private funding increased. By 1987, public funding had been reduced relatively in all but one of 23 industrialized countries, with private funding increased as a share of the total. Private funding, of course, is linked to private earnings and the profit motive, with its many potentially harmful impacts on the quality of health service.

The degree of decline in the share of public spending after 1980, however, was relatively small. In 20 of the 23 industrialized countries, the share of public spending in 1987 remained substantially higher than it had been in 1960; in only three (Denmark, Great Britain, and Italy) was public spending relatively lower in 1987 than in 1960, and this was by very small percentages. An explanation of these changes does not seem elusive. In 1980, an economic recession, starting in the United States, spread throughout world capitalism. Previous economic downturns had led to an increase in public social spending, but this one led to a decrease. Government authorities in power in the United States, Great Britain, and elsewhere followed a policy of reduced public spending for social purposes (including health) and higher public spending only in military affairs. Such policies, as shown in Table 9.9, seemed to spread to all industrialized capitalist countries. As a result, health spending in the private market rose, which coincided with the prevailing political ideology in many large countries.

Trend data, such as shown in Table 9.9, are not available for most developing countries, but UNICEF has published information on the percentages of central government budgets devoted to health activities over the period from 1972 to 1986 in 19 developing countries. These data are shown in Table 9.10. It is clear that over this 14-year period the central government budget allocation for health declined in 15 of the 19 developing countries and rose in only four. The average change for all these countries was a decline from a health allocation of 5.5 percent of the central government budget in 1972 to 4.2 percent in 1986. As UNICEF points out, over this same span of years the military spending in these countries

Table 9.10. Government Health Expenditures as a Percentage of Central Government Budgets: Selected Developing Countries, 1972 and 1986

Country	Percentage 1972	Percentage 1986
Pakistan	1.1	1.0
Korea, South	1.2	1.5
Uruguay	1.6	4.8
Zaire	2.3	1.8
Turkey	3.2	2.2
Morocco	4.8	2.8
Bangladesh	5.0	5.3
Mexico	5.1	1.4
Uganda	5.3	2.4
Malawi	5.5	6.9
Oman	5.9	5.0
Botswana	6.1	5.0
Bolivia	6.3	1.4
Sri Lanka	6.4	4.0
Tanzania	7.2	4.9
Kenya	7.9	6.4
Chile	8.2	6.0
Burkina Faso	8.2	6.2
El Salvador	10.9	7.5

Source: United Nations Children's Fund, *The State of the World's Children 1989.* New York: UNICEF, 1989, p. 17.

increased from an average of 12.7 percent of the central budget to 15.2 percent. Thus central government expenditures for military affairs in 1986 were not only more than three times the amounts spent for health, but they were on the increase.

Multiple sources of expenditures for health systems are sometimes claimed to have the advantage of flexibility; if one source is reduced, another source can be increased. Where a single source accounts for nearly all health expenditures—as in the socialist countries, and, for that matter, in Great Britain—the overall percentage for health in the GNP is usually quite low. But there is nothing inevitable about this relationship. In Sweden, with nearly 80 percent of expenditures derived from general taxation, health expenditures can be high (some 9 percent of GNP in the 1980s). The crucial determinant is doubtless political will.

PURPOSES OF HEALTH EXPENDITURES

The purposes for which health expenditures are made are as numerous as the many aspects of national health systems. The sources of United States health expenditures in 1988 were given in Table 9.3, and the purposes for which this $539.9 billion were spent are analyzed in Table 9.11. The lion's share of U.S. health spending clearly goes to hospital and nursing home care, which accounts for 47.2 percent of the total. If the cost of physician services for inpatient care were added (as is conventional in most countries outside of North America), expenditures for inpatient care would surely exceed 50 percent, and hospital construction costs would make this still higher.

The U.S. spending of 7.8 percent for drugs and medical supplies refers to such commodities purchased outside of hospitals and nursing homes; inpatient drugs are counted in the expenditures for inpatient care. The 4.9 percent of spending for program administration applies to all health programs, but the major share of these costs is for voluntary health insurance administration. The 2.9 percent of spending used for public health work applies to such health activities that are largely preventive, provided by federal, state, and local governments.

The breakdown of purposes for national health expenditures in other industrialized countries is available along slightly different lines, and applies to the year 1975. This infor-

Table 9.11. Health Expenditures by Purpose: Amount in Billions of U.S. Dollars and Percentage Distribution: United States, 1988

Purpose	Billions ($)	Percent
Hospital care	211.8	39.2
Nursing home care	43.1	8.0
Physician services	105.1	19.5
Dental services	29.4	5.4
Other professional services	22.5	4.2
Home health care	4.4	0.8
Drugs and medical supplies	41.9	7.8
Eyeglasses and med. equipment	10.8	2.0
Other personal health care	9.3	1.7
Program administration	26.3	4.9
Public health activities	15.9	2.9
Health Science research	9.9	1.8
Facility construction	9.5	1.8
All purposes	539.9	100.0

Source: U.S. Department of Health and Human Services, *Health Care Financing Review,* 11(4):30, Summer 1990.

Table 9.12. Health Expenditures by Purpose: Percentage Distribution in Selected Industrialized Countries, 1975

Purpose	Australia	Canada	France	West Germany	Switzerland	Netherlands	Sweden	Italy	Great Britain
Hospital care	51.0	53.8	38.0	31.5	37.9	45.2	64.1	48.0	46.6
Physician and dental services	30.0	27.6	44.5	30.2	41.0	41.9	24.6	34.9	40.0
Self-medication	4.9	4.5	3.8	4.5	5.0	—	3.5	5.6	—
Program administration	2.1	1.7	9.3	6.0	—	4.4	0.4	6.4	4.7
Public health activities	3.1	3.2	1.1	3.2	3.8	1.1	—	2.2	2.4
Health science research	0.5	1.1	1.1	0.3	—	—	0.4	—	2.5
Facility construction	7.0	5.2	—	3.5	7.0	7.4	7.0	—	3.8
Education	1.4	—	.2	1.7	5.3	—	—	—	—
Other	—	2.9	1.0	19.1	—	—	—	2.9	—
All purposes	100.0	100.0	100.0	100.0	100.0	100.0	100.0	100.0	100.0

Source: Maxwell, Robert J., *Health and Wealth—An International Study of Health-Care Spending.* Lexington, MA: Lexington Books, 1981, pp. 83–85.

mation is given in Table 9.12. It is clear that in all but two of these nine countries, hospital care (not disaggregated from nursing homes care) accounts for most health spending. In France, Germany, and Switzerland, where hospital costs seem low, the reason is doubtless a statistical artifact; those countries (and, to some extent, others) exclude inpatient physician services from the costs of nonpublic hospital care, whereas most countries include them. The last three countries listed in Table 9.12 have comprehensive health systems, whereas the other six have welfare-oriented systems, but this does not seem to influence the distribution of spending for various health purposes.

Because record-keeping methods differ among these nine industrialized countries and also from the United States, comparisons of expenditures for any specific purpose must be made with great caution. Public health activities, nevertheless, are clearly of small proportions everywhere, in relation to the large outlays for personal medical care. Where certain countries report nothing in a specific category, it usually means that this item is included within some other health purpose. Regarding education, however, missing data may mean that the item is regarded as being outside the health system. The exceptionally large figure under West Germany for "other" is explained by the German practice of separate tabulation

of spending for spa treatment, false teeth, and rehabilitation services.

Limited data on health purposes are available for Japan in 1986–1987. These show the following percentage distribution:

Hospitalization	32.7%
Ambulatory care	31.2
Drugs and supplies	16.4
Other purposes	19.7
All purposes	100.0

Because of the Japanese policy of excluding from "hospitalization" any inpatient care in facilities with fewer than 20 beds, the figure for "ambulatory care" doubtless includes service that would otherwise be considered "hospitalization."

Expenditures for "self-medication" shown in Table 9.12 are limited to drugs that have not been medically prescribed. The latter are included within hospital care and, to some extent, physician and dental services. If these expenditures are disaggregated, we can see the national health expenditures for drugs, in several industrialized countries, as shown in Table 9.13. As a percentage of overall national health expenditures, the spending for drugs in the three countries with highest drug spending is more than double that in the three countries with lowest drug spending.

The distribution of purposes for health ex-

Table 9.13. National Expenditures for Drugs in Selected Industrialized Countries: Percentage with and without Prescription, 1974–1975

Country	Percentage		
	With Prescription	Without Prescription	All Drugs
United States	—	—	8.3
Switzerland	—	—	8.5
Sweden	5.5	3.5	9.0
Canada	5.9	4.5	10.4
Great Britain	9.3	3.4	12.7
Australia	8.4	4.9	13.3
West Germany	13.4	4.5	17.9
Italy	14.4	5.6	20.0
France	17.3	3.7	21.0

Source: Maxwell, Robert J., *Health and Wealth—An International Study of Health Care Spending.* Lexington, Mass.: Lexington Books, 1981, p. 71.

penditures in the industrialized socialist countries is not as well understood. Data reported by the Soviet Union for 1985 indicated simply the following percentages:

Personal health care (hospitals, polyclinics, etc.)	86.4%
Sanitary–epidemiological activities (public health)	3.8
Physical culture	0.7
Other recurrent expenditures	3.4
Construction	5.8

Whether drugs, research, and education are included within these percentages is not clear.

In the developing countries, data on the purposes of health expenditures are also scarce.

Considering overall spending, Israel has reported the percentage distribution for 1978–1979 as follows:

Hospitalization	44
Organized ambulatory care	33
Dental clinics	15
Private physicians	3
Drugs privately purchased	4
Government administration	1

In a very different developing country, China, the purposes of overall health expenditures were distributed in 1981 as follows:

Hospitalization (except salaries)	13.0
Salaried health personnel	20.3
"Barefoot doctors" and auxiliaries	3.9
Medical equipment	4.9
Western pharmaceuticals	48.7
Traditional herbal medication	9.2

The very high expenditures for Western pharmaceuticals in China reflect the prices paid for imported products and even the cost of manufacture of Western drugs in the country. These data from only two developing countries show the great dependence of such analyses of expenditures on the scheme of classification of health "purposes."

In numerous other developing countries, the breakdown of health purposes can be reported only for government expenditures and private expenditures, analyzed separately. In Table 9.14, the purposes of Ministry of Health ex-

Table 9.14. Purposes of Ministry of Health Expenditures: Percentage Distribution in Six Developing Countries

Purpose	Country				
	Philippines (1982)	Thailand (1974)	Kenya (1981)	Brazil (1982)	India[a] (1980)
Hospitalization	53.4	67.0	72.9	84.2	41.8
Ambulatory care	28.9		11.8		7.3
Disease control	4.6	15.7	6.7	10.1	44.3
Environmental sanitation	—	6.2	—	—	0.4
Administration	3.4	7.3	6.4	3.1	6.1
Other	9.7	3.8	1.9	2.6	
All purposes	100.0	100.0	100.0	100.0	100.0

[a]Health expenditures in India apply to total government.
Sources: Derived from tables in Volume I, pp. 302, 287, 480, 330, and 536.

Table 9.15. Private Health Expenditures by Purpose in Developing Countries with Entrepreneurial Health Systems: Percentage Distribution, 1975–1981

Purpose	Country			
	Philippines (1975)	Thailand (1981)	South Korea (1975)	Kenya (1981)
Hospital and similar fees	30	40.8	8.4	27.6
Physicians and healers	25	55.3	33.5	43.1
Healers only	—	—	—	17.7
Drugs and supplies	45	5.1	57.3	9.9
Other	—	—	0.7	1.7
All purposes	100.0	100.0	100.0	100.0

Source: Derived from tables in Volume I, pp. 303, 288, 304, 481.

penditures are analyzed in three developing countries with entrepreneurial health systems and two with welfare-oriented systems. It is evident that except for India, the largest health expenditures in these developing countries are for personal medical care and, where reported, for hospitalization. The data for India apply to total government expenditures, rather than the Ministry of Health, with the largest percentage then going for environmental sanitation.

Analyses of purely private health expenditures are available for 11 developing countries. The distribution of private expenditures in four of these, with entrepreneurial health systems, is given in Table 9.15. The same distribution in six developing countries, with welfare-oriented health systems, is given in Table 9.16.

In all 10 of these developing countries private payments to physicians and healers were substantial, ranging from 25 to 60 percent of private health expenditures. In 7 of the 10 countries, private expenditures for drugs were also substantial—exceeding those for physi-

cians and healers in six of them. Expenditures on traditional healers were not separately identified in many countries, but in the two from Africa (Liberia and Kenya), this private spending was important. Private fees for the use of hospitals and other facilities, it may be noted, play a large role in three of the four entrepreneurial health systems, but in none of the welfare-oriented systems.

Information on private health expenditures is available on two developing countries, Costa Rica and Nicaragua, considered to have comprehensive health systems. This spending, analyzed by purpose, is shown in Table 9.17. In 1986, Costa Rica was at peace, and only 21 percent of its health expenditures came from private households. Nicaragua was at war with *contras,* and 46 percent of its health expenditures came from private households; drug importation was greatly impeded by an embargo. This may explain the differences in the relative importance of drug purchases in the two countries, although in both the largest share of private spending went for physician services. The very small percentage of private spending for

Table 9.16. Private Health Expenditures by Purpose in Developing Countries with Welfare-Oriented Health Systems: Percentage Distribution, 1975–1985

Purpose	Country					
	Brazil (1975)	Peru (1984)	Guatemala (1976)	Malaysia (1983)	Burma (1985)	Liberia (1984)
Hospital and similar fees	19.5	14.8	7.3	17.3	—	2.4
Physicians and healers	28.3	28.0	32.5	60.9	47	5.7
Healers only	—	—	—	9.1	11	38.1
Drugs and supplies	40.4	48.5	54.1	3.4	35	53.8
Other	11.8	8.7	6.1	9.3	7	—
All purposes	100.0	100.0	100.0	100.0	100.0	100.0

Source: Derived from tables in Volume I, pp. 330, 343, 361, 407, 517, and 550.

Table 9.17. Private Household Health Expenditures in Two Developing Countries with Comprehensive Health Systems, 1986

Purpose	Costa Rica (%)	Nicaragua (%)
Physicians and dentists	48.1	58.6
Hospital care	3.3	4.3
Drugs	47.3	15.8
Other	1.3	21.2
All purposes	100.0	100.0

Sources: For Costa Rica, Abel-Smith, Brian, and Andrew Creese (Editors), *Recurrent Costs in the Health Sector—Problems and Policy Options in Three Countries.* Geneva: World Health Organization, 1989. For Nicaragua, Volume I, p. 441.

hospital care in these health systems is also noteworthy.

PURPOSES LINKED TO SOURCES

In countries of all economic levels and with all types of health system, various purposes for health expenditures are generally linked to certain funding sources. Thus in modern times the construction of hospital facilities is usually dependent on funds from government taxation, even when a hospital has nongovernmental sponsorship. Organized preventive services, both environmental and personal, are also usually financed by government revenues. Such services in industrialized countries are often defined as *public health programs,* although in most developing countries that phrase also encompasses public medical care.

The general services of hospitals in nearly all countries are supported mainly by government funds derived from taxation or social insurance. In countries using both these methods of public financing extensively (e.g., Norway and Sweden), hospital services are supported mostly by taxation and the remaining personal medical costs rest mainly on social insurance. The United States is the only country in which less than half of hospital costs are met by public funds; even here, however, the private funds supporting hospital care are derived principally from collectivized private sources—that is, voluntary health insurance. Such private insurance also usually supports the substantial copayments for hospitalization required in France.

Health science research is supported almost everywhere predominantly by public funds. This may be in government facilities or by public grants to universities and other institutions that may not be governmental. The principal medical research supported by private sources is conducted or financed by pharmaceutical companies. Likewise the education of health personnel is supported in almost all countries mainly by public funds. This is true in the United States, where 42 percent of the medical schools are privately sponsored. In some developing countries, such as the Philippines and Brazil, private medical schools have greatly multiplied; the financial support of these schools, however, is meager, and the education of most health professionals still depends mainly on public funds.

Pharmaceutical products are less likely to be supported by collectivized methods of financing, public or private, than other elements in a health system. Even when drugs are included in a social insurance program, there are often copayment requirements; in many such programs there are no drug benefits. Also, some one-quarter or one-third of drug expenditures in many countries are for nonprescribed drugs, purchased entirely at private expense. Drug expenditures vary with the prescribing habits of doctors and the position of the pharmaceutical industry. These expenditures, therefore, vary greatly even among industrialized countries, ranging from 8 to 21 percent of total health expenditures in 1974–1975 (Table 9.13).

In developing countries, where drugs are predominantly imported, their costs generally occupy a still larger place in national health expenditures. We have noted how, in China (where many drugs are, indeed, produced domestically), Western pharmaceuticals account for 48.7 percent of overall health expenditures. A study in the very poor African country, Mali, in 1985 found drugs to involve 59.2 percent of overall health expenditures and 79.8 percent of private household expenditures. Focusing on purely private expenditures, drugs accounted for 35 percent in Burma (1985), 40.4 percent in Brazil (1975), 45 percent in the Philippines (1975), 48.5 percent in Peru (1984), 53.8 percent in Liberia (1984), 54.1 percent in Guatemala (1976), and 57.3 percent in South Korea (1975). In most developing countries, furthermore, the distinction between prescribed and nonprescribed drugs is not as sharp in daily practice.

METHODS OF COST CONTAINMENT

Throughout the world, as we have seen, national health expenditures have been rising for many years both absolutely and relatively—that is, in absolute monetary amounts (corrected for general inflation) and in the percentages of gross national product (GNP) or gross domestic product (GDP). This has naturally caused great social and political concern, especially as increasing shares of health spending have been derived through collective methods—tax revenues, social insurance, or even voluntary health insurance.

In the industrialized countries, where there are signs of medical extravagance and where the cost escalations have been especially high, the reactions have been strongest, and have led to various strategies for cost control. But certain methods of cost control or containment have been instituted in almost every country. When health systems absorb a significant fraction of government budgets, there is naturally concern about keeping this fraction as small as possible.

The various methods of cost control may be built into the organization of a health program at its onset or may be introduced over the years, as experience is acquired. These methods are of four main types and many subtypes, all of which may be employed in some countries, and only certain ones in others. Several types of cost containment depend on accurate medical records, which may be kept only in highly developed countries.

A major type of cost control is intended to influence the patient's behavior in seeking medical care. By requiring the patient to pay personally a fraction of the medical charge or even a flat amount for an initial medical service, it is expected that frivolous or "unnecessary" demand will be discouraged. Moreover, such copayment or cost sharing reduces the amount payable by an insurance fund, even if the volume of demand is not reduced. The size

of copayment, of course, must not be so high as to discourage "justified" demand, but this level varies with different persons; low-income families are bound to be inhibited more than high-income families. For this reason, copayments may be waived for pensioners and clearly indigent people. Copayments may be required for an initial medical consultation but not for subsequent visits in a period of illness. They may apply only to ambulatory care and not to hospitalization. The latter distinction is made in the copayments of the Scandinavian countries, but not in France where copayments apply to both ambulatory care and hospitalization. In Latin American social security programs for medical care, copayments are required only when the patient chooses to visit a private doctor rather than a polyclinic.

Another influence on patient behavior is to require referral by a general medical practitioner for access to a specialist, as Belgium does. Then, there is the whole field of prevention that affects the demand for medical care. This may be environmental, such as water fluoridation to prevent dental caries, or it may be educational, such as using strategies to reduce cigarette smoking. Education may also promote reasonable self-care to cope with minor ailments.

A second general type of cost control is the deliberate limitation of the resources available in a health system. It has long been recognized that under conditions of extensive economic support for hospital services, the number of hospital beds available is a major determinant of demand. For this reason, there are laws throughout the world requiring government approval of new hospital construction or enlargement of existing hospital capacity. In all countries, these laws are intended to maintain standards in hospital design, but in the industrialized countries, where hospital utilization has risen steeply, the controls are concerned also with the quantity of beds being established. If the ratio of beds to population is being increased, the local hospital sponsor (even if it is local government) must prove the objective *need*.

Similar limitation of resource production is done on the output of physicians. After an initial consultation, the physician determines the need for diagnostic tests, prescribed drugs, further medical visits, admission to hospital, and so on. Enlarging the number of physicians, therefore, ordinarily means a greater volume of medical services to be paid for. This has led most industrialized countries to set upper limits on the number of students admitted to medical schools. Such limitations have long been in effect in the medical schools of Norway, Germany, the United States, Australia, and other industrialized countries, but Belgium—with a staunch free market ideology—had an "open admissions" policy until recently. In developing countries, medical school enrollment quotas are mainly the result of limited school capacities (teachers, equipment, etc.). The decision of Egypt in 1982 to reduce medical school admissions, as a response to its perception of an excessive number of doctors, was unusual among developing countries.

Limitation of the number and types of drugs imported into a country is another form of controlling resources to contain costs. This has long been the policy in Norway, mainly as a measure for quality control, and has recently been done in Bangladesh as part of the strategy for use of only "essential drugs." In many public programs for medical care, the general use of *generic* versus *brand-name* drugs is a policy for controlling costs as well as ensuring quality.

A third approach to cost control is in the method of remunerating providers of service. When conventional fees are used, a schedule of their amounts is usually negotiated between officials and representatives of the health professions. This has been the policy in Western Europe, Australia, Japan, Canada, and elsewhere. The payment of general practitioners by capitation, for the number of persons enrolled with each doctor, as in Great Britain, Denmark, and the Netherlands, is another method; the doctor then has no financial incentive to maximize his services, and yet he must keep his patients satisfied. The payment of physicians or dentists for their time, by salary, is now the most widespread method of remuneration throughout the world. It is the dominant method for specialists in hospitals almost everywhere, and is becoming increasingly applied in ambulatory care.

Payment for hospital services is much more complex, and requires careful cost accounting to be both fair and economical. Almost everywhere the payment of fees for each hospital service has been replaced by other less costly methods. Payments for each patient-day of care or *per diem* are widely used for private hospitals, and periodic global budgetary payments are increasingly used for public hospitals; sometimes global payments are made to all hospitals. In the United States, a compromise between these two methods is used by paying hospitals prospective amounts for each diagnosis. To simplify matters, all diagnoses have been classified into some 200 or 300 *diagnosis related groups* (DRGs).

A fourth approach to cost containment is by influencing the performance of physicians. Many programs with organized financing of medical care have set up methods of *peer review*—that is, the review of each doctor's performance by a committee of peers. A physician identified as giving perfunctory or, more often, superfluous service is investigated and perhaps disciplined in some way. The doctor may be ordering excessive laboratory tests or X-rays, prescribing too many drugs, or having patients return too often. Full discussion with the doctor and at times a hearing with right of appeal must, of course, precede any disciplinary action; this might include mandatory continuing education. Requiring a prior authorization by some medical official, before elective surgery is undertaken, is another commonly imposed constraint on medical performance.

Closely related to this strategy is the requirement in organized programs for a second opinion before elective surgery. This requirement provides a restraint on questionable operations.

Perhaps the most effective strategy for cost containment is the influence on professional performance of establishing an organized framework for providing health services. When physicians and others are organized as a team, in which there is a reasonable division of labor, both economy and quality can be protected. This has long been recognized in hospitals, and it is increasingly being recognized in ambulatory care. Less costly auxiliary personnel can be assigned tasks that they can do perfectly well, and the doctors' time can be preserved for tasks that require their skill and judgment. The staff can be preparing one patient for examination while another patient is being examined. The economies of such organization explain why most developing countries in Latin America and the Middle East have chosen these patterns for delivery of medical care in their social insurance programs.

Among industrialized countries, these several methods of cost containment are being applied more widely and thoroughly in Europe than in the United States. The payment of hospital specialists by salary and the use of a negotiated fee schedule or capitation to pay for out-of-hospital doctor's care in Europe are the most obvious differences from the U.S. pattern. These differences are doubtless a major reason why European countries spend less than 9 percent of their GNPs on health, whereas the United States spends more than 11 percent, with much less economic protection of its people.

COMMENTARY ON METHODS OF FINANCING

Each of the methods of economic support for health systems has different human and social consequences. The oldest method, payment by individuals and families, is clearly the least adjusted to individual or social needs. Illness is generally greater among the poorest people, who can least afford to pay for its care. Moreover, in a family of any income, the occurrence of sickness or injury cannot be predicted, so that it cannot readily be planned for by savings. Aside from having less money to pay for it, the poor have less access to transportation to obtain care.

Charity is a benevolent method of supporting health system costs, but it is usually very limited in quantity and restricted to certain purposes—often to the care of certain persons. Hospitals benefited greatly from charity, when they were frugal places, but as they improved in technology and amenities, the relative role of charity has declined. As overall health systems have developed, the overall contribution of charitable funds has become less important.

Meeting the costs of sickness through voluntary insurance was a great social innovation

to cope with the lack of predictability of health need in any individual. It has serious limitations, however. First, it helps only those who have paid premiums into the insurance fund, and many low-income, unemployed people cannot do so. Second, premiums are typically a flat amount—not adjusted to each person's income; hence, the premium is more difficult for low-income persons to pay. (Flat premiums for families of any size may introduce some progressivity.) Third, voluntary insurance programs, usually being small, suffer from fiscal instability, and many have gone bankrupt. Fourth, as long as enrollment is optional, persons of low illness risk may disenroll, whereas high risk persons stay on; this adds to the financial instability of voluntary health insurance.

For these and other reasons, voluntary insurance in most countries has led to social insurance under law. This has been the sequence in all the European countries, in Australia, and in Canada, although not in the developing countries. As noted earlier, some 70 countries have enacted social insurance legislation for medical care, and in 35 of these more than 90 percent of the population are covered. The various political advantages of fund raising through social insurance, as against the general taxation, have been discussed in Chapter 6. Here it may be noted that in contrast to voluntary insurance, social insurance premiums can be based on a percentage of earnings, rather than being the same for everyone. Under social insurance, employers typically contribute to premiums, whereas under voluntary insurance this depends on collective bargaining. Most important, by mandating population coverage, social insurance overcomes the problems of adverse risk selection. Both types of insurance have the advantage of providing the same health care benefits during sickness, regardless of the amount of premiums paid in.

Put in another way, social insurance is simply an indirect but earmarked tax imposed on all consumers. The contributions of money from the wages of workers and the payrolls of employers is only the last link in a chain of economic transactions. These contributions come from earnings for the sale of commodities or services by an enterprise. These products may be purchased by various middlemen or merchants who, in turn, sell them to consumers. The money derived from the sale of the products is used to pay wages to workers, and a certain percentage of these wages constitutes social insurance *contributions.* Ultimately, the financial source of insurance contributions, therefore, is the total population that purchases the products of each enterprise.

In terms of equity, general taxation as a method of fund raising has the great merit of basing inputs on ability to pay, and providing services on the basis of health needs. Yet there are obvious weaknesses. General tax revenues are required to support the entire machinery of government, so that the health system must compete with many other sectors; the whole military establishment, public education, and multipurpose ministries of interior are strong rivals. In developing countries and to some extent in all countries, taxes on personal incomes may be difficult to collect, especially from rich families. Endless political debate surrounds the determination of proper rates of taxation, in relation to funds needed in the economy for private investment and private consumption. General tax revenues are subject to the hazards of wasteful management and sometimes of corruption.

In developing countries, foreign aid may be an additional source of health system funding, and this can be especially useful in supporting contruction costs. Aid from bilateral sources, however, is more abundant than aid from multilateral international agencies, and the motives of such aid are often suspect. The donor country, it may appear, is imposing its priorities, rather than supporting the policies of the recipient country. Certain construction projects may entail future recurrent costs that a developing country cannot afford.

Thus every method of supporting the costs of national health systems has its strengths and weaknesses. The most appropriate strategies in any country at a particular time must depend on the economic and political circumstances.

CONCLUSIONS

Certain conclusions emerge from the data and analysis in this chapter regarding the relevance and importance of economic analyses of national health systems:

1. For national health planning and associated policy decisions, it is important to know and understand all expenditures in a nation's health system—both the sources from which funds are derived and the purposes for which they are spent.

2. Such information requires, first of all, a clear definition of the composition and boundaries of the health system—which functions it should or should not include. Almost everything in society and the environment contributes to health directly or indirectly, but the health system should be regarded as including only those activities whose *primary* objective is the advancement of people's health.

3. Calculation of total health system expenditures, as a percentage of GNP or GDP, gives a useful indication of the importance a nation attaches to health, especially in comparison with other nations of similar economic level, and with other sectors in the same nation. Trends in this percentage over time can offer valuable guidance for policy decisions.

4. It is essential that calculations of total health system expenditures include funds coming from all public and private sources.

5. In collecting data on public expenditures for health, information must be obtained from all branches of government, with identifiable health functions, in addition to Ministries of Health. Data should also be gathered from all jurisdictional levels of government, with caution to avoid *double counting.*

6. It is crucial to collect information on private health expenditures from organized sources—voluntary insurance, charity, and industrial enterprises—as well as individuals and families. The relative proportions of household spending for health care reflect the level of people's satisfaction with public services, as well as having implications for equity.

7. Collection of information on private family health expenditures is always difficult, but the household survey is commonly

used. A less costly strategy is the indirect method of estimating gross provider income from private patient fees.

8. Because of technical advances in medicine, many countries appear to spend too much on costly technology serving few people, compared with primary health care for everyone. This must be documented to achieve balance in health policy.

9. In most developing countries, enlargement of health system financing would be necessary to attain the WHO goal of "health for all by the year 2000." For maximum equity, such enlargement should come mainly from a prudent combination of social insurance and general tax revenues.

10. At the local level, private donations, voluntary labor, building materials, and community health cooperatives may help to strengthen health services.

11. Whether or not increased health spending is feasible, efficiency in the use of funds should be maximized. This involves prudent health manpower policy, use of appropriate technology, nonbureaucratic management, and the coordination of diverse health programs.

12. Prudent use of health funds requires deliberate measures for cost control. Health resources (personnel, facilities, equipment) should not be developed beyond the best estimate of needs. Pharmaceutical purchasing should be guided by an *essential drugs* policy. Deviant medical performance should be identified and corrected. Effective organization should characterize ambulatory as well as hospital care.

13. The presentation of health economic data should clarify the gaps that frequently exist between the policy declaration and realities. The findings of health expenditure analyses should be widely disseminated, especially to those who make policy decisions.

14. To conduct studies of health system financing, on an ongoing basis, Ministries of Health should be staffed with competent economists and accountants. Records of health system activities should be orga-

nized in a manner that permits their economic analysis.

These conclusions, adjusted to each country's realities, may help to clarify the economic foundations of the national health system.

REFERENCES

Abel-Smith, Brian, "Why is the odd man out?: The experience of Western Europe in containing the costs of health care?" *Milbank Memorial Fund Quarterly,* 63(1):1–17, Winter 1985.

Abel-Smith, Brian, "The World Economic Crisis. Part 1: Repercussions on Health." *Health Policy and Planning* 1(3):202–213, 1986.

Abel-Smith, Brian, and Andrew Creese (Editors), *Recurrent Costs in the Health Sector—Problems and Policy Options in Three Countries.* Geneva: World Health Organization, 1989.

Carrin, Guy, "Community Financing of Health Care." *World Health Forum,* 9:601–606, 1988.

de Ferranti, David, *Paying for Health Services in Developing Countries—An Overview.* Washington, D.C.: World Bank (Staff Working Papers No. 721), 1985.

Ewen, C. L'Estrange, *Lotteries and Sweepstakes: An Historical, Legal, and Ethical Survey of Their Introduction, Suppression and Re-establishment in the British Isles.* London: Heath Cranton, 1932.

Field, Mark G. (Editor), *Success and Crisis in National Health Systems.* New York: Routledge, 1989.

Glaser, William A., *Health Insurance Bargaining: Foreign Lessons for Americans.* New York: Gardner Press, 1978.

Hoare, Geoff, and Anne Mills, *Paying for the Health Sector: A Review and Annotated Bibliography of the Literature on Developing Countries.* London: London School of Hygiene and Tropical Medicine (EPC Publication No. 12), Winter 1986.

Hogarth, James, *The Payment of the Physician—Some European Comparisons.* New York: Macmillan, 1963.

Hu, The-wei (Editor), *International Health Costs and Expenditures.* Washington, D.C.: U.S. Department of Health, Education, and Welfare, 1978.

International Hospital Federation, *Cost Containment.* London: International Hospital Federation, 1980.

Lee, Kenneth, and Anne Mills, *The Economics of Health in Developing Countries.* Oxford: Oxford University Press, 1983.

Mach, E. P., and B. Abel-Smith, *Planning the Finances of the Health Sector.* Geneva: World Health Organization, 1983.

Musgrove, Philip, "The Economic Crisis and Its Impact on Health and Health Care in Latin American and the Caribbean." *International Journal of Health Services,* 17(3):411–441, 1987.

Navarro, Vicente, "The Public/Private Mix in the Funding and Delivery of Health Services: An International Survey." *American Journal of Public Health,* 75(11):1318–1320, November 1985.

Organization for Economic Cooperation and Development, *Health Care Systems in Transition.* Paris, 1990.

Pfaff, Martin, "Differences in Health Care Spending Across Countries: Statistical Evidence." *Journal of Health Politics, Policy and Law,* 15(1):1–14, Spring 1990.

Schweitzer, Stuart O., *Policies for the Containment of Health Care Costs and Expenditures,* Washington, D.C.: U.S. Department of Health, Education, and Welfare, 1978.

Simanis, Joseph G., and John R. Coleman, "Health Care Expenditures in Nine Industrialized Countries." *Social Security Bulletin,* 43(1):3–8, January 1980.

Stevenson, Gelvin, "Profits in Medicine: A Context and an Accounting." *International Journal of Health Services,* 8(1):41–54, 1978.

U.S. Department of Health and Human Services, *Health Care Financing Review* ("International Comparison of Health Care Financing and Delivery"), Annual Supplement, 1989.

United Nations Children's Fund, *The State of the World's Children 1989.* New York: UNICEF, 1989, p. 17.

Winslow, C-E. A., *The Cost of Sickness and the Price of Health.* Geneva: World Health Organization, 1951.

World Bank, *Health Sector Policy Paper.* Washington, D.C.: World Bank, February 1980.

World Bank, *World Development Report.* Washington, D.C.: World Bank, 1988.

World Health Organization, Regional Office for Europe, *Control of Health Care Costs in Social Security Systems.* Copenhagen: WHO (EURO Reports and Studies 55), 1982.

Zschock, Dieter K., *Health Care Financing in Developing Countries:* Washington, D.C.: American Public Health Association, 1979.

CHAPTER 10

Health Planning and Administration

Just as every national health system requires economic support, in the modern world it also requires management. In earlier centuries, when health needs were so great that almost any health service was its own justification, deliberate management may not have been necessary. But as the resources, organization, and services for health purposes grew larger and more complex, the need for prudent health system management became widely recognized.

In the modern era—defined, let us say, as the last 50 years—health system management can be considered to include four main activities: planning, administration, regulation, and legislation. In this chapter we will discuss the worldwide scene in health planning and administration. The next chapter will examine regulation and legislation in health systems.

HEALTH PLANNING

Planning, of course, has many meanings, but in the context of health systems, we refer to decision making about the future development of resources and services, adjusted to meet estimated future health needs. In the absence of planning, the production and allocation of resources are the results of economic markets, functioning through the dynamics of supply and demand, price and competition. Thus planning, as a means of resource allocation, is ordinarily contrasted to market mechanisms.

Historic Development

Comprehensive health planning or the planning of overall health systems became prominent throughout the world in the period of World War II. This was the time of the Beveridge Report, leading to the postwar enact-ment of the British National Health Service in 1946, the Bhore Commission designing a comprehensive health system for India, the discussions leading to the *Servicio Nacional de Salud* in Chile, and the studies leading eventually to the national Comprehensive Health Planning Act of 1966 in the United States.

The origins of more focused health planning, however, can be traced to much earlier times. When hospitals were established by the Christian Church in twelfth century Europe, planning was required to determine their location, size, functions, and staffing. When universities were founded in the Renaissance, and medical schools within them, planning was necessary to acquire teachers and students. Organized public health services to prevent epidemics and guard against environmental hazards required a great deal of planning in the early nineteenth century, as did governmental social insurance to finance medical care in the late nineteenth century.

Perhaps the greatest early milestone in *comprehensive* health planning was the sequel of the Russian Revolution of 1917. Marx and Engels had not written about planning, but in 1928 the new Soviet Union launched its first Five-Year Plan, including strategies for complete transformation of the health system. This was not only comprehensive in scope, but highly centralized in its formulation. For the next 20 years or so, centralized planning was linked to Soviet communism and therefore avoided, at least explicitly, by most Western nations. When the Constitution of the World Health Organization was drawn up in 1946, it avoided completely the term *planning*. Instead, it called on the Executive Board to submit to the World Health Assembly "a general program of work covering a specific period."

Nevertheless, the essence of planning—intervention in the free market of health services with deliberate *programs of work*—was undertaken in many ways. Even before the formal Soviet Five-Year Plan but soon after the Russian Revolution, the British Ministry of Health issued in 1920 its *Interim Report on the Future Provision of Medical and Allied Services.* The Dawson Report called for a sweeping transformation of British health services into an organized framework of hospitals and health centers with salaried staffs. In 1921 the United States adopted the Sheppard–Towner Act, which through federal grants to the states initiated a nationwide network of maternal and child health clinics; the program was, indeed, attacked as "an entering wedge for socialized medicine," and was terminated in 1929. In 1928, France became the last western European country to establish social insurance to pay for medical care. In 1931, the League of Nations held its European Conference on Rural Hygiene, which explored numerous strategies for preventive health services that the free market could not be expected to provide.

The more comprehensive type of health planning after World War II was especially conspicuous in the developing countries. This was a period when so many colonies of European powers were emancipated, and the time was opportune for planning in every sector of society. Almost every newly independent country in Asia and Africa established a central office or ministry of social and economic planning, and within Ministries of Health various units for planning health manpower and facilities were set up. In Latin America such initiatives came a little later, but the Cuban Revolution of 1959 served to hasten planning actions. In 1961, the Alliance for Progress, launched at Punta del Este (Uruguay), generated plans for health resource development and improved health services in every Latin American country. The strategy of health planning undertaken in a country was related largely to the general characteristics of its national health system.

Planning in Entrepreneurial Health Systems

In the *United States,* serious though not explicit, health planning of national scope began in 1928, outside of government, with the establishment of the Committee on the Costs of Medical Care. The name of the committee was much more restricted than its scope of work (probably intentionally), because it actually addressed not only medical care costs, but also questions of health manpower, facilities, public health, modes of organization of health services, and just about every aspect of the U.S. national health system. The final report in 1932–1933 requried 27 volumes. One of these on *The Fundamentals of Good Medical Care* attempted to estimate the "service required to supply the medical needs of the United States" by measuring the incidence of illness, and judging the volume of medical and hospital services required (with the technology of 1930) to treat it. The recommendations of voluntary health insurance and group medical practice, although now seemingly modest, were greeted by the American Medical Association at that time as "socialism, communism, inciting to revolution."

The earlier U.S. Sheppard–Towner Act (1921) on maternal and child health services has been noted. In 1946 the Hill–Burton Hospital Survey and Construction Act required state planning of all facilities as a condition for federal grants. Two further sweeping national reports were issued under President Harry Truman—*The Nation's Health: A Ten-Year Program* in 1948 and *Building America's Health* in 1952. The first explicit legislation on *comprehensive health planning* (CHP), however, was passed only in 1966, a year after Medicare and Medicaid had brought the federal government significantly into medical care financing. This legislation authorized federal grants to state and local health agencies for various planning purposes, most prominent of which was the planning of hospital construction. Under the extremely free-market ideology of President Ronald Reagan, these CHP grants were terminated in the 1980s, although many states continued planning with state funds.

Health planning in a developing country of a transitional economic level, with an entrepreneurial health system, may be illustrated in *Thailand.* In the 1950s, steps were taken to establish a provincial infrastructure of preventive health services, but the first formal 5-year plan was initiated in 1962. In that year the National Economic and Social Development Board formulated a general 5-year plan, and the Thai Ministry of Health prepared a second plan for hospital and health center construction and for communicable disease control. The third plan stressed maternal and child health services and family planning, and the fourth plan (1977–1981) adopted primary health care (PHC) as the central MoH strategy. The fifth 5-year plan (1982–1986) in Thailand reinforced the PHC strategy with major efforts to stimulate community participation and intersectoral collaboration at the local level.

In 1972, the MoH of Thailand had established a formal Division of Health Planning, and organized selected "working groups" to tackle specific health problems. One of these groups, for example, recommended widespread training of "village health volunteers" and mandatory 2-year rural service for new medical graduates, both of which recommendations were implemented. Most Thai health planning, however, is limited to MoH programs, which constituted (as of 1983) only 20 percent of the national health system, as measured by expenditures. In spite of the alleged priority for PHC in rural areas, tax exemptions are granted to encourage the construction of high-cost private hospitals in the main cities. Rural medical salaries in the MoH are so low that private practice is actually encouraged despite its resultant inequities. A study of ambulatory health care utilization in 1981 found that only 33 percent of visits were made to governmental units, and 67 percent were made to private drugstores, private doctors, or traditional healers.

Health planning in a very poor developing country with an entrepreneurial health system may be illustrated in *Ghana*. Soon after gaining independence in 1957, planning was started at the national level. In the words of a high Ghanaian health official in 1973:

> In 1963 a Planning Commission including two doctors was set up, and a comprehensive national development plan was written. This plan, which . . . was not implemented, was very ambitious. It aimed to provide for very rapid development of

hospital services and at the same time for expansion of promotive, protective, and preventive services—an almost impossible task. . . . After the coup of 1966 this plan was shelved. . . . [A new Committee], reporting two years later stated that the emphasis should be on the promotive and the protective services . . . and training of health personnel. Nothing was done to implement this committee's report. In 1971 another committee was set up [for] devising a health-sector plan. . . . This committee reported towards the end of 1971 . . . when the Government which ordered it was overthrown by another military coup. . . . Thus the latest attempt to produce a health plan can be regarded as stillborn.

Examining Ghana's central government expenditures for health, between 1975 and 1982 they declined from 8.3 to 5.8 percent of the total budget. If adjustments are made for inflation, a World Bank analysis found the decline to be substantially greater. Within these government expenditures, much the greatest proportion has continued to be spent on hospitals. A World Health Organization report, published in 1983, states that 88 percent of the central health budget was used for curative services. The difficulty in a very poor country such as Ghana, with an entrepreneurial health system, is not only the severe shortage of resources, but also the lack of effective political will.

Planning in Welfare-Oriented Health Systems

In welfare-oriented health systems of industrialized countries, health planning seems to be built into regular operations, rather than being specially demarcated. Management of the large national health insurance programs seems to permit whatever directive strategies the leadership considers necessary. Thus Germany has no comprehensive health planning authority, nor does Belgium. In the Netherlands, planning is assumed to be incorporated within the normal regulation of hospitals (including hospital beds) and the financing of medical schools.

France does some very general economic

and social planning, but develops no specific plans for implementation. For example, the French Seventh Economic and Social Development Plan (for 1975–1980) formulated broad objectives as follows: (1) to prevent difficulties associated with pregnancy and to promote medicosocial services for children; (2) to maintain the elderly in their homes as long as possible, through the development of domiciliary care, day centers, and local health services; (3) to promote voluntary preventive and social work, particularly health education; (4) to improve hospital conditions, especially by increasing the nursing staff; (5) to develop medical research within the wider framework of scientific research; and (6) to improve the functioning of the occupational health services.

In 1970, a French Hospital Law incorporated many concepts of planning. It designated each of the country's administrative regions as a "hospital service region," each of which would have a principal regional hospital, usually connected with a medical school. The regions were divided into health sectors with local hospitals for (1) short-term cases, (2) medium-term convalescence, and (3) long-term care. In the 284 sectors, both public and private hospitals were included in the planning. In *Canada,* health planning was focused initially on hospitals, and then mainly on the supply of physicians. After 1975, the number of doctors seemed excessive, so that health manpower commissions were set up in the provinces and the immigration of foreign doctors was curtailed.

In *Malaysia,* a transitional level country with a welfare-oriented health system, health planning has focused on the rural areas. Even before independence in 1957, the colonial government had started a Rural Health Services Scheme. This was explicitly in response to an antigovernment guerilla movement, which had arisen from the poverty of the rural population. The plan was launched in 1954 to develop an extensive network of rural health centers and clinics. Accomplishments were impressive. Rural health centers increased from 16 in 1960 to 331 in 1982; rural clinics expanded from 26, with limited midwife functions, in 1960 to 1,518, with much broader health functions, in 1982. Malaysian infant mortality decreased from 76 per 1,000 live births in 1959 to 24 in 1976. Little was done in Malaysia to affect the large volume of private medical practice in the cities, but the development of a strong public infrastructure of health services in the rural areas had substantial impact on the national health record.

The countries of Latin America are largely of transitional economic levels, with welfare-oriented health systems, and *Colombia* may be taken as illustrative. In 1975 a broad National Integration Plan was legislated and assigned to the Ministry of Health for implementation. The MoH formed a National Health Council, representing also the Ministry of Education, the Social Security Institute, and the National Planning Agency. This council formulated a national health plan with seven objectives that were intended to be reached by 1990:

1. An increase in health care coverage, with priority for rural and poor populations, and within these mothers and children.
2. Improvement in the status and use of health facilities, through their regionalization at three levels: local, regional, and university.
3. Strengthening the administrative infrastructure of all health services.
4. Integrated development of the types of health manpower needed.
5. Increasing and strengthening all environmental protection programs, to ensure clean water, proper waste disposal, occupational safety and hygiene, and so on.
6. Development of all social institutions in the health system in accordance with a unified health care plan.
7. Coordination of health activities with those of other sectors to promote balanced socioeconomic development of the entire nation.

Translation of these broad objectives of Colombia into specific and concrete plans obviously required a great deal of further planning. Noticeably absent from these objectives was any strategy for raising the necessary financial support, but some would respond that "where there's a will, there's a way." Colombia is not unique in omitting economic considerations from its health plans. This 1975 roster of health planning objectives in Colombia was the outcome of a methodology known as *coun-*

try health programming, after disappointment with the results of an earlier strategy.

In the early 1960s, the Center for Development Studies (CENDES) in Caracas, Venezuela, with the support of the Pan American Health Organization (PAHO), had worked out a health planning methodology, known as the PAHO–CENDES method. This was a strictly logical and highly sophisticated method of measuring the health problems in a country or region, and then determining the appropriate actions (prevention, treatment, or both) to cope with them. Health problems were defined by disease categories and their rates of mortality. For each disease, the magnitude (rate of deaths), importance (years of productive life lost), and vulnerability (availability of effective prevention or treatment) were calculated to determine the best priority among the diseases for control efforts. Then the costs of various control strategies would be estimated. Each of these cost estimates would be related to the value of estimated outcomes, expressed in years of life saved, to arrive at a cost–benefit analysis. The resulting sequence of ratios would provide guidance for health planning.

The PAHO–CENDES health planning method was taught to hundreds of Latin American personnel, especially at a Latin American Institute for Economic and Social Planning in Santiago, Chile. After several years, however, not a single Latin American country was able to apply the method. Reliable mortality data were not available, especially for deaths occurring outside of hospitals. Even when diagnoses could be identified, age levels were often missing. The future costs of various control options in a country could not be estimated. Most preventive efforts (sanitation, nutrition, etc.) could not be linked to one specific disease but affected many diseases. Determination of cost–benefit ratios by different planners were grossly inconsistent.

After several years of frustrating experiences with the PAHO–CENDES planning methodology, it was abandoned. The World Health Organization then adopted the more down-to-earth and essentially political strategy known as country health programming, illustrated above for Colombia. This approach called for assembling the country's top decision makers and furnishing them with all the information available on national health problems and resources. The objective was to achieve consensus on feasible steps that could be taken promptly to make headway toward a goal of improved health services for the general population. Political commitment was essential— far more important than quantitative calculation of the weight of problems and the value of various corrective actions.

India is the best example of a very poor developing country with a welfare-oriented health system. National health planning has played a large part in the development of its health system, starting in 1943 when the British still ruled. In that year the Health Survey and Development Committee was appointed, under the chairmanship of Sir Joseph Bhore. Its sweeping recommendations were issued in 1946, and called for (1) the development of a nationwide network of primary health center complexes; (2) provision of integrated preventive and curative services for everyone; (3) extensive health education, with full participation of the people; (4) provision of all needed medical care, regardless of the individual's ability to pay; (5) training of all necessary health manpower and construction of all necessary facilities; and (6) the implementation of all proposals to be entrusted to the Ministers of Health of each of the Indian states.

An initial Five-Year Plan (1951–1955) incorporated all the Bhore recommendations. The plan called for each *primary health center* to serve 100,000 people, with a staff of one physician, one nurse, and various other personnel. In addition, the plan called for fighting malaria, extending preventive services to mothers and children, increasing the domestic output of drugs and equipment, disseminating family planning advice, and improving water supplies and sanitation. A Second Five-Year Plan (1956–1960) put greater emphasis on constructing and staffing health facilities, so that by 1960 there were 2,800 health centers, theoretically covering 63 percent of India's large population. It was realized, however, that only a fraction of 100,000 people could actually reach a primary health center.

Meanwhile another Health Survey and Development Committee had been appointed under the chairmanship of A. L. Mudaliar. This report, issued in 1961, recommended no further construction of primary health centers, but much better staffing of those already built. It recommended mobile clinics to extend services and a mandatory rural service period for all new medical graduates. The latter two recommendations were not accept. but instead thousands of subcenters were built, staffed only by auxiliaries. In 1963, 1968, and 1970, further reports were issued, with major stress on family planning to cope with India's rapid population growth. In 1973 a special national planning committee was devoted to the training and use of multipurpose health workers.

In 1978, still another planning group was formed as a joint committee of the Indian Council of Social Science Research and the Indian Council of Medical Research (ICSSR/ICMR). The report of this joint committee, incorporated in the Sixth Five-Year Plan (1980–1985), called for much greater decentralization of health responsibilities to 408 district authorities. Voluntary local agencies would be encouraged, with still greater emphasis on health promotion, disease prevention, and family planning. Financial support of the health system would have to be increased from about 3 percent of GNP in the mid-1980s to 6 percent by the year 2000.

India's health planning has obviously corresponded to *country health programming* even before that particular phrase was used. As a result of successive planning commissions, by 1988 India had established some 8,000 primary health centers, each staffed by physicians to serve 30,000 people. In addition there were 103,000 subcenters staffed by medical assistants. In spite of criticism of each commission by its successor, the planning resulted in stepwise health system improvement.

Planning in Comprehensive and Socialist Health Systems

In the comprehensive health systems, planning has also been in very broad strokes, rather than by use of refined measurements. The *British Inter-Departmental Committee on Social Insurance and Allied Services*, chaired by Sir William Beveridge, was appointed early in World War II, and issued its famous report in 1942. This was really a statement of policy goals for a "comprehensive national health service" to cover everyone, rather than a prescription of organizational strategies. It was left up to the Ministry of Health to develop the four-part structure for management of (1) ambulatory services, (2) hospital and specialist care, (3) medical education, and (4) local public health and social services. This ministry had the knowledge and capability to build this structure from legacies of the past, and to make it operational for the future.

In 1974, after 26 years of experience, the time was ripe for administrative reorganization of the National Health Service (NHS) to attain greater efficiency and effectiveness. Discussion of plans to achieve greater integration of NHS services had been started in 1968, with the issuance of a *green paper* on the matter. With a change of government (from Labour to Conservative Party), a second green paper for discussions appeared in 1971. Finally a *white paper* was issued by the government in 1974 to outline the scheme for reorganization. Basically, responsibilities for all parts of the NHS would be integrated under some 200 Health Districts.

The Beveridge Report of 1942 and the green papers of the early 1970s were essentially planning documents translated into political strategies. In the late 1970s, much attention was being called to inequalities in service among different geographic districts. A Resource Allocation Working Party (RAWP) was appointed to propose methods of reducing the inequalities. The formula for allocation of central funds, recommended and adopted, included measurements of existing health resources, the percentage of aged in the population, and the infant mortality rate. The RAWP formula increased allocations to the less favored regions.

Another British report, issued in 1980, was devoted to exploration of "Inequalities in Health". This working group, chaired by Sir Douglas Black, examined the trend of mortality rates in each of the five social classes recorded on British death certificates for more than a century. Although declines were clear in all social classes, their rate was greater in the upper classes than in the lower. As a result, after 30 years of the NHS, the degree of inequality was actually greater than at the outset. This provoked a great deal of discussion, but it really only demonstrated, as stated in the Black Report, that the material conditions of life are greater determinants of health than specific health services. The implications for planning, of course, vastly transcend the health system.

Norway is another industrialized country with a comprehensive health system in which planning has been built into normal operations. Norway has no network of local planning agencies, but the construction and staffing of all hospitals are regulated by the National Directorate of Health Services, and financial access to health care is ensured to everyone through the National Insurance Institute. Geographic availability of primary health care is assured by a nationwide planned network of Commune Health Officers or *district doctors.* The construction of community health centers, programs of health education, care of the elderly and chronically ill, and so on are planned by local commune governments, with approval from higher levels.

Within the Norwegian central Directorate of Health Services (in the Ministry of Social Affairs) there are five principal departments for (1) primary health care, (2) hospitals, (3) pharmaceuticals, (4) environmental control, and (5) general administration. There is no department for health planning, as each of the departments does planning, and also regulation, in its own field.

In the socialist health systems of industrialized countries, explicit planning has occupied a special role; this was true at least until the cataclysmic political changes of 1989. With markets largely eliminated, the allocation of resources was mainly a central government responsibility, based on various methods of determining need. The methodology of the *Soviet Union* has been carefully described by Soviet writers in monographs published by the World Health Organization. Both the determination of need and the organization of responsive actions differ substantially from such processes carried out elsewhere.

In contrast to techniques for measuring health needs in other countries, the Soviet health leaders did not conduct household surveys of morbidity or even disability. They regarded *perceived* need as the crucial question. The significant rate of morbidity was defined as the rate of *first consultations* sought by a given population during a certain time period, such as 1 month. It was assumed that—given the occurrence of illness, the personal feeling and behavior of individuals, the transportation available, family health care resources, and so on—the patients coming to a facility for health service constituted a measure of health needs. The various environmental conditions that determine whether a given symptom will lead to the seeking of health care naturally differ among large cities, small towns, and rural areas, and they differ in various regions of the country and various seasons of the year. Therefore studies of first consultations were conducted under these diverse circumstances, at different times and places. In all sites, there had to be an adequate supply of health care resources available, so that there was no constraint on the *supply side,* just as the lack of any charges eliminated economic constraint on the *demand side.*

Soviet health planners were aware, of course, that much serious illness may be present, without causing symptoms to stimulate the seeking of care. They were also sensitive to the need for preventive services in children and adults who may be perfectly well. Therefore, adjustments in the "need" for health care were made for unrecognized disease and for preventive services.

To translate the findings on health needs into estimates of resources necessary required the judgment of medical experts, along with observations in clinics and hospitals on the average number of patients that could be properly served per hour by various specialists. Equivalent calculations were made on the need for hospital beds. All these calculations provided the *technical* foundation for various standards or norms to be used in health planning.

These norms then had to be adjusted for practical realities, such as the time required to train additional personnel or to construct facilities. There were obvious constraints in the availability of teachers, building materials, and so on. These calculations constituted *economic* adjustments to the technical estimate of resource needs. Both the technical and economic phases of planning were carried out by the central Ministry of Health, through its Department of Planning Expertise and Estimates. Here, future changes in resource needs had to be forecast to take account of expected changes in the demography of population, the spectrum of morbidity, and levels of technology.

Even these adjusted estimates did not yield the final determination of standards for the health system. A third essential step was *political*. The health system was only one of several social sectors requiring education, construction, and so on. To reach the final decisions on the allotment of national resources to the health system required submission of all MoH plans to the central State Planning Commission (GOSPLAN). This agency was a technical arm of the cabinet or Council of Ministers of the USSR. GOSPLAN made recommendations to the Council of Ministers, which made the final decisions on standards. These standards became the basis for the preparation of budgets throughout the country. Since 1928, when the first Soviet Five-Year Plan was formulated, this process has been repeated every 5 years. Over the years, however, the process has become less mechanistic and less centralized. Under conditions of war and Cold War, the orderly planning steps could hardly be followed in detail. With the sweeping political changes occurring in the Soviet Union, especially since 1991, market dynamics may be expected gradually to replace central planning, but the effects of 60 years of such planning will surely linger on.

The health planning process in a developing country with a socialist health system may be illustrated by that used in *Cuba*. As of 1991, in fact, that middle-income (transitional) developing country had decided not to abandon its general socialist political ideology.

Health planning in Cuba simply drew on the experience and policies of other socialist countries. The country's principal health advisers were from Czechoslovakia, which, by 1959 (the year of the Cuban Revolution), had fully established a Soviet-style health system. In one

matter—the retention of medical education in the universities—Czechoslovakia differed from the Soviet Union, and in this feature the Czech model was initially followed in Cuba. The organization of the health system into health provinces, health regions, and municipalities was similar to the administrative structure in all the socialist countries, and laid the foundation for establishing the Cuban national framework of polyclinics and hospitals.

Regarding standards for the number and types of personnel to be trained, Cuba did not conduct any studies of *first consultations* in cities and rural areas. It simply set about to increase the existing supplies of health manpower as rapidly as possible. The flight of many private physicians and pharmacists set an initial goal of replacing those who left, but the output of personnel went far beyond this. Polyclinics and health posts had to be in easy reach of everyone, and these units had to be staffed with proper teams of physicians and others. An essentially political decision was to refrain from using any auxiliary health personnel for medical care or even maternity service; the people who made a revolution, they said, were entitled to be served by fully trained doctors.

After a socialist health system was well established in Cuba, the leadership decided to send Cuban doctors and nurses to other developing countries. *International cooperation* was a policy of the Cuban Revolution, and this was a concrete way of expressing it. To train the large number of doctors, medical schools were increased from one to four, and enrollments were gradually expanded. Private practice has not been forbidden, but it is frowned on—even after official duty hours. After retirement, a physician or dentist may see private patients, but there is very little market for such service; the public services are satisfactory to nearly everyone.

China is a very poor developing country with a socialist health system, in which health planning is highly political. Major policy decisions are made at the top, such as having general hospitals in every county, health centers in every township, health stations in every village cluster, training health auxiliaries, mounting health campaigns against disease vectors such as snails, and so on. Plans and strategies to carry out these policies allow wide variations among provinces and within provinces among counties.

At the central headquarters of the Ministry of Health of China, there is a Division of Planning and Finance. In this there are sections for statistics, for location planning, for capital construction, and for materials. This division gives technical guidance to the provinces, which in turn help the counties. The population of each of China's 21 provinces is so large that for most resources needed in the health system the planning can be done within the borders of the province.

The great influence of politics on planning in China is illustrated by the impact of the Cultural Revolution (1965–1975) on the health system. Chairman Mao's dramatic call for much greater attention to rural health services was the opening shot. Massive training of *barefoot doctors* and establishment of health stations in *production brigades* (later, village clusters) followed. In the drive against elitism, all directors of hospitals and health centers were replaced by *revolutionary committees.* The duration and content of training barefoot doctors—later upgraded to *village doctors*—have been highly variable. China takes pride in the decentralized implementation of its health policies, but it is obvious that all health activities are heavily influenced by health planning decisions in the national capital.

In all, then, health planning has come to play a part in all types of national health system, and in countries of every economic level. It may be explicitly identified in various ways or may simply be implicit in the management process. According to certain observers, central planning approaches should sometimes be debunked as "myths," because they seldom solve problems as totally as one would hope. Health planning seems to be most influential in comprehensive and welfare-oriented health systems, and somewhat less so in entrepreneurial systems. Regardless of political ideology, however, there is no country that entrusts health system implementation entirely to market dynamics.

HEALTH ADMINISTRATION

The term *administration* is sometimes used interchangeably with *management,* but here we use it in a more restricted sense to apply to the exercise of various forms of control within an organization. Hence, administration is a major component of management, along with planning, regulation, and legislation. In health systems, administration refers to various controls within health organizations.

The development of sophisticated methods for the organization of work—to maximize productive efficiency—is usually traced to American industry in the early twentieth century. Frederick Taylor (1856–1915) was an American industrial engineer who wrote about *scientific management.* This consisted of the subdivision of work into smaller parts, the delegation of responsibilities, the alignment of elemental human movements on assembly lines, monitoring outputs, and so on. Taylor was the analyst and organizer of work, and later students of management, as a production process, emphasized the behavioral aspects. Chester Barnard of the large American Telephone and Telegraph Company wrote of *The Functions of the Executive,* stressing the personal relationships between the worker, the foreman, middle management, and top management. It is mainly this aspect of management that we define as *administration* and discuss here.

The organization of clinics and health centers for ambulatory care in America was influenced to a significant extent by the scientific management movement. Although this movement arose within industry, the principle of attaining efficiency through the organization of personnel and their services could be readily applied to ambulatory health care. The early book of Michael Davis and Andrew Warner on *Dispensaries—Their Management and Development* took full advantage of the efficiency movement in its advocacy of organized clinics for out-of-hospital care. The same was true in the later advocacy of community health centers.

In Volume I, health administration was defined as a process including nine activities: (1) organization of resources, (2) staffing, (3) budgeting, (4) supervision of performance, (5) consultation on problems, (6) procurement of supplies and equipment, (7) records and reporting, (8) coordination of services, and (9) evaluation. Other conceptual analyses of administration, of course, are possible but, in any case, we could not hope to consider each of these elements separately. Instead, we can identify certain general characteristics of administration as a whole, and how these affect administrative methods or administrative style in different types of national health system. These characteristics or attributes may be considered along five principal dimensions, definable as follows:

1. The exercise of authority, ranging from highly authoritarian to very democratic.
2. The site of responsibility, ranging between centralized and peripheral or decentralized.
3. The type of administrative control, ranging from wholly governmental to wholly private.
4. The degree of uniformity, ranging from complete uniformity to very pluralistic.
5. The criteria for appointments, ranging from technical merit to political ideology or family nepotism.

These ranges of attributes are bound to overlap to some degree, but their recognition may help in analyzing the administrative features of a health system. The place of a health system, or even a specific health program, along each of the five ranges is determined largely by each country's history, but there are also other influences. For example, the geographic size and the population of the country, the recent election to power of one or another political party, the current level of economic development of the country, religion and cultural values, and a critical event, such as the discovery of penicillin or the occurrence of the AIDS epidemic, may all influence health administration. Here we select a few countries with each of the major types of health system, and probe the characteristics of administrative practice within them.

Entrepreneurial Health Systems

The health system of the *United States* has many administrative characteristics associated with its entrepreneurial character. The exercise of authority puts great emphasis on democratic, as against authoritarian, decision making. Even when central authority is strong, every effort is made to promote inputs from the periphery. The site of responsibility is highly decentralized to 50 states and even to more than 3,000 counties. The U.S. Constitution grew out of opposition to strong central power, and it established the separation of powers between legislative, executive, and judicial branches of government. As social problems, including health services, have grown more complex, greater authority has actually been vested in the central government, but the implementation of programs is still mainly by the states. Many programs even lodge responsibility in private entities—hospitals, health insurance schemes, planning bodies—under general public guidelines. As a result administrative procedures are very pluralistic rather than uniform. To guard against ideological favoritism, appointments are widely based on civil service merit systems.

Thailand is a transitional-level developing country with an entrepreneurial health system, but a history of monarchy and more recently military control. The latter circumstances have established rather firm authoritarian rule, with relatively little democratic input from the periphery. Responsibilities are retained largely in the central government, and officials at provincial and district levels are centrally appointed to carry out central policies. Administrative controls are kept in government hands except in special fields, such as family planning, where the government chooses to avoid visible responsibility. Because of the centralized authority, administrative practices everywhere are quite uniform. Appointments to various posts are often based on ideological persuasion rather than technical merit.

Kenya is a former British colony that, after independence, developed an entrepreneurial type of health system. As in many former colonies, there was a strong legacy of central government power that corresponded with the viewpoint of the ruling political party. Hence all significant authority is exercised at the central government level. There are provinces and districts for administrative purposes, but their health directors are appointed by the central Ministry of Health. There is very little participation of local residents in the management of health programs. Private enterprise is encouraged and, throughout the health system, there are church-sponsored private hospitals, entrusted with many public responsibilities. A special hospital insurance program has been developed to facilitate the maximum use of private hospitals. Within government, administrative practices are strictly uniform. Appointments of supervisory personnel in the MoH program are theoretically governed by a civil service merit system, but tribal affiliations generally play a large part in such selections.

Thus, within the category of entrepreneurial health systems, there are quite diverse styles of administration in different countries. Differences in the historic background and current economic levels of these countries are apparently of crucial importance.

Welfare-Oriented Health Systems

In *France,* the welfare-oriented health system has administrative practices that are greatly influenced by a history of strong monarchies and an early nineteenth-century period of imperial Napoleonic Law. Policies toward hospitals, health insurance, preventive public health service, and so on are centrally determined, and even the administrative officers in each of the country's 95 *départements* or provinces are centrally appointed. The French Revolution (1789) put an end to church-sponsored hospitals, but purely private proprietary hospitals abound; major administrative responsibilities for health insurance are delegated to the nongovernmental sickness funds. Methods of public administration of health programs are quite uniform, and official appointments are made under the constraints of a civil service code.

Germany's administrative policies are quite different from those of France. Under Adolf Hitler, Germany may have seemed like a pow-

erful and despotic monarchy, but its traditional structure has granted major authorities (especially in health and education) to the *länder* or provinces. In West Germany there were nine provincial governments, exercising authority over the entire health system. The federal Ministry of Youth, Family Affairs, and Health has had little authority outside of establishing certain technical standards for disease prevention. The important health insurance program is administered by semiautonomous sickness funds, regulated by the Ministry of Labor and Social Affairs in each province. The sickness funds represent local consumers of medical care, so that a form of *community participation* is inherently built into the administrative mechanism. Administrative procedures, nevertheless, are quite uniform, and since the defeat of fascism, appointments to government posts are made under a merit-based civil service code.

Canada has a welfare-oriented health system in which administrative methods are decisively determined by the federated nature of the entire nation. Each of the 10 provinces has established and operates its own programs for hospitalization and physician's care, with partial federal support coming through earmarked grants. The mechanism of tax collection and the exact combination of benefits are determined by each province, so that administrative practices are pluralistic rather than nationally uniform. Some provinces formerly delegated administrative responsibilities to private nonprofit organizations, but all appointments to public posts are based on civil service selection. The permissive type of administrative pluralism seen in Canada is evident also in other federated countries, such as Australia with its six states and Switzerland with its 23 cantons.

In *Japan,* on the other hand, a welfare-oriented health system comes principally under central authority. The tradition of a strong hereditary monarch has been retained in government, with much the greatest power at the top. Certain administrative functions, such as social insurance tax collections for small firms and the self-employed, are delegated to local units of government, but the procedures are nationally uniform. The local health centers in a national network all offer a similar range of preventive services. Yet small health facilities, with fewer than 20 beds, are not subject to hospital regulation and are free to be operated as part of private medical practice. Appointments to government posts are rather strictly based on proof of the individual's technical merit.

In all the industrialized countries with welfare-oriented health systems, the basic parliamentary form of government is highly sensitive to popular opinion. The executive branch of government is chosen by the majority of elected representatives, and may be changed (by parliamentary vote) at any time. Unlike the U.S. pattern, all cabinet members must have won an election; Mr. Aneurin Bevan, who, as Minister of Health, presided over the introduction of the British NHS, was a former Welsh coalminer.

Among middle-income developing countries with welfare-oriented health systems, *Peru* may serve as an example. As in other welfare-oriented health systems of Latin America, authority for policy determination is concentrated largely at the top. There is a divided framework of responsibility, however, for the Ministry of Health and the Social Security Institute. Under the MoH, each of the country's 17 health regions is headed by a Regional Health Director, but these officers are centrally appointed and obligated to carry out central policies. Each region is divided into three or four health areas—57 in all—in which a health center doctor is supposed to be in charge. The hierarchy of the Social Security program is entirely separate, with its own subdivisions. Peru has had several military governments, which did not encourage community participation at the area or regional levels. The scope of responsibility in the health areas and regions, as well as at the center, is limited to the MoH services and does not include Social Security or the private sector. The threat of an antigovernment guerilla movement in the Andean Mountain sections of Peru has served to increase the concentration of power at the top.

India is a very poor developing country with a welfare-oriented health system. Because of the country's great size (more than 800,000,000 people), its historic background of princely domains, and its Hindu philosophy of nonviolence, India is now a federated nation

of 22 states and 9 "union territories." Although general health policies are supposed to be determined by the central government, the all-important implementation of policy is left to the states. About two-thirds of financial support for governmental health services comes from the states and one-third from the national government—the latter mainly for family planning to limit population growth. A very large private sector for medical care is (except for medical licensure) essentially without regulation by either state or central governments.

Because of large variations among the states and territories in per capita wealth, there are substantial differences in their health programs. National policies have influenced the construction of certain types of primary health centers and subcenters, and the training of various types of auxiliary health worker, but the extent of development of these resources is highly variable. Even within one state, there are vast differences between urban and rural resources. Some states have elected to power political parties that put a high priority on public education and health—for example, Kerala and West Bengal; other states, such as Uttar Pradesh, have resources much below the average. In the central as well as the state governments of India, many administrative procedures have been carried over from the British, but these seem only to have multiplied bureaucratic paperwork. Perhaps the large numbers of clerks and clerical assistants employed in every governmental office of India are intended to provide employment to these generally impoverished people.

Comprehensive Health Systems

Great Britain has had a comprehensive health system, covering its entire resident population, since its enactment of the National Health Service (NHS) in 1946. This legislation and the reorganization in 1974 were actions of a strong central government that is fully accepted by its constituent parts—England, Wales, Scotland, and Northern Ireland—which make up the United Kingdom.

Although great authority is held at the top, the responsibility for carrying out health programs is distributed widely to health regions, health areas, and health districts throughout the country. The members of Regional Health Boards are centrally appointed, but the selections are made after consultation with the main health professions and local government authorities in the region, as well as with trade unions, voluntary bodies, and universities. At the level of the 90 Area Health Authorities, the chairman is appointed by the national Secretary of State for Health and Social Security; the members are appointed partly by the Regional Health Board of the region in which the area is located and partly by local government authorities and perhaps a local university.

The major site of concrete NHS administration is still more local, in some 200 health districts. In each of these there is a District Management Team, composed of an administrator, a community physician, a nursing officer, and a finance officer—all appointed centrally under a civil service merit scheme—and two elected representatives of local hospital consultants (specialists) and local general practitioners. This District Management Team (DMT) of six members is assisted by various technical officers on construction matters (a District Works Officer), on pharmaceutical services, and so on.

In each district there is a Community Health Council, intended to ensure a voice for consumers in NHS management. Half of the council members are appointed by local authorities, one-third by voluntary health organizations, and the remainder by the Regional Health Board. Although this council is purely advisory, its members may attend all DMT meetings and have access to the press to broadcast any complaints about the management of local health affairs. Members of the general population are free to bring any problems to the attention of the Community Health Council.

Thus the establishment of the British National Health Service was dependent on strong central authority, and key administrative officials are centrally appointed, but responsibility for its daily management is greatly decentralized. As noted earlier under health planning, any major proposals for organizational change are widely discussed, through various governmental *green papers* before they are finalized.

Administrative procedures are nationally quite uniform, but local wishes and attitudes may be expressed through appointments by local public authorities and elections of professional representatives.

Norway is a much smaller country than Great Britain, with a comprehensive health system. Central authority is strong in the Norwegian health system, with a broad scope of responsibility vested in a National Directorate of Health Services within the Ministry of Social Affairs. In each of the 19 provinces (also called counties), there is a Provincial Health Director, who is centrally appointed and expected to carry out national health policies. The provinces are subdivided into some 450 communes or municipalities, each of which has a locally elected Commune Council. This council appoints a Commune Health Officer, whose preventive work comes under the supervision of the Provincial Health Director. (Some years ago, the Commune Health Officer was also centrally appointed, but the more decentralized pattern was developed in the 1970s.)

Central authority is reinforced in the provinces by national government financing of about 50 percent of provincial health costs. In the communes, 75 percent of costs are met by national and provincial grants, so that only 25 percent must be raised locally. Administrative procedures are quite uniform nationally, and any disparity among the communes is due mainly to difficulties in recruiting professional staffs for some of the isolated areas in the far north. Aside from this, there is remarkably equal access to both ambulatory and hospital services throughout Norway.

Among the few developing countries with comprehensive health systems, *Tanzania* may be taken as illustrative. Being a very poor country, Tanzania's health resources are quite limited, and its policies attempt to adjust for these handicaps. In the national government, very broad authority is exercised by the Ministry of Health at the top. In the MoH, there are three major directorates for preventive services, for hospitals, and for health manpower development; the third directorate trains many types of personnel and has indirect control of the training of physicians and pharmacists in the universities.

There are 20 governmental regions in Tanzania, each of which has a Regional Medical Officer (RMO), who is centrally appointed. The RMO supervises the District Medical Officers (DMOs)—in about 100 districts in all—who are also centrally appointed. All these medical officers in the field are required to carry out the policies of the central MoH. In fact, the DMOs have little time for administration, since they face heavy demands for purely clinical work in district hospitals and, more peripherally, divisional health centers. Administrative procedures throughout the country are quite uniform.

Socialist Health Systems

Until the late 1980s, the administrative style in the *Soviet Union*—in comparison with that in most other industrialized countries—had to be characterized as highly authoritarian. The Ministry of Health at the top was not a very large organization, but its policies were applied with great uniformity throughout this large country. In each of the 15 constituent republics, there was an equivalent MoH, but the crucial administrative units were the 150 provinces *(oblasts)* into which the republics were divided. These contain populations of about 1,000,000 to 5,000,000, which are subdivided into some 3,100 districts or *rayons,* with populations of 40,000 to 150,000 people. There are many differences in the ratios to population of health personnel and facilities in the districts and provinces, but the key policies of free services (except for drugs) for everyone, government control of resources, integration of personal prevention and treatment, and so on, were followed everywhere.

The achievement of uniformity in the implementation of Soviet health policies was formerly through various governmental directives, backed up by the disciplinary power of a nationwide Communist Party. Parallel with the structure of government in the provinces and districts were branches of the Communist Party of the USSR. Since the 1917 revolution, through the years of the World War II and after, the Soviet Communist Party had acquired increasing influence over all aspects of society, including the health system. Until the great changes of the late 1980s ushered in with *perestroika* and *glasnost* (restructuring and openness), the Communist Party exercised constant surveillance over the operations of the Soviet health system.

Centralized control did not mean a very complex bureaucracy. On the contrary, the very small proportions of the private sector—without such elaborate complexities as fee-for-service remuneration of doctors—made administration relatively simple. Hospitals and polyclinics were financed by prospective budgets, which are much simpler than any other method of economic support. Administrative paperwork was minimal. This did not eliminate problems, however, which became evident in the mid-1970s, when declining measurements of health status appeared. But solutions were also relatively simple—to increase budgets in order to enhance salaries (and work incentives), purchase modern equipment, and elevate morale throughout the health system. These were, indeed, the intended strategies of *perestroika,* which were unfortunately impeded by the basic difficulties of the entire Soviet economy after 1990.

The pattern of authoritarian central control and broad surveillance by a Communist Party was adopted by the other countries installing socialist governments after World War II. It characterized the countries of Eastern Europe (with modification in Yugoslavia) and the socialist developing countries in other parts of the world. In *China,* partly because of its enormous population, "local self-reliance" was emphasized, but central policies were still respected everywhere; the *barefoot doctor,* for example, was used throughout the rural areas, although his or her exact regime of training was quite variable. In socialist countries taking shape later, such as in Cuba or in Vietnam, centralized control and pervasive Communist Party influence were clearly established. Even after the Leninist model of a single dominant political party was challenged in Eastern Europe, it was maintained in Cuba. In all the socialist countries, political ideology was the principal criterion for appointment of individuals to high positions in the government hierarchy.

COMMENTARY

This review of administrative practices in various national health systems does not easily lead to generalizations. There may be greater pluralism in entrepreneurial health systems and greater uniformity in comprehensive and socialist systems, but there are various deviations from this. Welfare-oriented systems differ in their administration between federated and nonfederated countries. In all developing countries, with any type of health system, there tends to be greater concentration of authority at the top, if only because local government has not yet become well developed.

Decentralization of responsibilities from the center to the periphery is carried out in diverse ways. They range from the simple assignment to peripheral posts of central government appointees to the delegation of full authority to locally elected officials or even private agencies. To some extent there seems to be a changing scenario in countries: those with a history of great local autonomy are acquiring greater centralized authority, and those with a history of central authority are taking steps to build up peripheral local responsibilities. In all health systems, disease control programs traditionally managed through *vertical* lines of authority, from top to bottom, are being transformed into programs managed and coordinated at the local level through *horizontal* exercise of authority.

Administrative costs have led to debates about how much a country is willing to pay for local autonomy and pluralism. Exact calculation of such costs is difficult—that is, achieving agreement on which activities should be considered "administrative." In Switzerland, where there are hundreds of small autonomous sickness funds, administrative costs have been deemed to be high; this is also the judgment on such costs in the United States, with its hundreds of voluntary insurance programs paying fees to private providers. In Canada, where there is a single governmental payer in each province, administrative costs are substantially reduced. In socialist health systems, the administrative costs of financial transactions are also low.

A tool of health administration in every system is the written record, which requires deliberate effort to produce. Medical records were first kept on patients cared for in the earliest hospitals of Europe in the twelfth century. In the seventeenth century, St. Bartholomew's Hospital in London established a library, which contained full accounts of interesting cases. When William Harvey became the physician in charge of St. Bartholomew's Hospital, he was instructed to keep written records on the patients. The early study of vital statistics by John Graunt in 1661 was based on the "bills of mortality" or lists of deaths and burials. By about 1800, medical records in hospitals became somewhat standardized, with information on the patient's age and sex, appearance, diagnosis, treatment, and progress notes. In the late nineteenth century large teaching hospitals, such as the Massachusetts General Hospital in Boston, began to keep a classified collection of records on all previous patients.

Extension of medical records beyond patients, to yield information on the general operation of national health systems, occurred in the twentieth century. With the recognition that health systems as a whole had difficulties, and some planning—explicit or implicit—was needed to address them, information had to be gathered on system features beyond the individual patient. Information was needed on health personnel and facilities (their numbers and ratios to population), on health services and their utilization by different people, on health expenditures, and on the health status of the population and its trends. In the United States of the 1920s, when health planning was only implicit (e.g., the Committee on the Costs of Medical Care), the demand for such health system information was especially strong. Compilations were made on doctor–population ratios, the rate of utilization of hospitals, the expenditures for drugs, and the mortality from tuberculosis. Similar information was soon produced in other industrialized countries of Western Europe. In the developing countries, data usually became available only after national independence. The sparsity of health system information in such countries is one of the many obstacles to sound planning. Yet *informatics* and computer technology are gradually spreading to all countries.

Difficulties in health system operations, especially in developing countries, are often attributed to incompetent management. Sometimes this is a political cover-up for inadequate financing, but it also may be partially true. The solution in many countries has been to develop training programs for health managers. Various short courses are organized for managerial personnel, already employed, to acquaint them with new techniques for achieving efficiency. A popular course, promoted by the World Health Organization discusses (1) planning and management at the district level, (2) supervision of health personnel, (3) management of drug supply distribution, and (4) financial planning in health systems. Periodic training sessions provide a general opportunity for communication between central headquarters and peripheral field personnel.

Because of the technical complexities of health service, top administrative roles are usually assigned to physicians, many of whom lack administrative experience. In response, management training is sometimes fashioned specifically for physicians. Also, trained managerial personnel are widely used in health organizations as administrative assistants to the medical director of a program. In the opinion of some, administrative medicine should be regarded as a specialty, equivalent to other specialties in the medical profession.

Whatever the style of health administration in a country at one time, it is likely to change with social circumstances. The occurrence of war, serious economic depression, the emergence of a great scientific breakthrough, or a devastating new epidemic—such developments are bound to affect any style of administration. In countries with government takeover by military coups, such as Argentina or Chile, authoritarian administration can be abruptly established. Community participation is seldom feasible under military governments. Even after resumption of democracy, authoritarian attitudes may linger on. It may be most prudent to say that administrative methods are determined by the total social situation at any time and place.

REFERENCES

Anderson, O. W., "Styles of Planning Health Services: The United States, Sweden, and England." *International Journal of Health Services,* 1(2):106–120, 1971.

Barnard, Chester, *Functions of the Executive.* Cambridge, MA: Harvard University Press, 1964.

Beveridge, William, *Social Insurance and Allied Services,* American Edition. New York: Macmillan, 1942.

Blum, Henrick, *Planning for Health,* 2nd ed. New York: Human Sciences, 1981.

Davis, Michael M., and Andrew R. Warner, *Dispensaries—Their Management and Development.* New York: Macmillan, 1918.

Deodhar, N. S., "Primary Health Care in India." *Journal of Public Health Policy,* 3(1):76–99, March 1982.

England, Roger, "More Myths in International Health Planning." *American Journal of Public Health,* 68(2):153–159, February 1978.

Escudero, Jose Carlos, "Democracy, Authoritarianism, and Health in Argentina." *International Journal of Health Services,* 11(4):559–572, 1981.

Evang, Karl, "The Position of the Medically Trained Person in the Administration of Health Services." *American Journal of Public Health,* 56(10):1722–1733, October 1966.

Freund, Paul J., and K. Kalumba, "Information for Health Development." *World Health Forum,* 7:185–190, 1986.

Heady, Ferrel, *Public Administration: A Comparative Perspective.* Albuquerque, NM: University of New Mexico, 1984.

Health Survey and Development Committee, *Report, Volumes I–IV.* New Delhi, India: Manager of Publications, 1946.

Henderson, Gail E., and Myron S. Cohen, "Health Care in the People's Republic of China: A View from Inside the System." *American Journal of Public Health,* 72(11):1238–1245, November 1982.

Hilleboe, H. E., A. Barkhuus, and W. C. Thomas, *Approaches to National Health Planning.* Geneva: WHO (Public Health Papers No. 46), 1972.

Horlick, Max, "Administrative Costs for Social Security Programs in Selected Countries." *Social Security Bulletin,* 31–56, June 1976.

Huffman, Edna K., *Medical Record Management.* Berwyn, IL: Physicians Record, 1972.

League of Nations, Health Organisation, *European Conference on Rural Hygiene.* Geneva, 1931.

Lee, K., and Anne Mills, *Policy-Making and Planning in the Health Sector.* London: Croom Helm, 1982.

Lee, Roger I., and Lewis W. Jones, *The Fundamentals of Good Medical Care.* Chicago (Committee on the Costs of Medical Care Publication No. 22): University of Chicago Press, 1933.

Levitt, Ruth, *The Reorganized National Health Service.* London: Croom Helm, 1976.

Liebler, Joan Gratto, *Managing Health Records: Administrative Principles.* Germantown, MD: Aspen Systems, 1980.

Mandil, Salah, "Health Informatics." *World Health Forum,* 2–5, August–September 1989.

Mills, Anne, J. P. Vaughan, D. L. Smith, and I. Tabizzadeh, *Health System Decentralization: Concepts, Issues and Country Experience.* Geneva: World Health Organization, 1990.

Ministry of Health, Consultative Council on Medical and Allied Services, *Interim Report on the Future Provision of Medical and Allied Services.* London: H.M. Stationery Office, 1920.

Molina-Guzman, Gustavo, "Third World Experiences in Health Planning." *International Journal of Health Services,* 9(1):139–159, 1979.

Navarro, Vicente, "Planning for the Distribution of Health Services." *Public Health Reports,* 84(7):573–581, 1969.

Okubagzhi, Gebre Selassie, "Ethiopia's Success Story (training health managers)." *World Health,* 21–22, May 1989.

Pacey, Arnald, "Taking Soundings for Development and Health." *World Health Forum,* 3(1):38–47, 1982.

Pan American Health Organization, *Health Planning—Problems of Concept and Method.* Washington, D.C.: PAHO (Scientific Publication No. 111), April 1965.

Pan American Health Organization, *Health Goals in the Charter of Punta del Este: Facts on Progress.* Washington, D.C.: PAHO, March 1966.

Pan American Health Organization and U.S. Department of Health, Education, and Welfare, *Health Planning—An International View* (Copenhagen, Denmark). Washington, D.C., 1977.

Pattison, Robert V., and Hallie M. Katz, "Investor-Owned and Not-for-Profit Hospitals." *New England Journal of Medicine,* 309:347–353, 11 August 1983.

Popov, G. A., *Principles of Health Planning in the USSR.* Geneva: World Health Organization (Public Health Papers No. 43), 1971.

Reinke, William A. (Editor), *Health Planning for Effective Management.* New York: Oxford University Press, 1988.

Rodwin, Victor G., *The Health Planning Predicament: France, Quebec, England, and the United States.* Berkeley: University of California Press, 1984.

Roemer, Milton I., "Planning Health Services: Substance Versus Forum." *Canadian Journal of Public Health,* 431–437, November 1968.

Roemer, Milton I., *Cuban Health Services and Resources.* Washington, D.C.: Pan American Health Organization, 1976.

Rosenfeld, Leonard S., and Irene Rosenfeld, "National Health Planning in the United States: Prospects and Portents." *International Journal of Health Services,* 5(3):441–453, 1975.

Rotem, A., *Managing Systems for Better Health: A Facilitator's Guide.* Manila (Philippines): World Health Organization, Western Pacific Region, 1988.

Shonick, William, and Ruth Roemer, "Private Management of Public Hospitals: The California Experience." *Journal of Public Health Policy,* 3(2):182–204, 1982.

Vacek, Milos, and Emidie Skrbkova, "Methods of Planning Health Services in Czechoslovakia." *Milbanh Memorial Fund Quarterly,* 44(3):307–317, 1966.

Vaughan, Patrick, Anne Mills, and Duane Smith, "The Importance of Decentralized Management." *World Health Forum,* 5:27–29, 1984.

Vukmonovic, C., "Decentralized Socialism: Medical Care in Yugoslavia." *International Journal of Health Services,* 2(1):35–44, 1972.

Walt, Gill, and Patrick Vaughan, "Politics of Health Planning." *World Health Forum,* 7:44–49, 1986.

Working Group on Inequalities in Health, "Inequalities in Health." *World Health Forum,* 3(1):68–73, 1982.

World Bank, *Colombia Health Sector Review.* Washington, D.C.: World Bank (Report No. 4141-CO), December 1982.

World Health Organization, *National Health Planning in Developing Countries.* Geneva: WHO (Technical Report Series No. 350), 1967.

World Health Organization, *Modern Management Methods and the Organization of Health Services.* Geneva: WHO (Public Health Papers No. 55), 1974.

World Health Organization, Regional Office for Europe, *Health Services in Europe—Vol. 2: Country Reviews and Statistics.* Copenhagen: WHO, 1981.

World Health Organization, *Managerial Process for National Health Development.* Geneva: WHO, 1981.

World Health Organization, "A Management Approach to Health Systems Development." *World Health Forum,* 3(1):64–67, 1982.

CHAPTER ELEVEN

Health Regulation and Legislation

The supervision of activities within a health organization is an important aspect of health administration, as discussed in Chapter 10. When some sort of central authority exercises control over activities in the open market of a society, it may be termed *regulation.* When that type of control is embodied in a law enacted by government (at various levels), it constitutes one category of *health legislation.* Pursuant to certain broad public authorities established under health legislation, an official agency may issue further detailed instructions, which are also known as *regulations.*

HISTORIC BACKGROUND

The earliest enactment of law by government specifically for the protection of a population's health occurred in the cities of Medieval Europe to control epidemic disease. Bubonic plague was believed to come from infected goods, carried by ships from the Orient to Europe. The major port of entry was believed to be Venice, where a "council of overseers of public health" was appointed in 1348. In 1374, Venice and Milan—both in northern Italy—took action to deny entry into those cities of any traveler or merchant with the plague or under suspicion of carrying the infection. The ordinance in Venice required ships to wait in the harbor for 40 days before unloading goods or passengers—hence giving rise to the word *quarantine.*

When the plague occurred later in Rome, mandatory legal action was taken in a city of the greatest importance. In 1656, a health *commisary* under the Roman Pope issued an edict to protect the city from this dreaded disease. Sanitary guards, placed at the city gates, required a certification of health from all travel-ers. The edict also called for regular cleaning of the streets and public sewers, the inspection of aqueducts, the disinfection of the clothing of deceased persons, and the prohibition of popular gatherings. In 1684, a book was published containing 245 sanitary edicts issued in Rome during the campaign against the plague.

Even earlier than society's legal battles against the plague had been the long struggle against leprosy, which started in the early Middle Ages. This action, however, was taken by the Christian Church rather than by civil government. In the sixth century, the Church Council of Lyons (France) restricted lepers from associating with healthy persons. In the seventh century leper houses were built outside city limits throughout Europe. After the tenth century, these places of isolation expanded greatly and by the end of the twelfth century there were estimated to be 19,000 leper houses on the European continent.

Regulations governing the isolation of lepers spelled out the procedures in detail. To symbolize the finality of the isolation, a simulated "funeral service" was enacted, in which the unfortunate leper, clad in a shroud, was conducted by priests to a hut or leprosarium outside the city. The brutal regulations enacted to suppress this ancient infectious disease (although of low communicability) were, in the long run, effective, but at an untold price in human rights.

The vast field of environmental sanitation was the subject of much early local legal action by European cities, in the form of edicts and decrees. Each city had some sort of governing council, the duties of which included the supervision of street cleaning and environmental sanitation. Water was brought into the city through pipes and distributed at public fountains, but municipal edicts had to be issued to

prevent drinking water from becoming polluted. In the fourteenth century, Milan had
several ordinances dealing with sewers and
cesspools. In London, regulations were passed
to forbid people from throwing rubbish into
the Thames River, but they were not well enforced. In Bruges (now in Belgium), the cus-
todian of the "water house" had great authority to guard it against pollution.

Many regulations concerned urban marketplaces, where food and clothing were sold. In
Medieval Florence, marketplaces had to be
swept clean every evening, and all refuse had
to be discarded more than "one thousand
paces" away; there were severe penalties for vi-
olation of this rule. There were also detailed
regulations about the sale of leftover fish or the
meat of sick animals. The officials appointed
to enforce these sanitary regulations were not
physicians, but generally respected citizens.

Of the many early subjects of health legislation, the saga leading to compulsory vaccination laws is especially interesting. In the early
eighteenth century, smallpox was endemic in
the cities and towns of Great Britain and continental Europe. For centuries it had been
known that a previous attack of this febrile disease protected a person from further attacks,
and in 1714 the inoculation of material from a
person with a mild case (variolation) was
found to give similar protection. In 1798, Edward Jenner, an English country doctor, reported that inoculation with cowpox matter
(from the hand of a milkmaid) left only a small
scar but also gave protection against smallpox.
Application of this *vaccine* (from a *vax* or cow)
became known as vaccination.

The social value of this finding was immediately appreciated in Bavaria, Germany,
where in 1807 the first law was enacted to
make vaccination compulsory. In Great Britain, where the discovery had been made, the
issue of a law compelling anyone to be vaccinated was debated for decades because of British concepts of individual rights. Finally the
British Vaccination Act of 1853 made it compulsory for parents to have their infants vaccinated by 4 months of age. There were no enforcement powers, however, and many
children went unvaccinated. It was many years
later, when vaccination and then other im-

munizations were required for attendance at
school (and education was compulsory), that
legally mandated protection against certain
communicable diseases became effective.
Compulsory notification of "febrile diseases"
to local health authorities in London was not
required until 1889.

Legislation to license physicians also arose
early in the history of western civilization. In
1140 the Norman King Roger II (who had
conquered regions of Italy) issued an order
stating

> Who, from now on, wishes to practice
> medicine, has to present himself before
> our officials and examiners to pass their
> judgment. Should he be bold enough to
> disregard this, he will be punished by im-
> prisonment and confiscation of his entire
> property. In this way we are taking care
> that our subjects are not endangered by
> the inexperience of the physicians. No-
> body dare practice medicine unless he has
> been found fit by the convention of the
> Salernitan masters.

The "Salernitan masters" referred to the faculty of the earliest medical school, which had
been founded at Salerno, Italy in the ninth
century.

Eventually this policy spread through Europe, with training being required in universities, and examinations being administered by
the professors. Representatives of the government were also present at examinations, and
the license to practice medicine was issued by
the monarch or his representative. When a
physician moved to another city, he had to ask
permission to settle there and then be examined by the faculty of the local university, if
one existed. If there was no university, credentials were reviewed by the municipal council or
its committee on public health. In London, the
Royal College of Physicians was chartered in
1518, and this body was authorized to grant li-
censes to physicians settling there. Over the
years, medical licensure has come to depend
on the approval of universities alone or universities combined with a government body.

Legislation to control the production and
distribution of drugs has great current importance and early origins also in Medieval Eu-

rope. In the fifteenth century, the guilds were given authority to maintain the purity of products sold by their members. In 1429, the English Grocer's Company was empowered to inspect certain foods and drugs, and to confiscate any that seemed adulterated. In 1540, King Henry VII proclaimed the first act to control drugs, by authorizing physicians to inspect apothecary shops. This act was amended in 1727 to permit apothecaries to accompany physicians making these inspections. Apothecaries had become separated from grocers in 1606, but their vendetta with physicians continued until the nineteenth century.

The first edition of the *London Pharmacopoeia* was published in 1618, but subsequent editions did not acquire legal status in Great Britain until 1858. At this time the pharmacopoeia's standards for quality control in drug production acquired the force of law. By 1875 the first British Food and Drugs Act was passed, designating penalties for the adulteration of drugs. Such food and drug control legislation was not enacted in the United States at the federal level until 1906.

The history of health legislation has many more chapters, but we should proceed to review the characteristics of this feature of national health systems in the current world.

FORMS OF HEALTH LAW

Health law, concerned with protecting or advancing the health of populations and also with improving the structure and operation of health systems, may take several different forms. First, in many countries there are Constitutions, established when the nation was founded or following some crucial change of authority; the latter change may sometimes have been the result of social revolution or the achievement of national independence after a period of colonial domination. Constitutions usually contain broad statements of principles, intended to establish the power of government and the rights of individuals. Health protection may be explicitly defined or, more often, implicitly contained within some broader concept such as *social welfare* or the *public good.*

A second form of health law is the vast diversity of statutes or laws enacted for a health purpose. Pursuant to a health statute, a governmental administrative body may issue detailed instructions in the form of *official regulations,* which have the force of law. A statute on public water supplies, for example, may be extended by official regulations on the exact concentration of chlorine to be maintained in water to ensure its purification.

A third form of law consists of judicial decisions on controversial matters, often involving interpretation of a statute. The decision of the United States Supreme Court in 1973 on *Roe* v. *Wade,* for example, established the legality of abortion under specified circumstances; this invalidated many laws of the states on the same subject. Decisions of the U.S. Supreme Court are typically based on interpretation of the U.S. Constitution, but those of courts within a state may be based on state Constitutions or even state statutes.

Any of these three forms of health law may concern the functions of government at different levels: national, provincial, or local. National legislation affects a whole country, such as the law establishing the Chilean National Health Service in 1950, effective in 1952. A law at the provincial level might be illustrated by the 1946 statute in the Canadian province of Saskatchewan, establishing the Saskatchewan Hospital Services Plan, which led to the eventual enactment of Canadian national health insurance legislation. At the local governmental level, there are various municipal laws or ordinances that prohibit smoking cigarettes in public places, such as those in Buenos Aires, Argentina (1984) or in São Paulo, Brazil (1980).

Quite outside of any unit of government, there may be voluntary or private organizations endowed by law with certain public responsibilities. The national health insurance legislation of Germany and France, for example, delegates to nongovernmental sickness insurance funds the function of carrying insurance and making payments to providers of service. In the medical profession of most countries, specialty status surveillance and certification are entrusted to nongovernmental medical associations. Legally mandated emergency services may be provided by hospitals under private as well as public sponsorship.

The scope of health legislation may vary from very broad to very narrow. In Kenya, for example, the early health legislation, after national independence in 1963, was simply carried over from the colonial period. Then in 1972 the Kenyan Public Health Act was extensively revised, establishing a very wide range of authority for the Ministry of Health. Under this broad legislation, many specific regulations are issued by the MoH. On the other end of the range, very specific laws are always being enacted by countries to address certain health problems that have arisen and attracted attention. In Thailand, the 1943 law controlling the use of human excreta as fertilizer or the 1974 law controlling the sale of cosmetics illustrates the countless specific laws enacted to protect health. An example between these extremes is the New Zealand Social Security Act of 1938, that provided for an extensive program of national insurance for medical, hospital, pharmaceutical, and related services.

In exploring health legislation, we should take note of a related legal domain. Referred to sometimes as *legal medicine* or *medical jurisprudence,* it is the element in health systems related to the legal pursuit of justice. When a murder is suspected, the medical examination of the victim's body is done by a coroner or *medical examiner.* The techniques used to acquire evidence of the guilty party are regarded as *forensic pathology* or legal medicine. The legal and medical foundations of this field, including the performance of autopsies, are traceable to Germany in the early sixteenth century, and the field has become increasingly sophisticated since then. This discipline, however, is outside the scope of our review of health law in the world.

The several types of health legislation in countries may now be considered. Any categorization of these laws is somewhat arbitrary and depends on one's objectives. The *International Digest of Health Legislation,* published by the World Health Organization, uses a schema of 22 categories that perhaps reflect priorities in WHO analysis of health systems. These are as follows:

1. General provisions (health codes, organization of care, economic aspects, health research, etc.)
2. Health manpower
3. Disease control and medical care (communicable disease, noncommunicable disease, etc.)
5. Dental health
6. Family health
7. Human reproduction and population policies
8. Care of the elderly and rehabilitation
9. Mental health
10. Control of smoking, alcoholism, and drug abuse
11. Ethical issues and professional responsibility
12. Death and related issues
13. Nutrition and food safety
14. Consumer protection
15. Pharmaceuticals and medical devices
16. Poisons and other hazardous substances
17. Occupational health and safety
18. Environmental protection
19. Radiation protection
20. Accident prevention
21. Sports and recreation
22. Health information and statistics

The following somewhat more inclusive categories are used in this chapter to cover the same range of subjects:

1. Protection of populations
2. Regulation of health personnel
3. Health facility regulation
4. Promotion of health
5. Financing health care
6. Regulation of health systems
7. Assuring individual rights

Although some overlapping of these categories is unavoidable, they permit us to review a very wide diversity of health laws in countries.

PROTECTION OF POPULATIONS

The earliest types of legislation on the control of epidemics and the reduction of risks from an unsanitary environment concerned the health protection of populations and the reduction of external hazards.

Communicable Disease Control

Virtually all industrialized countries have laws on the mandatory immunization of school children and the isolation of cases in acute stages of serious communicable diseases. In Ontario, Canada, for example, 1982 legislation set forth a detailed schedule of immunizations required for protecting all school children against diphtheria, tetanus, measles, mumps, poliomyelitis, and rubella. Because of the special hazards of rubella in pregnancy, Czechoslovakia enacted a law in 1982 to require girls in the sixth year of primary school to be vaccinated with a live rubella vaccine.

Legislation for the control of malaria in developing countries is extensive. In Malaysia, legislation in 1975 provided for various measures, such as the control of mosquito vectors through spraying houses with insecticides, drainage of swamps, the detection of cases through medical and laboratory examinations, treatment of infected persons, and so on. A Costa Rican decree of 1973 provided for the issuance of malaria surveillance cards, to ensure the reporting of detected cases. Compulsory reporting of malaria had been required in Italy since 1901. To improve control measures, Venezuela in the 1940s exempted from customs taxes a certain type of cloth, sufficiently fine to stop passage of the dominant mosquito vector.

The global campaign of smallpox vaccination, leading to the eradication of smallpox from the world in 1978, was a great triumph for international health organizations, led by WHO. Yet in back of this achievement, the national legislation in the developing countries, authorizing compulsory smallpox vaccination, was important. As recently as 1967, not more than 1 percent of cases in most of the world were reported to health authorities. WHO began its worldwide campaign in 1958, but it did not move into high gear until 1967. A rigorous and systematic policy of *epidemiological surveillance* (case reporting, contact tracing, rapid immunizations, etc.) had to be implemented, but it met many obstacles. From time to time strategies had to be changed, including monetary rewards for case reporting. Each of the procedural changes in specific countries could be launched only on a foundation of authority vested in the national health agencies. The treatment of the last case of smallpox in August 1975 was an achievement for WHO leadership and international cooperation, but it rested also on a body of national health legislation and the popular respect for governmental authority that it promoted.

Control of sexually transmitted or venereal diseases is the subject of special health legislation in many countries. Since such diseases may be highly disruptive of family life and are associated with issues of personal morality and social welfare, they have led to special laws and regulations over and above those for communicable diseases in general. The control of venereal diseases has become such a complex process that in a world survey of such legislation in 1975 WHO classified the legal measures under the following 12 headings:

1. Diagnoses included in venereal diseases (VD).
2. Obligation of patients to be treated and of physicians to so inform patients.
3. Compulsory notification of public health authorities.
4. Notification of authorities about any patient refusing or discontinuing treatment required.
5. Identification of sexual contacts.
6. Laboratory obligations to report positive VD tests.
7. VD testing in premarital and prenatal examinations.
8. Limitations on employment of persons with VD infection.
9. Persons allowed to treat VD and advertisement of anti-VD remedies.
10. Treatment of minors or mentally incompetent patients.
11. Compulsory hospitalization of uncooperative patients.
12. Organization of VD clinic services and availability of care without charge.

In most industrialized countries of the world, with all political types of health system, legislation on several or all of the above subjects is in effect. Specific VD control measures are especially well developed in France, Italy, Greece, Spain, Australia, and the numerous states of the United States. Among socialist industrialized countries, legal measures were especially well developed in Poland and East Germany. In Latin America, Argentina and Brazil have strong VD control laws. In the 1975 WHO survey, VD control legislation was identified in only a few countries of very poor economic level: Upper Volta, Senegal, Madagascar, and Fiji.

A very different type of sexually transmitted disease appeared on the world scene in the early 1980s. The acquired immunodeficiency syndrome (AIDS) and human immunodeficiency virus (HIV) infection became subjects of intense international interest in this period. In 1983, Sweden was the first country to introduce legislation on AIDS—with regulations mandating the reporting of confirmed and suspected AIDS cases to the National Bacteriological Laboratory. By 1988 more than 60 countries had legislation on one or more aspects of this pandemic disease.

Since the isolation of the HIV virus, some countries have simply added this serious disorder to their list of sexually transmitted diseases, but most have enacted special forms of mandatory legislation. Such laws differ significantly from those on other sexually transmitted diseases because of the lack of a vaccine or an effective treatment. An important focus of all AIDS legislation has been the issue of individual privacy and protection against discrimination. The widespread fears about this major pandemic are leading to new laws in countries of all economic levels and with all types of national health system.

Sanitation and Water

Legislation on environmental sanitation, to protect people from the risk of communicable disease, is found in every country. Laws on the sanitary disposal of human excreta and other waste, as we have noted, started in Medieval towns and cities, and they are still largely on a local, municipal basis. Countless local ordinances have governed human and other waste disposal up through the late eighteenth and nineteenth century development of public sewerage systems.

Legislation on the maintenance of sewers and garbage disposal is now found in cities throughout the world. Ordinances and regulations of large cities on sewerage, garbage disposal, food establishments, public nuisances, and related matters may be assembled as *sanitary codes* or *health codes.* The *New York City Health Code,* 1981 edition, is a volume of several hundred pages. In a federated country such as the United States, the state government Departments of Health often issue regulations that define standards for proper sanitation, leaving to local government the task of implementation. Unitary governments may issue national standards, which provincial and municipal governments are then expected to apply. Increasingly, the enormous problems of environmental pollution have led to national legislation governing air and water quality, solid waste disposal, and hazardous wastes, as well as other environmental issues.

In developing countries without a long history of active local government, legislation on environmental protection is most likely to be passed at a national level. A comprehensive statute of Algeria in 1983 is illustrative. The law provides requirements for the control of air pollution, water protection, waste disposal, control of radioactivity and noise, and other environmental matters. It provides that local communities represent various agencies, responsible for implementing environmental measures, and requires that details be specified in legislative or regulatory texts. Local communities are entitled to conduct studies and to undertake public utility works necessary to control water pollution.

In 1981 Cuba enacted a comprehensive law on environmental protection, encompassing surface and ground waters, soil, mineral resources, marine resources, air, agricultural resources, human settlements, and tourist resources. The central government was made responsible for directing and supervising all activities concerned with natural resources. Local governments were made responsible for a range of activities involving inspection and regulation of the environment and natural resources. Standards were to be issued by the central government and applied by local government agencies.

Legislation to ensure the availability and purity of water sometimes preceded and sometimes was coincident with legislation on waste disposal. Unlike sewerage, the provision of safe water was often contracted out to private companies in Europe and America. Such private performance of community service made legislation all the more necessary to establish standards. In the industrialized countries, the legal control of urban water supplies is still vested mainly in local municipal governments, although the larger management of water resources, as well as standards for purity, are handled at higher levels.

In France, for example, the general management of national water resources comes under the Ministry of the Environment, which established a framework for administration of six natural basins. Standards of water purity are established by the Ministry of Health, but the distribution of water and the collection of user fees are handled by local communes or water companies. In Spain, water supply programs are also a municipal responsibility, although this is carried out within the guidelines of a "national water supply and sanitation plan" made in 1967 by the Ministry of Public Works and Urbanism. In the Netherlands, likewise, water supply is a local government responsibility, carried out under the general surveillance of the Netherlands Association of Water Supply Companies; ultimate governmental authority comes legally under the Ministry of Housing, Planning, and Environment.

Thus in several industrialized countries—probably the majority—insofar as higher levels of government have authority for water supply, it is usually in ministries of public works or the environment. Such ministries are involved in managing large national resources, such as water. Ministries of Health may formulate standards of purity for human health, and sometimes monitor performance through testing water samples. Local management and distribution of potable water, however, usually are entrusted under law to local government.

In developing countries, the legal responsibility for safe water is much more heavily concentrated in central government. As in the industrialized countries, however, major legal responsibilities are usually vested in ministries of works, of local government, of natural resources, or in ministries devoted entirely to water supply and sewerage. In small villages and rural areas, however, water supply development is often legally assigned to the Ministry of Health.

In Peru, for example, the Ministry of Works, Housing, and Construction has 90 percent of the personnel concerned with water and sanitation. In 1981, this ministry established a National Drinking Water and Sewerage Service, with its own officials stationed throughout the country. Meanwhile, the Ministry of Health, with its nationally appointed personnel, is legally in charge of developing water supplies in rural communities with less than 2,000 population. Malaysia also vests national legal authority in its Ministry of Works, under a Water Supplies Branch. Rural villages, however, construct and operate local water supplies with the financial and technical assistance of the Ministry of Health. In Indonesia, the national Ministry of Public Works is responsible for all piped water supplies—urban, semiurban, or even in small villages. When a rural water supply is from a single source, without pipes, the Ministry of Health is legally responsible. Local governments in developing countries are generally too weak to be entrusted with significant environmental responsibilities.

Drug Control Legislation

Another important type of health legislation, designed to protect populations from harm, regulates the production and distribution of drugs in a country. We have noted the Medieval origin of laws on apothecaries and apothecary shops, but current legislation is concerned mainly with the pharmaceutical industry and the sale of its products. A *pharmacopoeia* on the composition and production of drugs acquired legal status in England in 1858, and most European countries established similar official compendia by the late nineteenth century. Subsequent regulation was concerned with the protection of consumers against drugs that were adulterated or labeled with fraudulent claims about their curative powers.

Norway, which has had to import nearly all of its drugs, was one of the first countries to enact national legislation on the safety and efficacy of drugs brought into the country. This was in 1928; Sweden followed in 1934. In these countries, the national government evaluates the safety, efficacy, accuracy of promotional claims, and even the pricing of all drug preparations, issuing official lists of a few thousand registered pharmaceuticals that could be imported and sold. A law passed in the United States in 1906 prohibited any adulteration of food and drugs, as well as fraudulent labeling, but considered neither efficacy nor the claims made in advertising. It took the death of more than a hundred children from a lethal "elixir of sulfanilamide" to lead the U.S. Congress to enact the much more rigorous amendments of 1938. This law required the testing of drugs for safety before marketing, appropriate warnings on drug labels, and the regulation of all advertising.

France enacted a strong regulatory drug law in 1941, but it took still another drug tragedy to induce many nations to take equivalent legal action. The German drug *thalidomide* was a simple sedative, sold without prescription and widely used in the 1950s, until it was found to cause severely deformed babies when taken by the mother in early pregnancy. This led to further amendments on precautionary drug testing in the United States in 1962. West Germany finally strengthened its regulatory drug law in 1971 and again in 1976; these laws controlled the clinical investigations performed to determine drug safety and registration before marketing. Eventually all industrialized countries enacted drug control laws or regulations to ensure the safety of new drugs before marketing. In some countries, complaints have arisen on the "lag" between the time of discovery of a promising new drug and its availability for use, because of the time required for careful testing.

Laws controlling drugs in industrialized countries, in contrast to sewage disposal and water supply, are enacted mainly at the national level. Drugs move so rapidly in commercial channels that no other approach could be effective. Even in a wholly federated country, such as the United States, the nationwide regulation of drugs is based principally on the Constitutional powers of the central government to regulate *interstate commerce.* Within the borders of a state or province, other legislation may influence the distribution of drugs, such as their use in a local program for medical care of the poor. Nevertheless, at the national level, prevailing political philosophies have an impact on regulatory controls. A 1980 study, comparing drug control legislation in the welfare-oriented health system of West Germany and the socialist system of East Germany, found much greater permissiveness in the West German law and greater restriction along scientific lines in the East German law.

In developing countries, the drug control legislation on paper usually resembles that in Europe and the United States, but in practice the effects are far different. In most such countries there are very few government personnel to enforce the regulations on the books, concerning both drug production and distribution. The great majority of drugs consumed in developing countries are imported from abroad, but grossly exaggerated claims are often made about their therapeutic value. Adverse drug reactions, recognized in the country of origin, are ignored or minimized in labeling and advertising. Many drugs exported to developing countries have exceeded their permissible age, and yet are "dumped" overseas. In some developing countries, legitimate and effective drugs from Europe or America have been counterfeited, with only a fraction of the active ingredient, and then packaged and sold as the genuine item. "Drug swindling" takes many ugly forms.

Perhaps the most ubiquitous deficiency in drug regulation is the extensive sale in developing countries of prescription drugs without a prescription from a physician or even an auxiliary health worker. Such dispensing may be done by a pharmacist or more often an untrained clerk in a drugstore, or it may be by a completely autonomous "drug seller". Such drug consumption, which is basically self-medication, may simply alter symptoms, without affecting the disease, and delay proper medical care, or it may be definitely harmful. Certain developing countries—India, China, Brazil, Egypt—have built up major domestic pharmaceutical industries, so as to be less dependent on imports.

The effective regulation of drug production costs, importation, and distribution is so complex and difficult that the World Health Organization has adopted a policy of promoting the use in all countries of a restricted list of *essential drugs*. In 1988, WHO estimated that of 104 developing countries studied, 24 had "low" coverage with essential drugs (under 30 percent of their population), 33 had "medium" coverage (30–60 percent of population), and 47 had "high" coverage (60–90 percent). Drug coverage is largely parallel to the GNP per capita of these three groups of countries, but there are numerous exceptions.

WHO does not issue any "model list" of essential drugs but calls on each country to prepare its own list, based on the judgment of its own physicians and pharmacologists. The emphasis is put on generic, rather than the more expensive brand-name drugs, and also on drugs required principally in the delivery of primary health care. Regarding legislation, an essential drugs policy does not usually require new statutes, but rather the adoption of suitable regulations under the established drug authority of the Ministry of Health.

Accident Prevention

Legislation for the prevention of accidents—or more accurately the prevention of human injury due to accidents—is another large category of law concerned with the general protection of populations. The many statutes concerned with traffic on public streets or highways, with the design of road, bridges, or other structures, the operation of elevators (or lifts) in buildings, or the entire process of production in factories or mines are in this domain. To protect children, there are usually special regulations applying in and around public schools. The design of automobiles and buses is also subject to much regulation to protect

their occupants against injury. Traffic accidents have been responsible for so many injuries and deaths in recent years that regulations on motor vehicle seatbelts and helmets for motorcyclists have acquired increasing importance, especially in the industrialized countries.

To prevent fires, there are laws on "safety matches," which will ignite only on certain surfaces. Night clothes for children must be made from fire-resistant fabrics in many European countries, Australia, and the United States. There are regulations on the construction of stoves and various electrical appliances, designed to prevent fires in the home. Since fires often occur in public buildings and hotels, there are legal requirements in many countries for convenient fire extinguishers or automatic sprinkler systems.

Because of traditions on individual freedom in several countries, such as Great Britain, there has been long debate on the compulsory wearing of seatbelts in automobiles. A law making seatbelt use compulsory took effect there only in 1982, and the beneficial effects in reduced traffic injuries and deaths were quickly demonstrated. Many European countries make it illegal to drive a vehicle after moderate alcohol intake, even if there is no accident; drivers may be stopped by police officers who take a blood sample to test for alcohol level. Seatbelt laws have been enacted in many developing countries, such as Senegal and the Ivory Coast, but they tend to be weakly enforced.

Legislation to protect against injuries in the workplace (later, against occupational diseases) has an especially long and contentious history in Europe. The earliest such legislation was in England and was designed to protect children who served as apprentices in textile factories. This was in 1802, but not until 1819 did the law stipulate a minimum age for working—9 years of age for not more than 12 hours a day. It was only in 1833 that this legislation was reasonably enforced with the appointment of *factory inspectors*. Even this timid legislation was passed only after overcoming the opposition of English factory owners, who objected to this government interference with private economic enterprise.

In France, legislation to protect workers was first enacted in 1813, prohibiting the employment in mines of children under 10 years of age. This prohibition was extended to any kind of child labor in 1841. In Germany, child labor was prohibited in factories in the 1830s, and in the United States the first such law against child labor was enacted in Pennsylvania in 1848. In some developing countries child labor is still tolerated today, especially in such village-based industries as the weaving of rugs.

In addition to children, women were identified for special protection in European industry, but only after the 1870s were all workers—adults and children, women and men—protected by safety legislation. For many years, the only recourse for a severely injured worker or the widow of a worker killed on the job was to bring suit against an employer in the courts to establish liability and receive compensation. A great change occurred in 1884, when Germany enacted the first *workmen's compensation insurance,* funded entirely by employers, to grant compensation to workers injured on the job, without regard to fault. This was initially limited to manufacturing and mining, but by 1887 was extended to all types of work.

In the last decade of the nineteenth century all industrialized European countries enacted similar worker's compensation laws to provide monetary and medical assistance to workers in case of on-the-job injuries. Most important was the policy of encouraging safeguards on dangerous machinery by reducing employer insurance premiums if safety measures were applied. Occupational safety is now reasonably ensured in most large enterprises of Europe, America, and other industrialized regions, although working conditions in small plants are still often hazardous. Factory inspection by government agencies, concerned with labor, industry, or manpower, is expected to identify severe safety violations and to have them corrected. New Zealand is unique in having social insurance for accidental injuries, not only at the workplace, but anywhere and for any type of person.

In developing countries, safety measures at the workplace are generally far less adequate, even in large establishments. Worker's injury compensation laws were in effect in 136 countries as of 1989, and these include a good majority of developing countries, but the associated programs of factory inspection are typically weak. In Thailand, for example, the Factory Act of 1969 and the Labor Act of 1972 require various types of protective equipment on dangerous machinery; the Department of Labor in the Ministry of Interior, however, has such a small staff that enforcement is virtually impossible. Even laws focused on large enterprises, requiring medical attendance or first-aid provisions, are seldom enforced.

Other types of legislation for the general protection of populations concern the contamination of food, the safety of various consumer products, the care of the elderly, and other issues to be considered below under "health promotion." The general scope of legislation to protect the well-being of populations is steadily expanding.

REGULATION OF HEALTH PERSONNEL

So many aspects of national health systems depend on the qualifications of health care providers that a large body of legislation has been developed in most countries to address these matters. As already noted, the licensure of physicians has a long history, and current legislation on health care providers is much greater than this in scope.

Professional Licensure

The laws for licensure of physicians may take one of three main forms. The authority may simply be vested in the central Ministry of Health, as in Sweden and in Japan; it may be vested in an independent quasigovernmental group that has been recognized under law, such as the General Medical Council in Great Britain and the National Council of the Order of Physicians in France; or it may be vested in various agencies of the provinces or states that determine licensure within their borders, which is the policy in federated countries such as the United States and Canada, and also in Germany with its *länder.* Procedures in the United States, with 50 state jurisdictions, have been simplified through the extension of *reci-*

procity for licensure among the states and through the recognition by nearly all states of examinations by the National Board of Medical Examiners.

Medical licensure authority in developing countries is predominantly in some subdivision of the Ministry of Health, as in Colombia or Thailand. In certain former British colonies, however, the British pattern is still followed, such as in Malaysia with its separate and quasipublic Malaysian Medical Council. In Indonesia, the central Ministry of Health has licensure authority, but that country's highly entrepreneurial type of health system is shown in the requirement of a favorable recommendation by the private Indonesian Medical Association before a license is granted.

In virtually all countries, the receipt of a university degree in medicine is the main basis for determining the qualification of a medical candidate. Since the great majority of universities are governmental, and nongovernmental institutions of learning have to be officially approved, passing university examinations is usually considered adequate proof of competence. In a few countries, however, such as the United States and Japan, the governmental licensure authority may require a second official examination and certain practical exercises (such as a hospital internship).

After World War II, when thousands of physicians and other health personnel moved extensively across national borders, recognition of the medical qualifications of foreign-trained physicians became a contentious issue. WHO conducted an international survey of legislation on the cross-national equivalence of qualifications to practice medicine; in 1967 some legislative provision for coping with this matter was found in 40 countries. In general, the affluent European countries set rather strict requirements for the recognition of foreign-trained physicians; this had also been true in the colonies of European powers (British, French, or Dutch). As the latter developing countries became independent, and strove to expand their medical manpower, the barriers to immigration of foreign physicians were greatly reduced.

After a doctor is certified by a specialty body, his or her designation as a specialist may be announced generally, and may also be registered with the governmental licensure body. In developing countries and in the previously socialist countries, the specialist designation is usually recorded in the registry of the Ministry of Health. In Western Europe, North America, and Australia, specialty status is not linked to licensure. It is recognized, nevertheless, whenever appropriate, such as in the many health insurance programs that pay higher fees or salaries to qualified specialists. This is true in the United States, even though the American Medical Association has no official legal standing.

A noteworthy aspect of specialization in the 1980s and 1990s has been its inclusion in many countries of specialty status for *general medical practice* or *family medicine.* This has helped to increase the professional attractiveness of a major component of primary health care in both industrialized and developing countries. In several industrialized countries the same specialty recognition has been accorded to public health work, preventive medicine, or *community medicine.*

Regarding the licensure of nurses, pharmacists, and other health personnel, legislation is patterned largely on that of physicians. The categories of health personnel subject to licensure differ among countries. Much of the content of these laws concerns the authorized scope of practice of various categories. A trend in most countries is to expand the legal scope of practice of nurses and other health personnel.

Service Obligations

Another legal aspect of medical practice concerns obligations imposed on the medical graduate after qualification. In Mexico in the 1930s a law was passed to require every graduate of a Mexican medical school to spend 6 months in a period of *social service* in a rural area, under the supervision of the local public health authorities (Secretariat of Health and Social Assistance). Soon other Latin American countries adopted similar policies, and by 1990 nearly all these countries had such laws or regulations.

Early in the 1930s the Soviet Union required

all new medical graduates to spend 3 years at a rural post. Virtually all graduates became attached to the Ministry of Health, but they were not entitled to work in a city (with certain exceptions) until they had served in a rural district. Similar policies were adopted by the several other countries that became socialist after World War II.

In the 1960s, as national health systems became increasingly organized in Asia and northern Africa, the policy of mandatory rural service for new medical graduates became widely adopted. Egypt required 2 years of employment in the Ministry of Health, usually at a rural health unit. Tunisia had a similar policy. Iran made use of military service as a method of getting rural medical coverage. Indonesia, in spite of its very privately oriented health system, carried over a policy from the Dutch colonial government that required new medical graduates to work for 3 years in the Ministry of Health. Burma passed a mandatory rural service law in 1964, but decided in 1969 that the same objective was being achieved through the normal public employment of graduates.

In some countries of sub-Sahara Africa, such as Ghana or Kenya, the shortage of physicians is so great that no requirements are imposed on new medical graduates; evidently it is felt that they are needed wherever they go. In Tanzania, on the other hand, private medical practice has been legally forbidden, so that all medical graduates remaining in the country must work in the Ministry of Health or some other organized program. In Zimbabwe, all new medical graduates are legally required to work for the Ministry of Health.

In the British National Health Service, there is an ingenious policy directed toward achieving a balanced distribution of physicians. The general practitioner, who is typically in private practice, may not settle in a local area designated as "overdoctored"; practitioners who do are not entitled to acquire a list of capitation patients under the NHS. Therefore, general practitioners must go to an "underdoctored" area. Regarding specialists, virtually all NHS posts are in public hospitals, so that the staffing of such hospitals automatically determines the distribution of specialists. Hospital construc-

tion or extension, in turn, has been done according to broad planning guidelines.

Medical Ethics

Closely related to medical licensure is the "regulatory" influence in almost all countries of nonstatutory codes of medical ethics. Such codes are usually established by medical associations or *orders of physicians,* which new graduates may be legally obligated to join. In Western European and North American countries, the ·basic principles of medical ethics have been traced to the *Oath of Hippocrates* originating in classical Greece, and modified in countless details over the centuries. The *Declaration of Geneva,* adopted by the World Medical Association in 1948, is probably the closest to an international code of ethics that exists. Yet modern leaders in medical ethics have criticized these codes in various countries for their exclusive focus on the individual patient (rather than society), their failure to recognize the role of patients in medical decisions, and the usual failure to include in ethical codes some consideration of costs and competition for scarce resources. Other ethical codes have, in fact, been applied in the Soviet Union, China, Islamic countries *(Islamic Code of Medical Professional Ethics),* India, and Japan.

The regulatory process, through which ethical codes are enforced, is typically outside the framework of government bureaucracy. The administrative complexity of these arrangements in a western European country may be illustrated by the process in Belgium. (Belgian procedures have been modeled essentially after those in France, but they are described here for the smaller country.)

In each of Belgium's nine provinces there is a Provincial Medical Commission; the chairman and vice-chairman of each commission are appointed by the Ministry of Health, the Secretary is always the Provincial Health Officer, and the members are elected by the physicians in each province. On showing proof of medical school education, the candidate's name is submitted to the central MoH, where it is registered (no further examination is given). Before being authorized to practice, however, every physician must enroll with the Order of Physicians, which is a separate body. Among the officers of this Order, 6 are appointed by the King from medical school faculties and 10 are elected by all physicians. The Order of Physicians is responsible for formulating *Codes of Medical Ethics,* which define the general duties of doctors, relations of doctors with third parties and also with each other, the doctor–patient relationship (including medical records, confidentiality, and fees), and the continuity of care.

In Belgium, accusations of unethical behavior against doctors, alleged by pharmacists, patients, or other doctors, are brought before the Provincial Medical Commission. After preliminary review and screening, if the charge is serious, it is brought by the Commission before the Provincial Order of Physicians. The Order decides if the physician should be expelled and hence lose his right to practice. In the 1970s there were about 500 cases of allegedly unethical behavior in Belgium per year, but only about 1.0 percent of them ended in disciplinary action—these being mostly for drug addiction (in the physician). There are still other organizations of physicians in Belgium that may debate questions of medical ethics, but have no implementing authority. These are the medical syndicates, which bargain with government agencies about fee schedules, and medical associations (separately for general practitioners and specialists), which do continuing education. There is also a Belgian Academy of Medicine for the advancement of medical research.

Medical ethics in Great Britain and in many other countries of the British Commonwealth of Nations (mostly former colonies) are formulated in codes and monitored somewhat differently. The British General Medical Council, which handles licensure of physicians, is also responsible for monitoring medical ethics through its Disciplinary Committee. (The Council, as noted earlier, is a private body of physicians that has been granted quasiofficial status.) Disciplinary Committees function in London (for England), Edinburgh (for Scotland), and Dublin (for Ireland). These committees have the authority, rarely exercised, to withdraw approval by the General Medical Council and therefore terminate the right to

practice. This pattern of enforcing medical ethics is followed in several other countries in the British Commonwealth of Nations.

In Germany a *Chamber of Physicians* functions along lines similar to the Belgian or French *order* and the British *council.* In each of the provinces or *länder* (about 15 since the reunification of West and East Germany) there is a Chamber of Physicians, to which every physician must belong; the chamber's officers are elected by the physicians. The chamber is responsible for the content of medical education, the requirements for specialty status, and the monitoring of medical ethics. If a physician's behavior has been found to be unethical, the chamber can recommend to the Ministry of Youth, Family Affairs, and Health that licensure be terminated. All policies of the chamber are, in fact, enforced by the Health Office within that ministry.

The monitoring of medical ethics in the United States is a function of the nongovernmental American Medical Association (AMA) and its affiliates in the 50 states. Within the AMA and in most of the state societies there is a *Council on Ethical and Judicial Affairs* or its equivalent. A finding of unethical behavior by a physician may lead to a recommendation to terminate licensure, but the final decision rests with the authority in the state government. Sometimes such a finding may relate simply to an allegation of "unfair competition" (not considered by the state body to be illegal) and the recommendation is rejected.

The countries of Eastern Europe that, until recently, had socialist economic systems have codes of medical ethics that are remarkably similar to those in western capitalist countries. Principles of dedication to the welfare of patients, doing no harm, respecting the confidentiality of medical information, and so on are quite the same as in other industrialized countries. Abortion, however, is not barred, since it is legal. The basic context of medical care is obviously different in socialized health systems, but the ethical principles are the same. In the 1970s, philosophical discussions in Eastern Europe health systems centered around achieving improved quality of service, in contrast to previous emphasis on the quantitative output of health resources.

In most developing countries procedures for surveillance of medical ethics are modeled after those in European countries. Malaysia, with its heritage as a British colony, has a Malaysian General Medical Council with ethical functions, among others. In Thailand, although it was not a British colony, British ideas were influential and there is likewise a Thailand Medical Council; this Council monitors medical ethics and also registers doctors for practice and designates requirements for specialization. There are 25 members of the Thailand Council, of whom 10 are elected by the doctors and 15 are appointed by the Ministry of Health. In Brazil there is a nongovernmental Federal Council of Medical Ethics with disciplinary powers.

In dentistry, pharmacy, nursing, and other health professions, there are sometimes codes of ethics, designed to approximate those in the medical profession. Outside of medical practice, however, ethical issues arise very rarely—although somewhat more often in the industrialized than in developing countries. In the professions or occupations allied to medicine, the ethical issues usually concern actions that are considered outside the legal "scope of practice" of the person.

The substantive content of ethical codes encompasses a very wide range of issues, which cannot be discussed here. However, it might be noted that over the centuries since ancient Greece, ethical precepts have focused mainly on the behavior of doctors in relation to individual patients. Only in recent decades have general social and economic considerations even been proposed in ethical codes. Ethicists have come to consider questions of equity in the provision of health services—to the poor, to the elderly and the dying, to prisoners, to the recalcitrant patient, and to meet health needs in the face of limited resources.

To reflect the broad range of societal considerations in a physician's performance, it is worth taking note of some principles advocated in 1982. The World Medical Association Declaration of Geneva in 1948 started with "(1) I solemnly pledge myself to consecreate my life to the service of humanity." After this, there might be added the following clauses:

2. I will do whatever I can to help my patient and the whole community to prevent disease or injury and to maintain good health.
3. I will respect the dignity of all persons, serving them in accordance with their health needs, irrespective of their personal status or the pecuniary rewards involved.
4. Realizing the greater health problems of the poor, I will make a special effort to respond to their needs.
5. Conscious always that the cost of health care is borne by the people, I will do nothing wasteful or without justification.
6. In spite of the attractions of certain localities, I will serve the people where they live and work, wherever my skills are most needed.
7. I will serve cooperatively with other health workers, in the interests of effective provision of health service.
8. I will cooperate with public authorities in the implementation of health legislation that reflects the democratic decisions of the people.
9. With utmost effort I will attempt to keep myself well informed on advances in medical knowledge.
10. As a socially conscious citizen, I will be alert to health hazards of the environment, join with others to eliminate such hazards, and do everything possible to advance the welfare of all the people.

As of 1990, some of these principles had been included in the ethical codes of some of the developing countries, but none seems to have been adopted in the code of any affluent industrialized country.

Medical Malpractice

An aspect of medical and allied personnel practice, sometimes confused with the question of ethics, is medical malpractice. As medical technology has become more elaborate—with hazards of its misuse—and a democratic appreciation of patient rights has grown, the perceived risk of faulty medical performance has greatly increased. Legal actions against doctors, therefore, have become more frequent, and physicians in many countries have been led to seek insurance against the liability of medical malpractice suits. In the United States—where technology has been especially highly developed, where patients are especially aware of their rights, and where lawyers skillful at litigation are very numerous—liability for medical malpractice has become a prominent issue. Such law suits have become so numerous, and awards by juries to plaintiffs so high, that insurance against malpractice actions offered by commercial insurance companies has become extremely expensive. In some specialties, such as obstetrics and orthopedic surgery, medical malpractice insurance has required premiums of more than $2,000 per month—leading some specialists to change their specialty or quit medical practice entirely.

In the mid-1970s, U.S. malpractice insurance costs were so very much higher than those in Canada and western Europe that comparisons between the different settings of medical practice were invited. In a "letter to the editor" of a large newspaper in 1975, therefore, I offered the following reasons for the spiralling of these insurance premiums in America:

1. With greater sophistication of people, patients are more aware of their rights and no longer consider the doctor as a deity who can do no wrong.

2. Advances in medical science may lead some doctors to attempt procedures of which they are not really capable, and even conscientious medical and hospital policies do not restrict this; moreover, many hospitals are lax about their medical staff regulations.

3. Even the most diligent medical or surgical performance may occasionally lead to an untoward outcome in some patients, for reasons not yet understood by medical science.

4. The spiraling costs of medical care, and frequent inaccessibility of doctors to patients at times of need, has made many patients irritated at or angry with doctors. Studies of malpractice cases nearly always find that, for one reason or another, the patient has become angry with the doctor.

5. Lawyers have become more aggressive in this field of law, especially since medical witnesses for plaintiffs have been easier to find (in contrast to the "cover-up" attitude in the medical brotherhood of past years). Furthermore, contingency fees yield the potential of high earnings for successful lawyers—even if cases are settled out of court. Thus, lawyers find it profitable to fan the flames of patient anger, thereby helping the patient as well as themselves.

6. Trials by jury mean that the general social image of the medical profession is bound to affect the attitudes of jurors. The medical profession's image in recent years, for reasons noted above, has been poor, and this may often lead to extravagant awards against doctors. A correspondingly negative attitude toward large insurance companies doubtless contributes also to the magnitude of these awards. Apprehension about these attitudes often leads insurance carriers to settle claims with substantial awards, even when the likelihood of actual malpractice was very slight.

With respect to the basic framework of law in the United States, compared with that in other industrialized countries, many contrasts could be made:

1. There is a generally less litigious spirit in other nations, the result of more elaborate administrative mechanisms for solving problems.
2. Contingency fees for lawyers are illegal or considered unethical.
3. Jury trials are not used in noncriminal legal actions, such as malpractice.
4. Malpractice protection of doctors is usually provided not by commercial carriers but by *medical protective associations,* which always defend the doctor, if reasonable, and "settle" only when the doctor is deemed clearly culpable.

In combination, these several aspects of the U.S. medical–legal scene lead to the following conclusions about patient care in the U.S. health system, with major implications for malpractice insurance:

1. Much medical care in the United States is felt to be very impersonal, with poor doctor–patient relationships.

2. Surgical operations are performed (with general anesthesia) at very high rates—especially elective procedures—generally higher than in Europe or in previous U.S. history.
3. Most American hospitals have relatively loose medical staff organization.
4. Few formal channels exist in government or in voluntary health insurance programs for redress of grievances.
5. There are angry and often frustrated patients, when high medical costs are combined with failures to cure disorders (not to mention clear-cut harm).
6. The commercial insurance industry usually considers *settlement* of malpractice claims less costly than litigation, which might yield large awards to the plaintiff.
7. American lawyers can expect substantial earnings from either successful court actions for patients or generous insurance settlements.

It was easy to understand, therefore, why malpractice actions were rising rapidly in the United States, and why awards were large, whether by litigation or out-of-court settlement. The extremely high malpractice insurance rates in the United States could be contrasted with those in countries such as Canada or Australia, having comparable cultural heritages. In 1976 the malpractice insurance premiums paid by doctors in those countries averaged about $100 per year, compared to $2,000 to $50,000 per year in America. Some slight rise in premiums was occurring in the British Commonwealth countries and also in Germany, France, and Belgium, but the high premiums in America were unique in the world.

In response to the scandalous premiums for malpractice insurance—the costs of which most doctors simply passed on to their patients in the form of higher fees—many U.S. states undertook reforms of their legislation on torts. Various maximum awards were set, limitations were put on compensation for "general pain and suffering," and so on. No U.S. state, however, went so far as Sweden, which in 1975 converted medical liability into a risk governed by social insurance, that is, awards would be

given for any harm following medical or surgical service, regardless of fault. This is often called *no fault* insurance, and in Sweden it has resulted in a larger number of awards to patients with a smaller average amount of money in each award. New Zealand also has established such social insurance for *all* types of accidents, including those arising out of medical service.

In the late 1980s another medical malpractice insurance "crisis" developed in the United States, as awards to patients rose again and insurance premiums escalated. Studies of commercial insurance financing, however, showed that losses due to poor investment policies were the major cause of premium increases. Several U.S. states set new ceilings on malpractice awards, but fundamental reform of tort legislation toward no fault social insurance remained only a subject for medicolegal discussion. In Great Britain, France, and Germany, with *medical protective associations* rather than commercial companies carrying malpractice insurance, premiums are relatively low. Within these countries, premiums are lowest for doctors in public employment, where malpractice claims are fewer than in private practice.

Legal Status of Traditional Healing

The policies of countries regarding traditional healing or traditional medical practice are embodied in certain health legislation. Analysis of these policies by the World Health Organization, in relation to the status of modern scientific medicine, has identified four broad categories of policies: (1) exclusive policies, where only modern scientific medicine is recognized as lawful; (2) tolerant policies, where only scientific medicine is legally recognized but to some extent traditional practitioners are tolerated by law; (3) inclusive policies, in which traditional forms of medical practice are fully recognized as part of the national health system; and (4) integrated policies, where there is official promotion of integration of traditional and modern medical practice throughout the health system.

Many industrialized countries throughout the world have exclusive policies, which regard any mode of treatment outside modern scientific medicine as illegal. Such policies prevail in France, Italy, Scandinavian countries, Japan, Australia, Canada, and some U.S. states. During the first half of the twentieth century, the colonial governments of European powers often established similar legal policies in their colonies (before national independence). Some former colonies, even after independence, such as Algeria, continued these exclusive policies. In the 1970s, many newly independent countries changed these restrictive medical policies. In the Soviet Union and socialist countries influenced by it, the practice of medicine by unqualified persons has been specifically barred and is punishable under law.

Tolerant attitudes toward traditional forms of healing are found in a few industrialized countries and in several developing countries. In Germany, a tradition of *lay healing* has survived since prior to 1914 and was strengthened by a law passed in 1939 (under the Nazis) licensing *lay health practitioners.* (Such practitioners, however, were not permitted to be paid under the official health insurance program, or to treat communicable diseases or handle childbirths.) In Great Britain, only registered medical practitioners who are scientifically qualified may serve under the National Health Service, serve in public hospitals, and so on, but in the private sector homeopaths, acupuncturists, Ayurvedic practitioners, and others may practice. These alternative practitioners are barred from certain functions, such as treating children under 8 years of age or treating communicable disease in anyone. In many states of the United States, chiropractors are fully licensed, as long as their treatment is directed to disorders of the spinal column; naturopaths have also been permitted under the patient's Constitutional right to privacy.

In the developing countries, tolerant policies toward traditional healing have been permitted in practice—if not under specific laws—because of the general shortages of scientifically trained physicians. In Paraguay, the Ministry of Health must license *empiricos en salud* in any areas where this is deemed necessary. Argentina and Uruguay permit herbalists to sell their compounds, as long as their shops have been authorized.

In Africa, several countries have set up research institutes to test the benefits of traditional medications and, along with these, have been tolerant in granting traditional herbalists the right to practice. This is the policy in Mali, Burkina Faso, and elsewhere. In Mauritania, Togo, Burundi, Uganda, and Sierre Leone, traditional practitioners are explicitly authorized, if they "carry out treatments and administer drugs in accordance with usage and custom." In Lesotho, traditional practitioners are registered and then permitted to carry out "natural therapeutics," which is defined to encompass the practices of naturopaths, homeopaths, acupuncturists, chiropractors, and others; these practitioners are barred only from giving injections or performing surgery. Swaziland also registers "natural therapeutic practitioners," defining their scope of nonsurgical practice. Zimbabwe has especially comprehensive legislation, enacted in 1981, for registration and regulation of *traditional medical practitioners;* any illness of body or mind may be treated, including the use of "spiritual" methods, but excluding any surgical procedure. Several African countries have established national associations of traditional healers, which have even promoted ethical codes for their members.

Malaysia is one Asian country with tolerant policies toward traditional healers; such persons may practice "systems of therapeutics or surgery (sic) according to purely Malay, Chinese, Indian or other native methods and to recover reasonable charges in respect of such practice." This law was enacted in 1971 and was clearly responsive to the general interethnic group conflicts in that country.

The third category of health policies toward traditional healing has been termed *inclusive,* and is found in large countries of Southern Asia. Arising principally in India, special doctrines for diagnosis and treatment are not merely tolerated, but are recognized as entirely proper and legitimate features of the national health system, with a substantial role in every community and support from government. In addition to India, inclusive policies prevail in Pakistan, Bangladesh, Sri Lanka, Burma, Thailand, Indonesia, Hong Kong, and Democratic Kampuchea.

The major healing doctrine in all these Asian countries is based on Ayurvedic concepts originating in ancient Hindu culture, probably before the birth of Christ. Over the years, Ayurvedic doctrines have changed and given rise to modified forms, know as Siddha and Unani. Herbal medications now predominate in all the Hindu fields. These practitioners are educated in schools requiring 5 years of study (after primary or middle school); if the school meets Ministry of Health standards it is subsidized by the government, and the graduates are officially registered. Yet there are also thousands of unregistered practitioners. Legislation in all the Indian States regulates the practice, as well as teaching and research, of Ayurvedic medicine. Similar laws may apply also to homeopathy. To distinguish these practices from modern scientific medicine, the latter is often called *allopathy*. Inclusive policies in Indonesia are similar to those in India, although they are not supported by much explicit legislation.

The fourth type of health policy, which aims to integrate traditional and modern medicine throughout the national health system, is confined essentially to China, with some partial implementation in North Korea and Nepal. In the world's largest country, China, the official strategy is to employ both traditional and modern doctors in hospitals, polyclinics, and other facilities. The two types of doctor are expected to work together in treating patients. Even the secondary-level village doctors (formerly *barefoot doctors*) are taught about traditional drugs as well as modern drugs in their period of training. Health policies have changed significantly in China over the years, with changes in the larger political scene. The integrated policy still prevails officially, although since 1980 and the policy of *four modernizations,* it has had lesser emphasis.

In all countries that grant any legitimacy to traditional healing, and even in some of those that deny this, there is active discussion about the merits and problems that come from such legitimation. It is argued that modern scientific medicine is only one approach to disease, and other competing theories should be free to serve people. The elaborate technology of much scientific medicine has created the im-

pression that the human and personal needs of patients are often ignored, while the traditional practitioner takes a *holistic* approach. This issue of sensitivity to the personal feelings of patients has given rise to still other legislation, such as that for development of *family medicine* as a medical specialty, and the scientific training of various types of auxiliary health personnel.

One form of traditional practitioner, the traditional birth attendant (TBA), is the subject of much health legislation. A WHO survey in 1979 reported that 33 developing countries registered or licensed TBAs, including 8 in South Asia, 3 in the Middle East, 10 in Africa, and 12 in Latin America. In many of these countries, the Ministry of Health attempts to identify and train TBAs in hygienic methods as a prelude to registration. Even in developing countries without legislation, however, the delivery of babies by TBAs in rural areas is commonplace, and legal prosecution is rare.

In 1983 a more strictly legal review of actual laws on TBAs yielded a more restricted world picture. Under the "black letter" of the law, in most countries service by TBAs is illegal, but in practice their activities are generally approved "by custom and usage." Legal regulation, therefore, has usually been opposed by communities, and has in any case been almost impossible to enforce. The formal legislation on TBAs in countries has been found to fall under one of five patterns:

1. TBAs are illegal and have no right to practice under any circumstances; this pattern is found in Syria and Turkey.
2. TBAs are prohibited in any locality where a trained midwife is available—found in the Philippines.
3. TBAs have no legal status, but can practice in their own communities—the pattern in Nigeria, Rwanda, Zaire, and Zambia.
4. TBA practice is regulated by the government health authority, and practitioners are informally recognized. This pattern is widespread in Latin America (e.g., Belize, Brazil, Colombia, Costa Rica, Guatemala, Haiti, and Peru) and elsewhere (e.g., Chad, Malaysia, the Philippines, and Western Samoa).

5. TBAs have legal status, with authority to practice under prescribed conditions—as in Mexico and Liberia.

These five legal patterns should not be interpreted rigidly, because their exact meanings vary among countries. The meaning of terms such as *recognized, registered, certified,* and so on may be quite different in various countries. Perhaps the only valid generalization about legislation on TBAs would be that many developing countries have policies for *managing* TBAs that are intended to respond realistically to local health needs in light of the limited personnel resources available.

REGULATION OF HEALTH FACILITIES

Regulations and laws on facilities or structures, within which health service is provided, are not so abundant as those governing health personnel, but they have been expanding throughout the world. Most detailed is the legislation affecting hospitals, but there are also measures on facilities for long-term care, for ambulatory care (health centers), for laboratory work, and for other health purposes. Broadly speaking, these controls are concerned with (1) construction of facilities and their capacity, (2) the factors affecting quality of service in facilities, and (3) both quantity and quality aspects of facilities.

Laws on the licensure of hospitals, which exist in almost all countries, apply ordinarily to established as well as newly constructed facilities, although they tend to be more rigorously enforced for new buildings. The older such laws in European countries often applied only to public hospitals and focused on physical aspects, such as the space-per-bed and sanitation resources. Since about 1950, these laws have come to apply to both public and private facilities, and they are concerned with features of hospital operation (for example, laboratory equipment or resources for emergency care) as well as physical features. The main objective of such regulation, of course, is to protect patients served in the hospital.

A French ministerial order in 1982, for example, established a Commission on Stan-

dards for the Equipment and Operation of Public and Private Hospital Establishments. This commission was made responsible for developing minimum technical operating standards and minimum equipment standards, to be met by all hospitals, to ensure patients the quality of care required by their condition, and to ensure that hospital personnel were working in a proper environment.

In the United States, as well as other federated countries, hospital licensure laws are enacted by the various states. In New York State, for example, a 1969 law contains detailed provisions on hospital construction, financial reporting, and many aspects of patient care in both public and private facilities. Among other things, this statute requires complete evaluation of all patients periodically, full-time medical staffing in emergency departments, policies on surgical consultation, and prompt admission of patients in extreme need of care "without advance inquiry as to their ability to pay." Many other U.S. states have enacted similar legislation, so that hospital licensure laws have moved far beyond standards for bricks and mortar.

In developing countries laws on hospital licensure tend to be less demanding. In some, such as the Philippine Republic, the statutory language may be quite comprehensive, but the enforcement is weak. Enforcement is usually very weak with respect to public hospitals. In government facilities, conditions may be seriously overcrowded (with two patients lying in one bed), but enforcement is left up to the same Ministry of Health as operates the hospital, so that little is done to correct deficiencies.

Implementation of hospital licensure laws is ordinarily assigned to the major government health authority at national or provincial level. Personnel for making inspections, however—even in affluent industrialized countries—are seldom adequate in numbers and in background knowledge. Hence, effective enforcement usually occurs only when a deficiency in hospital performance has had a scandalous outcome, such as occurred in 1987 when 14 patients in an Indian hospital were fatally poisoned due to irresponsible management. Equivalent tragedies have occurred in many countries, and they often lead to more rigorous enforcement of hospital licensure standards— for a while.

In the strongly free-market economic setting of the United States, a contentious issue has developed around the question of the proper supply of hospital beds in a community. The issue is formulated as *competition versus regulation* as the major determinant of policy. Studies in the 1950s and 1960s showed, however, that in states with very different supplies of hospital beds the occupancy levels were approximately the same, that is, the hospitals in states with 3.0 beds per 1,000 people, for example, were not more crowded than were hospitals in states with 6.0 beds per 1,000. Under widespread economic support (through insurance or tax funds) for care, in other words, whatever hospital beds were built soon came to be used. This finding (often called Roemer's Law) led to state legislation requiring the establishment of "public need" for more hospital beds, before new construction was authorized by a state health authority. In 1966, such a policy became nationwide in the United States, so that regulation came to replace competition in determining a "proper" supply of hospital beds in each state.

As the costs of hospital care rose everywhere in the world, after World War II most industrialized countries established similar public controls over new hospital construction or the expansion of old hospitals. Such controls became necessary to safeguard the solvency of social insurance funds, and they were usually simply incorporated in the hospital insurance laws. In developing countries, where hospital beds were usually in short supply, such legal constraints on new construction were seldom applied.

Facilities and services for emergency care are mandated by law in certain industrialized countries. In France, for example, the Hospital Reform Law of 1970 specifies that public hospitals are responsible for *emergency care,* including mobile means of providing such care. Similar legislation in Belgium outlines the obligations of public ambulance services to transport persons to appropriate hospitals. The hospitals are also obliged to admit such persons promptly "without any prior formalities."

In Finland, the Act on Municipal General Hospitals specifies that such hospitals must send emergency teams to the place of an accident and transport victims to the hospital, as necessary. In Norway, the law requires that every hospital and maternity ward must have medical staff on duty at all hours of the day and night, to provide immediate emergency medical service if needed.

The British National Health Service initially included ambulance services in the responsibilities of established local units of government (counties, boroughs, and county councils). In the reorganization of 1974, ambulance services were transferred to *area health authorities,* along with the other types of health service. Ambulances are expected to contribute to normal outpatient as well as emergency care.

Other types of health facility regulation focus on special features, such as laboratories, or on special services, such as the intensive care of newborn babies. The Hospitals Act of the Netherlands, for example, requires a special license from the Ministry of Health for laboratories measuring radioactive isotopes. Legislation on clinical laboratories in Belgium has been designed to reduce commercialization of these services by requiring special qualifications of laboratory directors or operation on a nonprofit basis. Similar rather stringent rules for medical laboratories have been legislated in Morocco.

The establishment and design of health centers for ambulatory care have not been the subject of much formal legislation. Such facilities are established by countries simply under the general responsibility of governments to protect the public health. The same applies to worldwide policies on the regionalized planning and operation of health facilities. Regionalization has been a strategy for attaining efficiency in the provision of complex types of medical care to populations—especially when they are spread over large rural areas.

LEGISLATION ON HEALTH PROMOTION

In addition to laws on communicable disease control and environmental sanitation, the earliest legislation directed toward the general promotion of health in a population applied to pregnant women and small children. Special clinics for newborn infants, for distribution of safe cow's milk, and for the examination of expectant mothers were set up in Europe and North America for many years in the nineteenth century, before legislation on maternal and child health (MCH) service was enacted in the twentieth century.

Maternal and Child Health Services

As early as 1860, a French physician advocated a special branch of hygiene devoted to promoting the health of infants and children. Under the term *puericulture,* knowledge about the nutrition and development of small children was extended in France, Germany, and England. In France, infant consultation centers were widely established, growing to 497 by 1907. These clinics were set up under the authority of local (municipal) public health agencies. Great Britain enacted a Maternity and Child Welfare Act in 1918. In the United States the Sheppard–Towner Act of 1921 authorized federal grants to the states to finance the establishment of well-baby clinics and prenatal clinics for expectant mothers. Although this U.S. legislation was terminated in 1929 because of opposition from the organized medical profession, it was reinstated in 1935 as a section of the U.S. Social Security Act. Recognition of the importance of this MCH legislation was underscored by its definition as a special *title* within the Social Security Act, separate from all the other provisions for federal public health grants to the states.

Since the end of World War II, MCH legislation has become a standard feature of the health laws of virtually every country. Under official policies, the provision of routine examinations, with immunizations, nutritional counselling, and often treatment of minor illness, has become a prominent service given at community health centers and small health stations everywhere. Several countries have enacted legislation defining MCH services very broadly, to encompass not only the health protection of infants and mothers, but also the health of school children, adolescents, the ex-

tension of family planning, and the education of health personnel on these matters.

In Italy, for example, a Regional Law of 1979 calls for general preventive health services to mothers and children, multidisciplinary specialized services, emergency obstetric and neonatological care, refresher training for pediatric personnel, and encouragement of breast-feeding. Legislation in Bolivia details requirements for MCH services at primary, secondary, and tertiary levels. The quality of care by traditional birth attendants and *health promoters* is regulated. Agencies providing this care must be licensed and supervised by the national Ministry of Health. Mothers are ensured legal protection during their reproductive life and the "internationally recognized rights of children" are protected.

Family Planning Service

Since the post-World War II recognition of world population problems, legislation on family planning has acquired special importance. In certain countries, especially where Catholicism is a dominant religion, contraceptive practices were long considered immoral, and even prohibited by law. When Margaret Sanger organized a clinic in Brooklyn, New York, to offer women advice on *birth control,* she was arrested and sent to prison. This was in 1916, but by 1923 a U.S. National Committee on Federal Legislation for Birth Control was formed, and by 1937 laws permitting contraceptive education and practices were enacted in most U.S. states. Restrictive legislation on contraception continued in Latin America and other predominantly Catholic countries for many years. The French law of 1920, for example, prohibited the advertising of contraception and was held by a French court to bar the distribution of contraceptives as well. This law was not modified until 1967 and again in 1974 to permit the sale of contraceptives for certain cases. In all countries, the protection of the mother's health and of family welfare is the major reason for laws on family planning.

In most Francophone countries of Africa, the old French 1920 law restricting contraception has still remained technically in place, although it is not enforced. Tunisia legalized the sale of contraceptives in 1961. In Latin America, contraceptive practices were prohibited by law in Mexico and Brazil, until after World War II. Since 1950, Mexico, Chile, and Ecuador passed laws that integrate family planning (FP) services into the regular MCH programs.

In India the growth of population has been so great a problem that the very name of the National Ministry of Health was broadened around 1970 to Ministry of Health and Family Welfare. Indonesia, Sri Lanka, and Australia all promote FP services, but they still have laws restricting the importation or advertisement of contraceptives. The Philippines is a predominantly Roman Catholic country that only recently repealed a former legal ban on importing contraceptives. Legal changes to eliminate prescription requirements for oral contraceptives have broadened FP services in Pakistan, and contraceptive pill distribution by auxiliary personnel has been legalized in South Korea.

In Europe, a Swedish law of 1946 required all pharmacies to sell contraceptives. Laws in several European countries require medical prescriptions for oral contraceptives, and require that intrauterine devices be inserted only by a physician. Legal restrictions against the distribution of contraceptives were long in effect in Spain, Portugal, and Ireland. In the Islamic countries of the Middle East, there are no legal prohibitions of FP services.

Sound Nutrition

The hygienic aspects of food preparation and distribution are included in much sanitary legislation, but the promotion of a balanced diet and sound nutrition is not customarily a matter of law. Legal provision for maximum levels of food preservatives or the iodization of salt to prevent goiter are more common. In 1983, the World Health Organization adoption of an International Code on Marketing of Breast-Milk Substitutes led many countries to enact legislation implementing the code; these laws restricted the sale of infant formula products that would discourage breast-feeding. Although the International Code was issued in the form of a recommendation, rather than a regulation, it has had substantial influence on

the marketing of manufactured breast-milk substitutes in developing countries.

A comprehensive approach to national nutrition policy, embodied in law, was enacted in Norway in 1976. Pursuant to this, a Food Control Board was established in 1980, with representatives of several ministries on it. Also a National Nutrition Council was formed, composed of experts on nutrition, dietetics, food production, and the food industry. Working together, these bodies influence nutritional education, policies on food production, marketing of food to consumers, school feeding programs, and so on.

The general Public Health Law of Iraq devotes a major section to legislative intent and strategies for achieving a balanced diet for all citizens. The Ministry of Health is required, among other things, "to carry out surveillance of the nutritional components of meals served in creches, kindergartens, schools, factories, hospitals, convalescent homes, homes for the elderly, and other places specified by the Ministry." A similarly broad law in Zaire establishes a National Center for the Planning of Human Nutrition, with equivalent responsibilities.

Critical to improved nutrition, of course, is financial support for food needed by families of low income. The government provision of a ration of rice to all families in Sri Lanka in the 1950s and 1960s (later limited to low-income families) was an outstanding demonstration of such a policy. In the United States, the Food Stamp Program enabled low-income families to purchase selected foods at low prices from 1961 to 1975; later a similar strategy was followed in the Special Supplemental Food Program for Women, Infants, and Children.

Closely related to nutrition are legislative enactments on the fluoridation of water supplies to prevent dental caries. When this preventive measure was first introduced in the 1940s, based on epidemiological observations in the United States, it encountered great opposition. Laws or regulations on fluoridation of public water supplies became subject to popular referenda and, in the face of false and frightening propaganda, were often voted down.

A worldwide review of legislation on fluoridation of public water supplies in 1983 showed that about 50 countries had such laws affecting some parts of the their populations. In most of these countries, the legislation was enabling (authorizing governments to undertake water fluoridation), but in seven countries (or provinces within those countries) it was mandatory. The earliest statute requiring fluoridation of public water supplies throughout a country was in Ireland in 1960. Argentina passed a similar law in 1975, and such action has also been taken in certain provinces of Canada and states of the United States. Where many people are not reached by public water supplies, legislation has authorized the manufacture and distribution of fluoridated salt and other such strategies; this has been done in Switzerland, Hungary, Mexico, and Colombia. Still another approach has been to pass regulations authorizing the fluoridation of school water supplies or the topical application of fluorides to the teeth of school children; this has been done in the United States, Switzerland, and parts of Yugoslavia.

Legislation Against Use of Tobacco

The most extensive legislation for health promotion throughout the world has probably been that directed against the use of tobacco. Recognition of the injurious effects of smoking on health can be traced to 1938, but legislation to combat smoking for health reasons was not enacted until the 1960s. As summarized in the WHO study on *Legislative Action to Combat the World Smoking Epidemic,*

> Stimulated by mounting evidence of the relation between lung cancer and cardiovascular diseases and smoking, various countries then began to enact legislation. In 1962, Italy became the first country in Western Europe to prohibit advertising of tobacco—although this early law may have been dictated not so much by health considerations as by commercial considerations. . . . In 1965, the USA passed its federal cigarette Labeling and Advertising Act. . . . In 1970 and in the years that followed, country after country took action by legislation or voluntary agreement with the tobacco industry to require warning notices, to restrict advertising, to set upper

limits on tar and nicotine, and to ban smoking in public places.

Since 1970, the legislative attack on the "world smoking epidemic" has gained momentum in every part of the globe. The laws enacted fall into two main groups: those directed against the supply of tobacco and those seeking to reduce the demand. On the supply side, there are laws that (1) control the advertising and sales promotion of tobacco products, (2) require health warnings and disclosure of tar and nicotine contents on cigarette packages, (3) control the level of tar and nicotine in cigarettes, (4) put restrictions on places of sale to adults, and (5) abolish economic subsidies and encourage crop substitution.

On the demand side, antitobacco legislation attempts to modify smoking behavior by (1) imposing taxes and increasing prices, (2) restricting smoking in public places, (3) banning smoking in the workplace, (4) prohibiting sales to young people, and (5) mandating health education against smoking.

By 1990, legislation against smoking had been enacted in 91 countries. These included all of the industrialized countries and a large share of the developing countries. It is noteworthy that the earliest legislation of comprehensive scope—banning all advertising, smoking in public places, and so on—was enacted in Finland, Norway, and Iceland; these are all countries with comprehensive types of national health system. In general, the antitobacco legislation enacted before 1975 was categorical, with specific strategies. After 1975 this legislation was more comprehensive in scope and usually stronger in its impact. In certain countries, voluntary agreements with the tobacco industry had been relied on, but this policy has been largely abandoned everywhere except in Great Britain. Complete bans on all types of tobacco advertising have been established in 27 countries.

Since tobacco has been found to play a substantial role in the pathogenesis of cancer and cardiovascular disease, legislation against it is doubtless one of the major strategies for health promotion in the modern world. As the growth of new smokers has declined in the industrialized countries, the multinational tobacco companies have directed increasing efforts to spread the lethal smoking habit to the developing countries. With leadership from the World Health Organization, this irresponsible tactic is being opposed with education and national legislation.

Other Legislation on Health Promotion

Directly or indirectly other types of legislation contribute to the promotion of people's health. Regulations establishing bicycle lanes on city streets contribute to both safety and beneficial exercise. Regulations on the sale and advertising of alcoholic beverages have some effect on alcohol consumption—along with drunken driving, disease of the liver, and so on. In many countries there are laws that prohibit advertisements in which liquor is associated with attributes of virility, of femininity, or with generally pleasurable experiences. Policies on the education of children and youth about sexual behavior have many ultimate impacts on health.

Numerous laws and regulations affect the health and well-being of elderly people. There are laws creating national agencies to plan and implement a wide range of health-related services for the elderly. Legislation may establish *senior centers* to facilitate socialization among the aged, *meals on wheels* to enable frail elderly to live at home, special inpatient facilities for the elderly, and so on. A Mexican law of 1979 established a National Institute for the Elderly, and a similar 1978 law in Venezuela created a National Institute of Geriatrics and Gerontology. In France a decree in 1982 set up a National Committee on Retired and Elderly Persons to advise the Ministry of Health on such matters. An Italian Law in 1981 makes regional authorities responsible for special services to promote the well-being of persons over 60 years of age.

In the United States, legislation in 1974 established a National Institute on Aging for health research. In 1981 the Older Americans Act of 1965 was amended to provide financial support for coordinated long-term care for elderly persons with "special emphasis upon services designed to support alternatives to institutional living." A 1982 law of Japan defines a

comprehensive scope of health care for the elderly, including disease prevention, medical treatment, functional training, and domiciliary care. In Finland, legislation of 1983 on domiciliary care of the aged provides that the patient's surroundings "should be such that he feels secure, at home, and stimulated, and furthermore (should) permit privacy and promote his rehabilitation, initiative, and ability to cope."

LEGISLATION ON FINANCING HEALTH SYSTEMS

Legislation providing for taxation to support health activities is essential in all countries, although it is seldom earmarked or identified in this way. The strategies for collecting taxes on land, on personal or corporate income, on the general sale of products, on the sale of special products (e.g., liquor or tobacco), or on other economic transactions permeate the entire structure of national, provincial, or local law.

There are fundamental laws, of course, on tax collection and special laws on the allocation of funds for health purposes. Laws establishing social security or social insurance programs have special meaning for health systems, insofar as this form of taxation usually sets up special trust funds usable only for selected purposes, such as old-age pensions or health services. Money from these funds may be invested in other fields, from which the interest earned adds further financial support. Social insurance financing has the special attribute of setting aside money that is not in competition with other requirements of government, such as transportation or military defense.

In many countries the authorization of public expenditures for certain health purposes is the subject of one law, whereas the actual appropriation of money requires separate legislation each year. Government expenditures may be used for services provided in the public sector (i.e., by public providers) or in the private sector (by private providers). Regulation of the methods of payment or reimbursement tend to be greater when services are rendered in the private sector. Health expenditures from a social security fund, however, are usually regulated by policies of the social security organization, whereas expenditures made from general revenues are subject to parliamentary law or central government decree.

When a social security program operates, its major objects of support are usually the curative health services. General tax revenues are the commonest source of support for community preventive services, for medical and allied education, and for health sciences research.

Health expenditures have been rising throughout the world both absolutely and as a percentage of national wealth. In Chapter 9, we reviewed the various strategies employed for cost containment, and each of these is usually the subject of some regulation or legislation. On the supply side, there are regulations on the supply of health resources (such as hospital beds), on payment to hospitals by prospective budgetary amounts, on negotiated medical fee schedules, on the use of generic drugs, and so on. On the demand side, there are regulations imposing copayment obligations on patients, on requiring referral by a general practitioner for access to a specialist, and so on. In developing countries, the direct reduction of governmental health budgets is the customary means for reducing expenditures. Private spending may then compensate for government cutbacks partially but never completely.

HEALTH SYSTEM REGULATION

Many of the laws already discussed concern the regulation of aspects of health systems, and here we may note their general scope.

Reporting

To provide guidance to the national health leadership, virtually every country has laws and regulations on the reporting of several vital events and the collection of vital statistics. Most fundamental is the reporting of births and deaths, and often of the occurrence of marriages and divorces. All industrialized countries and many developing countries require the reporting to local authorities of many (though seldom all) communicable diseases, and similar requirements may apply to certain occupational diseases, to cancer, to gunshot wounds, to child abuse, and selected other disorders.

The procedures for collection and public reporting of vital statistics depend on the general structure of government in a country. Initial reporting is usually made to a local unit of government, from which the information is typically sent along to a higher unit. Most countries—whether they are federated or not—have provinces or other subdivisions that collect vital data, which is passed along to a central national authority. There it is typically analyzed and published, so that everyone can learn about the national population and its health. Successive reports show the trends over time for population and for specific causes of death and communicable diseases.

Laws may also define the requirements for a periodic total count or census of the population, and regulations may specify the type of information to be gathered in a census. In the United States the first decennial census was conducted in 1790, and this count was deemed so important that it was embodied in the U.S. Constitution. Earlier provisions for a national census were made in Canada in 1666 and in Sweden in 1749. Over the years almost all countries have enacted laws on census enumerations, and the specific information to be collected. This may include data on a physical disability such as blindness.

Laws or regulations generally define the information to be recorded on death certificates. Since the mid-nineteenth century, for example, death certificates in Great Britain have been required to record the occupation of the head-of-family, which has permitted epidemiological research on disease prevalence in relation to social class. The death certificates in developing countries usually provide important data on deaths occurring inside or outside of hospitals and deaths unattended by a physician. These requirements are often stipulated in the regulations of a Ministry of Health, and they may also be specified under the obligation of police authorities to report on deaths occurring in public places.

Planning

The planning of health resources and services is a further subject of health system legislation. Since the initiation of Socialist 5-year plans in the Soviet Union in 1928, many countries—especially the developing ones—have designed such periodic plans for the health system, but this strategy was seldom crystallized in legislation. After World War II, much health planning was included in legislation on hospitals and the numbers of beds to be constructed in an area. The incorporation of such controls over hospital bed supply in the facility licensure laws has been noted earlier.

Health planning legislation has played a larger part in developing countries since the late 1970s, when worldwide policy under WHO leadership shifted priorities to emphasize primary health care (PHC). Various administrative mechanisms were specified in law to ensure stronger budgetary provision for PHC and to train various types of auxiliary health personnel to render such care. The training of health guides in India and of various other types of community health workers in numerous countries has often arisen from the recommendations of health planning bodies, and has then been implemented by regulations of a Ministry of Health.

Decentralization

In developing countries, with a history usually of strong central colonial governments, democratization has often been implemented by a policy of decentralizing authority. Legislation to decentralize health system management to provinces or districts is often difficult to carry out. Local personnel must be educated for the tasks of governance, supervision, and handling and distributing money prudently. Regulations must be quite explicit to ensure equity and fiscal solvency to the end of each budget period. Decentralized decision makers must learn where to draw the line between the application of central policy and adaptations to meet local needs. In huge countries such as China or India, management of health affairs by the provinces or states is logistically neces-sary, but the issue of decentralization applies to governance even below the level of the province.

To implement decentralization of health authority and to enhance democratic inputs generally, the World Health Organization has advocated maximum participation by community people. In contrast to conventional domination of health systems by physicians and other providers of service, community participation stresses the voice of consumers in the formulation of policies and their implementation.

The 1974 reorganization of the British National Health Service established *community health councils* to offer advice to NHS administrators at all levels. In the health system of Yugoslavia, much authority was delegated to *Self-Managing Communities of Interest* (SMCIs), representing both health workers and consumers of health service. These SMCIs were responsible for coordinating hospitals and health centers, for planning new construction, and for allocating money from the social insurance fund or government revenue. Legislation has modified SMCI functions over the years, but the voice of consumers remains strong.

An especially significant example of legislation promoting community involvement is the 1983 New Zealand law on *area health boards* to coordinate hospital boards and district public health offices. The objective was to call on all agencies to be concerned with health promotion as well as the treatment of illness. The area health boards are required also to coordinate the planning, provision, and evaluation of health services rendered by public, private, and voluntary agencies. Most of the members of these boards are elected by the general population. In the health legislation of many countries on the care of the elderly or on services for the mentally ill, citizen advisory committees are required. In the 1980s, Mexico passed important legislation providing for decentralization of health services and facilities to the state governments.

Intersectoral collaboration—that is, cooperative relations between health and other social sectors—is another principle advocated by WHO in the management of health systems.

This is often shown in the multiministerial membership specified by law in various planning, coordinating, or policy-making bodies. It is conspicuous in the field of environmental health protection and in campaigns to combat complex social problems such as drug abuse, alcoholism, or prostitution.

LEGAL PROTECTION OF INDIVIDUAL RIGHTS

Legislation on the protection of populations, on health promotion, on financing health systems, and even on other matters has obvious implications for the protection of individual rights. Beyond such general legal assurances, there are a number of specific laws intended to protect individual rights in special circumstances, where they might be abridged.

The provision of medical care, especially in surgical interventions, is often associated with certain rights of the patient. A procedure that is nearly always helpful may sometimes result in harm, even death. To cope with this issue, the laws of many countries require that patients be properly informed of the possible consequences of any medical procedure and the degree of hazard involved. All industrialized countries have enacted such legislation, and it is gradually being introduced in the developing countries.

To ensure that this "informed consent" has been obtained, hospitals have routinely included consent forms in the patient's medical record. The legal requirement that the patient's informed consent must be given prior to a surgical or other intervention is expressed in various statutes. In Austria, for example, it is in the Basic Hospital Law; in Denmark, it is in the Practice of Medicine Act; in the Netherlands it is in the Health Provision Act; in Sweden it is in the Health and Medical Care Act for public patients and in the Supervision of Health and Medical Personnel Act for private patients. In Hungary the Public Health Act requires informed consent for surgery and invasive diagnostic techniques.

Closely related are legal requirements for protecting the patient's privacy and the general confidentiality of medical information. The confidentiality or secrecy of medical information is usually affirmed in ethical codes as well as in law, although in some countries—such as Great Britain and Ireland—it is only in ethical codes and court decisions. In France professional secrecy is governed by penal law and administrative regulations (a fact that has inhibited various attempts to monitor the quality of medical care in health insurance programs). Medical secrecy is also specifically mentioned in the criminal law of Germany and Greece. In the states of the United States, the courts generally respect the confidentiality of medical information, based simply on ethical principles, whether or not relevant statutes exist. The same is true in most developing countries, although there this issue seldom arises.

A highly contentious issue of individual rights in many countries is the legal status of *abortion* of an unwanted pregnancy. Since the interruption of pregnancy is contrary to certain religious doctrines, especially in the Catholic faith, the procedure was legally banned for centuries. During the last half-century, however, as women's rights have become more widely established, these policies embodied in laws have changed, and abortion has become legal under various circumstances.

As of 1990, a worldwide survey of 132 countries with over one million population showed that legislation on abortion had four degrees of permissiveness. The least permissive or most restrictive laws existed in 53 countries, where laws permitted abortion only to save the life of a pregnant woman. These countries—mainly in Africa, southern Asia, and Latin America—had 25 percent of the world's population. In 42 other countries, with 12 percent of the world's population, abortions were legally permitted for various reasons related to the woman's health. This included abortion for anticipated genetic defects in the baby and for pregnancies resulting from rape or incest.

Another 14 countries with 23 percent of the world's population had much more permissive laws, permitting abortion for social and sociomedical reasons; these typically involved family welfare. Finally, there were 23 countries, with 40 percent of the world population, with the most permissive laws—allowing abortion essentially on the request of the woman. These included the world's most populous countries, China, the United States, and the Soviet Union; they also included about half of the European countries.

The last two sets of countries, with the most liberal abortion legislation, reflect societies in which the law has shifted from a focus on criminality to a concern for the rights and health of women and family well-being. The statutes, of course, are seldom as simple as the above categories might suggest, because there are usually also provisions on the maximum weeks of pregnancy, the setting for abortion procedures, and so on. The trend, however, has been to eliminate previous requirements for approval by hospital abortion committees, to grant immediate permission during the first 12 weeks of pregnancy, and to cover abortion costs under health insurance or social security programs. In the United States, abortions have come to be widely performed outside of hospitals (reducing costs and increasing access), and this practice has been adopted in other countries. Once abortion laws are liberalized, attempts to reinstate restrictions have usually failed, although in the United States such regressive actions have succeeded at the national level and in selected states.

Another type of legislation affecting individual rights is that concerning *involuntary commitment of patients to mental hospitals.* Since mental hospital admission may deprive patients of freedom against their will, admission of persons to them was long a judicial process. Laws on involuntary commitment of patients to mental hospitals, stressing judicial procedures, had been enacted in the middle of the nineteenth century. When drug therapy and other psychiatric developments changed the whole medical environment of mental hospitals in the 1950s, laws in many countries were changed to transform commitment from a judicial to a medical process. Great Britain enacted one of the earliest such laws in 1959, when the British Mental Health Act converted the great majority of mental hospital admissions to *informal*—in the same sense as admission to a general hospital.

In the mid-1970s the World Health Organization conducted a worldwide survey of mental health legislation to determine changes influenced by the new methods of admission, the new psychotherapeutic drugs, and other new forms of psychotherapy. The emphasis in Europe and elsewhere was clearly shifting from large mental hospitals toward active mental health services in communities. Insofar as hospital admission was legally defined, it was to be an informal or a voluntary process for the great majority of cases in most countries. The concept of *commitment to an insane asylum* was changing everywhere to *admission to a mental hospital.* For the minority of cases requiring involuntary hospitalization, judicial procedures were provided, designed to protect the individual rights of the patient. Mental health legislation was inevitably becoming harmonized with the global movement—after the defeat of fascism—for the protection of individual human rights.

Finally, a general right of individuals to health care may be explicitly defined in law, although more often it is implied by the provision of health care resources, the enactment of social insurance programs, the existence of public assistance for medical care of the poor, and so on. In some countries, however, a right to health care is spelled out in the Constitution—as in Italy, Ireland, Hungary, Poland, the Soviet Union, and Yugoslavia. In the Netherlands a new Constitution was adopted in 1982, in which health care and environmental protection are formulated as fundamental social rights. This was done also in the Spanish Constitution of 1978. The United States Constitution makes no reference to health or health care, but legislation on health care may be enacted under the police power of the states, and at the federal level under two limited delegated powers—to regulate interstate commerce and to tax and spend for the general welfare.

Specific laws in Finland, Greece, and Morocco also guarantee citizens a right to health care. In Sweden, the Health and Medical Care Act of 1982 affirms that entitlement to health and medical care is a social right, and declares that county governments are obligated to provide such care. In the laws and Constitution of many developing countries, the right of citizens to health care is frequently stated, but this has come to be regarded as a general intention rather than a legal reality.

We have reviewed seven major types of health regulation or legislation that have been developed in national health systems, classified according to their main objectives: (1) protection of populations, (2) regulation of health personnel, (3) regulation of health facilities, (4) legislation on health promotion, (5) legislation on financing health systems, (6) health system regulation, and (7) legal protection of individual rights. In all of these fields, the worldwide trends have been toward increasingly explicit legislation to clarify and strengthen policies and their implementation.

The overall trends have been toward the enactment of laws that ensure equity in the operation of health systems. Beyond equitable distribution of services is the objective of ensuring high quality care through regulation of personnel, facilities, drugs, and other resources. As instrumentalities for attaining both equity and quality, there are countless legal strategies for health system financing. And when health expenditures have seemed excessive, other procedures have been introduced by law to control or contain the costs.

Some observers are cynical about the value of health legislation, pointing out that laws may be poorly enforced and that actions count most. But political will and public authority develop in time, and a firm legal foundation can help any health system to evolve in a desirable and intended direction.

REFERENCES

Ackerknecht, Erwin H., "Early History of Legal Medicine." *Ciba Symposia,* 11(7):1286–1289, Winter 1950.

Algeria. "Law of 5 February 1983 on Environmental Protection." *International Digest of Health Legislation,* 35(1):176–194, 1984.

Anon., "Comparative Approaches to Liability for Medical Maloccurrences." *The Yale Law Journal,* 84(5):1141 ff., April 1975.

Bankowski, Z., "Ethics and Health." *World Health* (Geneva), 2–6, April 1989.

Barker, R. A., "Health Services Reorganization—New Zealand's Area Health Boards Act." *International Digest of Health Legislation,* 35(3):697–700, 1984.

Bayer, Ronald, D. Callahan, A. L. Caplan, and B. Jennings, "Toward Justice in Health Care." *American Journal of Public Health,* 78(5):583–588, May 1988.

Bolivia. "Regulations on the Conduct of Family Health Activities, dated 15 March 1982." *International Digest of Health Legislation,* 34(3):510–512, 1983.

Bullough, Bonnie (Editor), *The Law and the Expanding Nursing Role.* New York: Appleton-Century-Crofts, 1980.

Burns, Chester R. (Editor), *Legacies in Law and Medicine.* New York: Science History Publications, 1977.

Castiglioni, Arturo, *A History of Medicine.* New York: Alfred A. Knopf, 1941.

Cook, Rebecca J., and Bernard M. Dickens, "International Developments in Abortion Laws: 1977–1988." *American Journal of Public Health,* 78(10):1305–1311, October 1988.

Cuba. "Law of 10 January 1981 on Environmental Protection and Rational Use of Resources." *International Digest of Health Legislation,* 33(1):102–114, 1982.

Curran, W. J., and T. W. Harding, *The Law and Mental Health: Harmonizing Objectives.* Geneva: World Health Organization, 1978.

DeVries, Raymond G., "The Content for Control: Regulating New and Expanding Health Occupations." *American Journal of Public Health,* 76(9):1147–1150, 1986.

Fattorusso, Vittorio, "Developing Country Perspectives—An Overview." In Institute of Medicine, *Pharmaceuticals for Developing Countries.* Washington, D.C.: National Academy of Sciences, 1979, pp. 250–259.

Finland. "The Social Care Ordinance No. 607 of 29 Jun 1983." *International Digest of Health Legislation,* 35 (3):588, 1984.

France. "Decree No. 82-697 of 4 August 1982 Establishing a National Committee on Retired and Elderly Persons." *International Digest of Health Legislation,* 34(1):78, 1983.

France. "Law of 28 October 1982," *International Digest of Health Legislation,* 34(1):65–66, 1983.

Frazer, W. M., *A History of English Public Health—1883–1939.* London: Balliere, Tindall and Cox, 1950.

Grad, Frank P., *The Public Health Law Manual, 2nd ed.* Washington, D.C.: American Public Health Association, 1990.

Harrison, I. M., *The Law on Medicines.* Lancaster, England: MTP Press, 1986.

Hayes, H.R.M., and J. K. Nelson, *The Medical Effects of Seat Belt Legislation in the United Kingdom.* London: Department of Health and Social Security (Research Report No. 13), 1985.

Henderson, Donald A., "The History of Smallpox Eradication." In Abraham Lilienfeld (Editor), *Times, Places, and Persons: Aspects of the History of Epidemiology.* Baltimore, MD: Johns Hopkins University Press, 1980.

Henshaw, Stanley K., "Induced Abortion: A World

Review, 1990." *Family Planning Perspectives,* 22(2):76–89, March/April 1990.

Hopkins, Jack W., *The Eradication of Smallpox: Organizational Learning and Innovation in International Health.* Boulder, CO: Westview Press, 1989.

Iraq. "Ordinance No. 1057 of 8 August 1981 Promulgating the Public Health Law." *International Digest of Health Legislation,* 33(2):201–223, 1982.

Isaacs, Stephen L., *Population Law and Policy.* New York: Human Sciences Press, 1981.

Italy (Compania). "Regional Law No. 37 of 1979." *International Digest of Health Legislation,* 33(2):267–270, 1982.

Japan. "Law No. 80 of 17 August 1982 on Health Services for the Elderly." *International Digest of Health Legislation,* 34(1):78–87, 1983.

Jayasuriya, D. C., "The Regulation of the Advertising of Alcoholic Beverages: A Survey of National Legislation." *International Digest of Health Legislation,* 38(4):721–745, 1987.

Joskow, P. L., "The Effects of Competition and Regulation on Hospital Bed Supply and the Reservation Quality of the Hospital." *Bell Journal of Economics,* 11(Autumn):421–447, 1980.

Lee, Philip R., and Jessica Herzstein, "International Drug Regulation." *Annual Review of Public Health,* 7:217–235, 1986.

Leenen, H.J.J., G. Pinet, and A. V. Prims, *Trends in Health Legislation in Europe.* Paris: Masson, 1986.

Malaysia. "An Act of 1975 to Provide for the Destruction and Control of Disease-Bearing Insects and for the Medical Examination and Treatment of Persons Suffering from Insect-Borne Diseases and for Matters Connected Therewith." *International Digest of Health Legislation,* 29(2):399–401, 1978.

Marty, Marie-Paule, and Alan T. Marty, "Medical Malpractice—the French Way" and "Malpractice Insurance in Great Britain." *Journal of the American Medical Association,* 233(11):1210–1211, 15 September 1975.

Mexico. "Decree of 20 August 1979, Establishing the National Institute of Aging." *International Digest of Health Legislation,* 33(1):29, 1982.

Nightingale, Stuart L., "Regulation of Food, Drugs, and Medical Devices in the USA." *World Health Forum,* 8:461–468, 1987.

Norway. Ministry of Health and Social Affairs, "Report No. 11 to the Starting on the Follow-up on Norwegian Nutrition Policy." Oslo, 1981.

Ontario, Canada. "An Act to protect the health of pupils in schools, 7 July 1982." *International Digest of Health Legislation,* 35(1):57–59, 1984.

Owen, Margaret, "Laws and Policies Affecting the Training & Practice of Traditional Birth Attendants." *International Digest of Health Legislation,* 34(3):439–475, 1983.

Page, Benjamin P., "History of Medical Ethics: Eastern Europe in the Twentieth Century." In W. J. Reich (Editor), *Encyclopedia of Bioethics,* Vol. 3. New York: Free Press, 1978, pp. 977–982.

Pan American Health Organization, *Policies for the Production and Marketing of Essential Drugs.* Washington, D.C.: PAHO (Scientific Publication No. 462), 1984.

Pellegrino, Edmund D., "Toward an Expanded Medical Ethics: The Hippocratic Ethic Revisited." In Robert M. Veatch (Editor), *Cross-Cultural Perspectives in Medical Ethics: Readings.* Boston: Jones and Bartlett, 1989.

Roemer, Milton I., and Max Shain, *Hospital Utilization under Insurance.* Chicago: American Hospital Association (Monograph Series No. 6), 1959.

Roemer, Milton, I., "One Doctor's Diagnosis of the Medical Malpractice Insurance Issue." *Los Angeles Times,* 16 August 1975.

Roemer, Milton, I., "Medical Ethics and Education for Social Responsibility." *World Health Forum,* 3(4):357–375, 1982.

Roemer, Ruth, "Legal Systems Regulating Health Personnel: A Comparative Analysis." *Milbank Memorial Fund Quarterly,* 46(4):431–471, 1968.

Roemer, Ruth, *Legislative Action to Combat the World Smoking Epidemic.* Geneva: World Health Organization, 1982.

Roemer, Ruth, "Legislation on Fluorides and Dental Health." *International Digest of Health Legislation,* 34(1):1–31, 1983.

Roemer, Ruth, "Legislation to Control Smoking: A Round Table." *International Digest of Health Legislation,* 37(3):447–474, 1986.

Roemer, Ruth, *Legislative Action to Combat the World Smoking Epidemic,* 2nd ed. Geneva: World Health Organization, 1991.

Roemer, Ruth, and John M. Paxman, "Sex Education Laws and Politics." *Studies in Family Planning,* 16(4):219–230, 1985.

Roemer, Ruth, and Milton I. Roemer, *Health Manpower Policies in the Belgian Health Care System.* Washington, D.C.: U.S. Department of Health, Education, & Welfare (DHEW Publication HRA 77-38), 1987.

Rosen, George, *A History of Public Health.* New York: MD Publications, 1958.

Rosenthal, Marilyn, *Dealing with Medical Malpractice: The British and Swedish Experience.* Durham, NC: Duke University Press, 1988.

Schiller, E. J., and R. L. Droste (Editors), *Water Supply and Sanitation in Developing Countries.* Ann Arbor, MI: Ann Arbor Science Publishers, 1982.

Schrifin, Leonard G., and Jack R. Tayan, "The Drug Lag: An Interpretive Review of the Literature." *International Journal of Health Services,* 7(3):359–381, 1977.

Schwartz, Daniel H., "Societal Responsibility for Malpractice." *Milbank Memorial Fund Quarterly/Health and Society,* 469–488, Fall 1976.

Shubber, Sami, "The International Code of Marketing of Breast-Milk Substitutes." *International Digest of Health Legislation,* 36(4):877–908, 1985.

Silverman, M., P. R. Lee, and M. Lydecker, *Prescriptions for Death: The Drugging of the Third World.* Berkeley: University of California Press, 1982.

Silverman, Milton, Mia Lydecker, and Philip R. Lee, "The Drug Swindlers." *International Journal of Health Services,* 20(4):561–572, 1990.

Sigerist, Henry E., "The History of Medical Licensure." *Journal of the American Medical Association,* 104:1056–1060, 30 March, 1935.

Sjovall, Hjalmar, "Liability and Compensation Independent of Medical Negligence: The New Swedish System." *Forensic Science,* 6:235–239, 1975.

Stepan, Jan, "Traditional and Alternative Systems of Medicine: A Comparative Review of Legislation." *International Digest of Health Legislation,* 36(2):283–341, 1985.

Teleky, Ludwig, *History of Factory and Mine Hygiene.* New York: Columbia University Press, 1948.

United States. "An Act to Extend and Revise the Older Americans Act of 1965 dated 29 December 1981." *International Digest of Health Legislation,* 33(2):274, 1982.

Unschuld, Paul U., "The Issue of Structured Coexistence of Scientific and Alternative Medical Systems: A Comparison of East and West German Legislation." *Social Science & Medicine,* 14B:15–24, 1980.

Varma, V. K., S. K. Verma, and T. W. Harding, "Mental Health Legislation in Ten Asian Developing Countries: The Perceived Need for Change." *International Digest of Health Legislation,* 35(2):284–304, 1984.

Veatch, Robert M. (Editor), *Cross-Cultural Perspectives in Medical Ethics: Readings.* Boston: Jones and Bartlett, 1989.

Venezuela. "Law of 28 August 1978 on the National Institute of Geriatrics and Gerontology." *International Digest of Health Legislation,* 30(4):923, 1979.

Vladeck, Bruce C., "The Market vs. Regulation: The Case for Regulation." *Milbank Memorial Fund Quarterly/Health and Society,* 59(2):209–223, 1981.

Wardell, William M., *Controlling the Use of Therapeutic Drugs.* Washington, D.C.: American Enterprise Institute for Public Policy Research, 1978.

World Health Organization, "Specialization: A Survey of Existing Legislation." *International Digest of Health Legislation,* 8(4):561–595, 1957.

World Health Organization, *Venereal Disease Control: A Survey of Recent Legislation.* Geneva: WHO, 1975.

World Health Organization, "Equivalence of Medical Qualifications and the Practice of Medicine." *International Digest of Health Legislation,* 18(3):459–503, 1967.

World Health Organization, *The International Drinking Water Supply and Sanitation Decade Directory—Edition 3.* London: Thomas Telford, 1987.

World Health Organization, *The World Drug Situation.* Geneva: WHO, 1988.

Zaire. "Ordinance No. 78-386 of 6 September 1978 Establishing a National Center for the Planning of Human Nutrition." *International Digest of Health Legislation,* 32(2):298–299, 1982.

PART FOUR

HEALTH SERVICES DELIVERY

CHAPTER TWELVE

Ambulatory and Primary Health Care

From the perspective of the individual, health services include three major types of intervention: (1) service to the ambulatory person, (2) modification of the environment, and (3) care in a special facility. Environmental protection and eventually broader public health programs demanded social action. Hospital facilities required organization to accumulate funds for construction, to mobilize personnel, to render care, and so on.

By contrast, the ambulatory health services, until recently, have been mainly individual and nonorganized. In Chapter 3, the early development of the dispensary as a type of organized ambulatory health service was reviewed. From the dispensary evolved the health center and the outpatient department of hospitals. But before the twentieth century, these facilities were oriented to the poor or other special population groups. The mainstream of ambulatory medical care was still represented by the individual doctor. A strong tradition has taken shape in most countries, especially the wealthier industrialized ones, about the privacy, even the sanctity, of the personal patient–doctor relationship.

When organized schemes for financing these ambulatory services evolved in nineteenth-century Europe—first voluntarily and then mandatorily under law—the money raised by social mechanisms was used initially to support the costs of private physician–patient contacts. Only later was social financing used to support ambulatory service in some sort of organized framework. Moreover, health service to the ambulatory person came to be appreciated as a more effective foundation of a national health system—more preventively oriented and less costly—than the high technology approach to serious sickness in

hospitals. The historic development of this insight should be reviewed, to help one appreciate the meaning of the current worldwide emphasis on primary health care.

HISTORIC DEVELOPMENT OF PRIMARY HEALTH CARE

The history of medicine has been a long and complex story of the acquisition of knowledge about disease and methods of coping with it—first by treatment and later by prevention. Physicians have been the principal carriers and appliers of this knowledge, and its complexity has shaped the characteristics of the medical profession.

Mounting Specialization and High Technology

Throughout most recorded history, the physician was a generalist in the diagnosis and treatment of disease in individual patients. As knowledge about disease became more abundant and elaborate, it grew beyond the ability of any single physician to master. Specialization became necessary. In Europe, where scientific medicine was most highly developed, medical and surgical specialties proliferated, particularly for the treatment of seriously ill patients in hospitals. Specialties, therefore, became closely linked to hospitals, and hospitals increasingly acquired the tools of advanced technology.

The stunning discoveries in bacteriology and organ pathology in the later nineteenth century led to an unprecedented aggrandizement of the popular image of doctors. The community general practitioner became warmly respected, and specialists, it was believed, could perform wonders. Industrialization led to the rapid growth of cities and, within them, large hospitals with many clinical departments and bewildering technology. Western Europe, where most of the scientific discoveries were made, became the undisputed center of scientific medicine, and remained so until World War I (1914–1918).

After the devastation of World War I, medicine's world center shifted gradually to the United States, where there had been great freedom in the health sector, as in everything else. Scores of medical schools—most of them with meager resources and quite mediocre standards—sprang up after the Civil War (1865). Between 1890 and 1910 hundreds of hospitals were established.

As the United States entered the twentieth century a reaction set in. In 1906, the U.S. Congress enacted the first Food and Drug Control Act. In 1910, the Carnegie Foundation issued the famous Flexner Report on *Medical Education in the United States and Canada.* In 1913, the American College of Surgeons was founded, and set out to raise the quality of general hospitals through its *standardization* movement. In 1916, the first American *specialty board* was established, in ophthalmology.

Before World War I, American physicians had traveled to Europe to learn about the latest medical advances. After World War I, European physicians came to America. In the 1920s Africa and Asia were mostly under colonial control, and their public leaders looked to both Europe and America for models of health care policy. Latin American countries—no longer Spanish or Portuguese colonies—looked for guidance to the United States. Then the worldwide economic collapse of the 1930s, followed by World War II, left the United States the preferred model in health care policy and many other fields. Emancipation of European colonies after World War II turned most developing countries toward America more than ever.

Emulation of U.S. health care patterns meant many things, most prominent of which was advanced technology and the construction of modern hospitals. Other hallmarks of American medicine, such as private medical practice, were not so readily copied by developing countries. Their people were too poor to provide a private market outside the main cities; moreover, the colonial governments had left the heritage of a salaried medical bureaucracy, weak as it was. In the cities, however, hospitals could be built—visible symbols of national pride.

The governments of the newly independent nations usually set out to give greater attention to the rural areas than had their colonial predecessors. Construction of health centers and health posts for ambulatory care, both preventive and therapeutic, were the response to rural needs everywhere. Still, the extent of these facilities, and particularly their staffing, was typically far less than the actual need. As indigenous upper classes arose in the former colonies, neocolonial ideologies emerged. The new national elite wanted to have *"the best"* in modern medicine available in the main cities, where they lived. When military coups took power in country after country on every continent of the developing world, neocolonialism did not diminish but increased. As a result, the composition of government health budgets was painfully similar almost everywhere: 65–70 percent for hospitals in the main cities, where 10–20 percent of the population lived, and 30–35 percent for health services in rural areas, where 80–90 percent of the people lived. These public disparities were usually further aggravated by a growing market for private medical resources, concentrated also in the cities.

Reaction against specialization and elaborate technology in medicine began to surface in the mid-1960s. In many developing countries, far-sighted public health leaders questioned the large investments in tertiary hospitals in the major cities, with millions of poor rural people going without simple prenatal care or basic immunizations. Plans to do something about these distortions in national health policy began to be explored by the World Health Organization in the early 1970s. As governments in the newly liberated countries matured, they looked increasingly to the World Health Organization for guidance.

Policy Development in the World Health Organization

When the Constitution of the World Health Organization was adopted in 1946, its signatories remembered well the demise of the League of Nations, along with its Health Division, in 1939. The lesson seemed clear. If WHO was to survive, it must be independent of, though in association with, the United Nations. Also it must avoid involvement in politics and political issues. Unfortunately in 1951 at the height of the Cold War, the Soviet Union and several of its allies left the Organization, to return only when political tensions declined. In the years 1952–1954, the Organization was also badly shaken by debate over the issue of birth control, or what is now called family planning.

To avoid issues with any political implications, therefore, in the 1950s WHO focused its attention on strictly technical matters. It offered advice to countries on the preparation of vaccines, on the curriculum for a school of nursing, on methods of purifying water, and so on. To be concerned about policies on the organization and distribution of health services in a country was considered inappropriate.*

The heavily technical, rather than policy-oriented, approach of WHO was reflected in the trend of its annual expenditures. Malaria control, for example, requiring major technical interventions, consumed 8.6 percent of the Organization budget in 1952, rising to 16.7 percent by 1962. The rubric *public health administration* included whatever activities concerned the organization or provision of

general health services, and in 1952 this work absorbed 15.8 percent of the WHO budget; by 1962, the proportion had declined to 10.5 percent.

By 1970, with, the enrollment of more newly independent nations in WHO, the votes of these poor countries in the World Health Assembly became dominant. Whatever the character of their governments, the vocal concern of these countries was for the problems of poverty. The plight of vast rural populations with high infant mortality rates and rampant disease was voiced in dramatic speeches. Resolutions called for greater support for the less developed by the more developed nations.

In the late 1950s, WHO had launched one of its greatest strategies of technical intervention—a program to eradicate malaria from the earth. For some years this program made progress, but in the mid-1960s the development of mosquito resistance to insecticides began to be recognized, and by 1968 the effort had to be declared a failure. The basic reason was the lack of a solid public health infrastructure to carry on with malaria control and other health work after national vector-control teams left each area.

A few years later, in 1971, the People's Republic of China—ostracized by most of the world since 1949—was recognized by the United Nations as the proper occupant of the seat of China in the U.N. Assembly and Security Council. The next year, the People's Republic of China regained its seat in WHO, replacing Taiwan. Suddenly the world learned what China had been doing since 1949 to make essential health services available to its huge population. Policy changes since China's second great upheaval, the Cultural Revolution of 1965, were especially significant for health. They included, among other things (1) major attention to the rural areas, (2) the training and use of *barefoot doctors,* and (3) a combination of modern and traditional Chinese medicine. China won the world's admiration for its coverage of hundreds of millions of rural people with the elementary but important services, preventive and curative, of briefly trained barefoot doctors.

*It happens that I worked personally on the staff of WHO from 1951 to 1953 and was instructed by a higher official to respond to the request of a sister U.N. agency (the International Labour Organization) for advice on the "medical aspects of social security." The Committee of distinguished international experts that I convened was chaired by Professor René Sand, who had also been Chairman of the Technical Preparatory Committee that drafted the WHO Constitution. Not surprisingly, the Committee advised the ILO that social security was an effective method for financing medical care, whereupon I was reprimanded for a serious indiscretion.

Primary Health Care and the Alma Ata Conference

The movement that led to the Alma Ata Conference on Primary Health Care in 1978 was clearly a response of the developing countries to the vast health problems of their rural populations. As dramatized in China, *community health workers* were seen almost everywhere as the means for providing essential health services to the people who lacked and needed them. The Alma Ata Conference set out to clarify the content and form of health services needed by all people, but especially by those whom conventional modern medicine had virtually ignored.

A few years before the Alma Ata Conference, WHO and UNICEF published a seminal report on *Alternative Approaches to Meeting Basic Health Needs in Developing Countries.* It was based on case studies of services to rural populations in 10 countries, in 8 of which the principal personnel were various types of community health workers. (Only in Cuba and Yugoslavia were physicians the main personnel.) This document was clearly the harbinger of the Alma Ata Conference, although as a WHO staff report, it could not constitute a statement of policies.

One special value of the Alma Ata Conference was its enunciation of a roster of specific services that should be ensured for all people. Quoting from the WHO Constitution, it reaffirmed that "governments have a responsibility for the health of their people." It goes on to say that

> a main social target of governments, international organizations and the whole world community in the coming decades should be the attainment by all people of the world by the year 2000 of a level of health that will permit them to lead a socially and economically productive life. Primary health care is the key to attaining this target as part of development in the spirit of social justice.

The Declaration of Alma Ata continues by stating that primary health care (PHC) must include at least the following services:

1. education concerning prevailing health problems and the methods of preventing and controlling them.
2. promotion of food supply and proper nutrition.
3. an adequate supply of safe water and basic sanitation.
4. maternal and child health care, including family planning.
5. immunization against the major infectious diseases.
6. prevention and control of local endemic diseases.
7. appropriate treatment of common diseases and injuries.
8. provision of essential drugs.

Since 1978, health leaders in the more developed countries have enlarged the meaning of "appropriate treatment of common diseases" to include specifically the identification and treatment of mental illness, simple rehabilitation of the physically disabled, and elementary dental care.

Beyond these specific health services, the Declaration of Alma Ata recognized that effective implementation of the broad concept of primary health care required a fundamentally new interpretation of national health system strategies. Although these had to be adjusted to the economic realities of each country, everywhere they demanded "political commitment." The expression of this commitment was formulated in a series of general principles that would apply in every country.

General Principles of Primary Health Care

These principles were formulated in the Alma Ata Declaration of 1978, and they have been further elaborated at other international conferences since then. They may be considered under seven headings—all interdependent in any one setting, but quite different under diverse settings.

Feasibility. First, the strategy of PHC must be economically affordable—within the capabilities of a country. The resource limitations of most developing countries have led to the recognition of briefly trained community health workers as major personnel for the delivery of primary health care. At the same time, supervision of these personnel must be provided. In more highly developed countries, with enough wealth and enough physicians, general medical practitioners are feasible providers of primary health care. In some transitional countries both auxiliary and professional personnel may jointly contribute to PHC delivery.

Acceptability. The CHW is socially and phychologically acceptable to most people in developing countries. Those who have seldom seen physicians would not usually demand them. In an affluent industrialized country, only physicians would be acceptable. Even the general practitioner needs the technical backup of specialists, to be fully acceptable. As the education of people advances, one may expect standards and expectations to rise also.

Community Participation. To ensure acceptability and to adjust PHC activities to local circumstances, the people being served should play a role in making policy decisions and their implementation. Such participation is often the best strategy to overcome medical or bureaucratic domination. It may be expressed in many forms. The participation or involvement of people in the development of PHC programs plays so great a part in their success that a large literature on this subject has been produced by the United Nations and the specialized agencies.

Over the centuries, major innovations in health systems have sometimes come from physicians, but mainly from the initiatives of other people. Hospitals were founded by religious groups, and their representatives still sit on hospital boards of directors. Boards of health were formed by municipal leaders to fight epidemics. Sickness insurance funds were first organized by groups of workers. Societies to combat tuberculosis or mental illness were started by patients who suffered from these disorders.

People's participation may be expressed through formal administrative mechanisms or through direct actions. A district health committee or a community health council may be appointed or elected to develop policies and priorities. The British National Health Service has its mandated Community Health Councils, Yugoslavia has its "self-managing communities of interest," Canadian provinces have their elected Regional Health Boards. With or without such formal channels, local people in developing countries may help to construct community health centers or posts, to dig wells for safe water or build latrines, and to promote family planning or mobilize children for immunizations. If health facilities are built by government, community people may determine their location, their hours of operation, and their style of service. Such involvement of community people early in health program development helps to ensure their continuing support in later years.

Appropriate Technology. The origins of the PHC strategy as a reaction against excessively high technology have led to a stress on *appropriate* technology. The laboratory and X-ray procedures needed in a tertiary-level hospital, or even in a secondary-level district hospital, are obviously not appropriate in a village health station. Likewise indoor flush toilets need not be expected where well-designed sanitary latrines are satisfactory and an improvement over previous conditions.

The principle of appropriate technology has shown that premature newborns, for example, can often be protected by the mother's body heat as well as by a sophisticated incubator—especially in a social setting where incubators break down and cannot be repaired. Simple body movements can have rehabilitative value exceeding that of many exercise machines. At the other end of the scale, however, in an industrialized country good X-ray equipment should be expected even in a rural health center. Prosthetic hip replacements should not entail a waiting time of several years. Appropriateness applies to PHC programs in both high-income and low-income countries.

Intersectoral Coordination. Since health is influenced by countless environmental and social forces, outside of health services, primary health care must attempt to mobilize other social sectors for the benefit of populations. This means concern for education, for improved agriculture, for industrial employment, for housing, for transportation, and for the entire physical and social environment that impinge on human health. The question is what can the health system or health personnel do to mobilize or strengthen these many other sectors in society?

Realistically, health personnel can try to work cooperatively with the major actors in education, agriculture, housing, and so on. Health leaders can be supportive of positive programs in these fields. Health services should, of course, be provided in schools and factories, water supplies for crop irrigation should be coordinated with water supplies for human use, and political support for low-cost housing should be mobilized along with support for health facilities. At the level of communes or districts or provinces, citizen groups in these several fields should work together in shaping social policy and programs.

Intersectoral relationships are not always positive and beneficial for everyone. A policy of price support for grain may help farmers but raise living costs for city workers. Price controls on manufactured products may stem inflation in the long run but reduce wages in the short run. Balancing interests in a complex society calls for leadership with awareness of all social sectors, including health.

As reported in Volume I, when simple correlations of basic variables were sought with life expectancies in 142 countries, the highest coefficients were found to apply to *female literacy* and *access to safe water.* Both of these variables are aspects of social sectors outside the health system, although they both also have distinct relevance within the health system. Broadly considered, one must conclude that countries having a high level of female literacy and good access to safe water are most likely to have the many circumstances that contribute to long life.

Comprehensiveness. Another general principle of primary health care applies to its scope. The 8 or 10 specific preventive and treatment services enumerated earlier are meant to define the scope of a PHC program. In view of past experience, any one of the specific elements of

PHC—immunizations, family planning, nutrition, or safe water—cannot be expected to generate the essential infrastructure in a community. Many experiences with selective elements of PHC have shown this approach to lack endurance. A campaign limited to polio immunization or malaria control or family planning leaves no enduring structure when the campaign is finished.

Therefore, a reasonably broad range of PHC services, adequate to yield an enduring infrastructure, is an essential principle of the PHC concept. If a specific intervention, such as malaria control or smallpox vaccination, is started in a community, it should be broadened to a full range as soon as possible. Only then can the specific intervention be maintained. Moreover, the treatment of ailments is an indispensable component of PHC, if only to win the confidence of people necessary for their cooperation in preventive services. A permanent infrastructure requires the development of local government or some type of decentralized authority for primary health care.

World Health Organization experience in the late 1980s pointed to the value of *health districts* as the feasible local units of PHC administration. Larger than a village and yet smaller than most provinces, the district should include health resources adequate to meet the needs of 90 percent of the local population. With around 100,000 to 200,000 people, it should have several units for providing the full range of PHC services, backed up by a district hospital for referral of cases. Only the unusual serious case should have to be referred outside the district for care. Integration of previously separate vertical programs becomes feasible at the local place of impact. A comprehensive range of PHC services provided in self-reliant health districts became the ideal model advocated by WHO in the 1990s.

Equity. The final general principle of primary health care is the most important: it should be available to all people in relation to their needs. Social class, purchasing power, or the societal importance of any individual should play no part in access to primary health care; it is for everyone. This basic principle, of course, must lead to consideration of how

PHC is to be financed in each national setting. If the country's economic level is low, services would have to be less thorough than in an affluent country, but they should be at the same level for everyone.

This discussion of general principles of primary health care can be concluded with the definition given in the Alma Ata Declaration:

> Primary health care is essential health care based on practical, scientifically sound, and socially acceptable methods and technology made universally accessible to individuals and families in the community through their full participation and at a cost that the community and the country can afford to maintain at every stage of their development in a spirit of self-reliance and self-determination.

PRIMARY HEALTH CARE IN PRACTICE

The enormous differences in health personnel resources, between the industrialized and the developing countries, have given primary health care a very different meaning in the two types of country. In the health systems of developing countries, primary health care has been closely associated with training and use of medical assistants and community health workers who could deliver the services. In industrialized countries, primary health care has mainly involved general medical practitioners and their functions in various settings.

Developing Country Experience

The use of health personnel, trained much less thoroughly than physicians, was extensive long before the movement for primary health care. In Chapter 2, we reviewed the early use of *native dressers* in African colonies of European powers, and the training of various types of hospital assistant or assistant doctor in colonies of Asia. Czarist Russia had trained and used *feldshers* for elementary medical care since the nineteenth century. Nurses and assistant nurses had long been entrusted to treat common ailments in rural areas. The special feature of community health workers (CHWs) trained during and after the 1970s was the rel-

ative brevity of their training and its focus on specific preventive and elementary treatment services.

The training program for China's *barefoot doctors* made an especially strong impression throughout the developing world. These were simple peasants, with previous education only to the level of literacy, and their training in a small hospital or health center lasted only 3 to 6 months. One or two weeks of continuing education was given each year. With this modest preparation, the barefoot doctor was capable of giving immunizations, promoting contraception, advising on water and sanitation, offering general hygienic education, and treating common minor ailments.

In most developing countries, the preparation of increasing numbers of modern physicians had done little more than scratch the surface of rural health needs. The vast majority of doctors settled in the cities, even if they had been legally obligated to occupy a rural post for 1 or 2 years after graduation. By contrast, auxiliary health personnel would be recruited from villages, and could be expected to remain in them after their training. The whole program was relatively inexpensive. In some developing countries, the CHW was not even paid, although a modest salary was generally found necessary to encourage diligent work.

Second only to China, India has attempted to apply the PHC approach on a massive scale. Through a series of national health plans, by the mid-1980s India arrived at a policy in which thousands of community health workers were serving rural people in health subcenters. These multipurpose CHWs staffed more than 100,000 subcenters by 1988, reaching 64 percent of India's population. Each unit was expected to meet PHC needs of 5,000 people, with back-up from medical staff at primary health centers. Enormous training efforts were necessary to convert former unipurpose health workers (for malaria control, smallpox vaccination, family planning, etc.) into multipurpose workers, male and female.

Papua New Guinea is a developing country in the South Pacific ocean, in which the health authorities have put major emphasis on primary health care. Each of 19 provinces has a general hospital, but in 1983 PHC was provided by 340 health centers and 194 aid posts, staffed by nurses and village health aides. With very low literacy levels and weak health education, however, many people still use untrained traditional healers and then go to provincial hospital outpatient departments, bypassing the PHC units.

In Thailand, a special demonstration project on primary health care was launched in 1974 in Lampong Province. Village health volunteers were trained only 10 days to provide simple medical relief, distribute oral contraceptives, and refer cases to a medically staffed health center. Traditional birth attendants were also given 10 days of training. With such limited preparation, it is not surprising that the PHC accomplishments were meager. Curative services provided at various health centers increased, but preventive services did not, and overall utilization rates were low. Analysis of work done showed that only 54 percent of PHC worker time was devoted to productive activity.

The program of community health worker training and deployment in Ecuador was like that in several Latin American countries. Chosen from primary school graduates, these young people were given two months of training by a registered nurse, and then returned to their communities of origin. Here they would try to educate people about mother and child health, environmental sanitation, and nutrition. They would provide first aid, do case finding, and make referrals to a health center. They would organize health committees and try to serve as the link between village needs and the government health services. A small supply of drugs was furnished to each CHW.

In practice, however, the Ecuador PHC program fell short of its goals. Shortages of drugs and supplies were frequent. Supervision and consultation were scarce; auxiliary nurses at health centers were supposed to supervise and assist, but they were incapable of doing this. Morale among the CHWs, therefore, was low and several discontinued working.

Experience with primary health care through CHWs in Africa has also been generally disappointing. Safe water is available to only a small fraction of the people, immunization levels are generally low, and family planning is practiced only in the better edu-

cated families. Maintenance of a few large urban hospitals still absorbs more than two-thirds of government health budgets. Food production per capita in Sub-Sahara Africa has actually declined below the level of 1961–1965. Many health centers and dispensaries for primary health care have been built, but their staffing with CHWs is weak and utilization levels are low. In Kenya, impressive plans for PHC coverage of the rural population were made in 1972; by 1982 the coverage had reached only 30 percent of the rural people.

An experimental PHC program in one district of Gambia showed that with fully trained doctors and midwives, infant mortality rates could be sharply reduced. This cast doubt on the whole approach of using CHWs, who were really unable to do what was needed.

A general evaluation of CHWs by a WHO/ UNICEF conference in 1980 concluded that (1) these personnel appear to be superficial and hasty in their work, (2) they spend almost all their time on symptomatic treatment of patients coming to the health post and little time on prevention or outreach to the community, (3) little was done to involve local people in operation of the PHC program, (4) the utilization rate of CHW services was very low, and (5) the attitude of CHWs was generally apathetic and physical conditions of the health post were usually unkempt and unsanitary.

In a few developing countries, the PHC approach has been implemented mainly with physicians directly supervising nurses and midwives. This is the pattern in Turkey, where health stations serving a few thousand people (staffed by auxiliary nurse-midwives) are backed up by medically staffed health centers. Under these circumstances, the auxiliary personnel are regularly supervised by and in touch with the doctors. Arrangements are somewhat similar in Malaysia, where rural clinics with auxiliary midwives serve 3,000–4,000 people, under the supervision of a health center doctor for each 20,000 rural people. In Malaysian towns there are many private general practitioners furnishing primary care, as well as busy outpatient departments of hospitals. Nicaragua has trained large numbers of doctors, so that health centers serving around 20,000 people could each be medically staffed; these units supervise auxiliary nurses at health posts serving about 5,000 people. All new medical graduates must devote at least 2 years to this public *social service,* even though private practice is also allowed.

These experiences in developing countries have led WHO to put greater stress on the careful training of community health workers, and their provision regularly of continuing education. Manuals of instruction in primary health care have been published in various languages to facilitate supervision. Special attention has been given to the development of health leadership at the district level.

Industrialized Country Experience

In the industrialized countries, primary health care has involved the evaluation of general medical practice and a variety of strategies to strengthen it. As specialization developed, in close association with hospitals, the general practitioner out in the community was sometimes regarded as a second-class doctor. In the 1950s, studies in England and North America reported detailed observations of numerous general practices, suggesting a great deal of superficial and mediocre performance.

In Europe, the strengthening of general practice (GP) was sought through (1) more continuing education, (2) modified fee schedules under insurance to increase the relative rewards for GP service, (3) inviting GPs to clinical conferences at the hospitals, (4) locating GP offices in community health centers, staffed with technicians, nurses, and social workers, and (5) developing a residency program leading to specialty status for general practice.

In the United States, a Specialty Board in Family Practice was launched in 1969. It rapidly stimulated the organization of scores of residency programs and attracted many new medical school graduates. The European countries developed specialization in general medicine about the same time. Departments of general practice were established in many European medical schools. Continuing education was promoted to upgrade the quality of general practice everywhere.

This reaffirmation of the importance and dignity of general medical practice was an appropriate reaction to the excessive specializa-

tion, but it did little to stem the tide of mounting medical care costs. Both public and private expenditures continued to rise in all industrialized countries, and another form of reaction in these affluent environments was to question the whole value of expensive technology. A strong *back to nature* movement grew in many countries, rejecting all scientific interventions. In 1975, Ivan Illich published *Medical Nemesis,* in which it was claimed that medical expenditures were an absolute waste, since medical care (including even immunizations) did more harm than good.

In the mid-1960s another reaction to technology and specialization took place in the United States, although not in other industrialized countries. The great lack of general practitioners in America has been noted, and a new strategy occurred to medical leaders during the Vietnam War. Among the returning Vietnam veterans were many medical corpsmen who had learned surgical procedures under battle conditions; why not train some of these young men as *physician assistants* (PAs) to give health service in places where doctors would not go? This meant rural districts and urban slum areas. PA salaries exceeded those of nurses, and before long *nurse practitioners* (NPs) were being trained at scores of medical centers. These *physician extenders* (both PAs and NPs) substituted for general medical practitioners in many low-income areas. By the late 1970s, however, the whole movement was slowing down, in the face of an enlarging supply of American general physicians. In other industrialized countries—and even in developing ones with relatively high ratios, such as Egypt or Turkey—the doctor-substitute movement did not arise.

Primary health care took on another significance in the industrialized countries, as health expenditures after 1970 soared to new heights. If population coverage was the main objective of the PHC approach in developing countries, cost containment became the main rationale in the affluent countries. Primary health care in these countries meant prompt service early in an illness, with less need for hospital care. This usually yielded substantial savings.

A social experiment in California in the mid-1970s dramatized the relationship between primary health care and hospitalization.

In the Medicaid program for the poor, officials considered the utilization of doctors to be excessive, and imposed a $1 copayment for each visit. The rate of office visits promptly declined, yielding savings, but after a few months the rate of hospital use increased (compared with a matched Medicaid population not making copayments). The cost of extra hospital days more than wiped out the savings from reduced ambulatory care. Discouraging primary care, in other words, was penny wise and pound foolish, so the copayment experiment was ended. A decade later, the opposite policy was explored in Cuba, with about half the population provided especially intensive primary health care. Hospital use by this population declined, compared with a matched group getting normal medical care.

Another significant study of two industrialized countries compared Sweden and Norway. Sweden in the 1970s stressed hospitalization and Norway stressed primary health care. Both countries had similarly good health records, but the per capita health expenditures of Norway were significantly lower. Then in the 1980s, Sweden increased its attention to primary health care, and Norway permitted greater sovereignty in hospital operations; as a result the per capita health expenditures of the two countries came closer together.

In addition to the role of general practitioners in containing health care costs, their value as gate keepers and coordinators of health services is crucial. As specialization complicates the health system, it becomes increasingly necessary for generalists to help their patients use the system. There are psychosocial aspects to every significant illness that require the understanding of a general practitioner. This role is important whether the GP is in a private office or in an organized health center.

Because of the importance of the doctor–patient relationship in primary health care, the method of paying physicians has long been a subject of debate in the industrialized countries. This has been an issue whether the money comes from public or private sources. Payment by fee-for-service is naturally expected to induce doctors to work hard, since each act yields a fee; on the other hand, the fees may induce superfluous services—unwar-

ranted diagnostic procedures or even unnecessary surgery. Salaries eliminate any incentive for overservicing, but they may lead to negligence or mediocrity. Protection against the latter is the influence of organizational discipline and the development of an *esprit de corps*. Incentives for personal advancement also have financial rewards. This is easily observable in the high quality work done in teaching hospitals, and it can be expected also in health centers for ambulatory care.

Payment of general practitioners by the capitation method, as in the British National Health Service, eliminates incentives for overservicing, but still encourages diligent work. Patients who are not satisfied can always change to another doctor's list. Some programs combine basic salaries with capitation payments (up to a certain maximum), to reward the doctor who attracts more patients. The amount of capitation paid, furthermore, can be greater for elderly patients who naturally require more service.

Regardless of the methods of providing health services and paying physicians, the dominance of the medical profession in all aspects of health systems is generally declining everywhere. As the population's educational level has risen, and as numerous other parties have entered the health care scene, the doctor's position has become modified. The doctor's decisions are subject to review, and consultation whenever possible is the norm. There is plenty of respect for doctors in all cultures, but this is as the captain of a team rather than as a monarch. Even in the role of captain, the physician is expected to respect fully the roles of other professional members of the team.

The decline of professional sovereignty has led some observers to see a trend of *proletarianization* of physicians. Doctors are said to be exploited by corporations or bureaucratic organizations that use their services. Even when doctors work for salaries, rather than individual fees, however, the salary levels are typically very high; to regard them as exploitative is far-fetched. The mobilization of resources and the organization of health services are necessary adjustments to the complexities of health science and technology; only through such organization can the health needs of populations be met.

Utilization of Ambulatory Physician's Care

The rate at which a population seeks ambulatory care from physicians is influenced by many features of the doctor–patient relationship. Economic access is basic; are visits to the doctor covered by insurance, with or without copayments by the patient? Is access to a specialist direct or only on referral by a general practitioner? Does the method of paying doctors provide an incentive to maximize contacts, as with the fee-for-service method, or to minimize contacts, as with capitation or salary? What is the influence of geographic proximity, of the educational level of patients, or of cultural attitudes about seeking medical care? How do these several features interact with each other?

Disentangling the effects of these diverse features on the rate of ambulatory care utilization in a country is virtually impossible. The net rates reported principally by health insurance programs in 22 industrialized countries are given in Table 12.1. One might speculate about the relatively high rates in Germany and Japan reflecting fee-for-service payment methods and the relatively low rates in Great Britain and the Netherlands reflecting capitation payment, but similar reasoning does not explain the low rate in New Zealand (where fees are paid) or the high rate in Italy (where capi-

Table 12.1. Ambulatory Physician Services: Rate Per Person Per Year in 22 Countries, 1980–1983

Country	Rate	Country	Rate
Turkey	1.2	Canada	5.5
Sweden	2.7	Switzerland	5.6
Netherlands	3.2	Ireland	6.0
Finland	3.4	Australia	6.4
Portugal	3.8	Belgium	7.1
New Zealand	3.8	Italy	8.3
Great Britain	4.2	Denmark	8.4
Norway	4.5	Germany	10.8
United States	4.6	Japan	14.2
Spain	4.7		
France	4.7		
Iceland	4.9		

Source: Organization for Economic Cooperation and Development, *Financing and Delivering Health Care.* Paris: OECD, 1987.

tation prevails). The relatively low rate in the United States would seem to reflect the general lack of insurance protection for ambulatory care, especially compared with the somewhat higher rates in culturally similar Canada and Australia, where health insurance is universal.

These data for the United States, France, and Switzerland apply to both primary care and specialist services, whereas for Great Britain and New Zealand they are doubtless limited to general practitioner care. Such disparities in definitions serve to emphasize the need for caution in these cross-national comparisons.

Similar difficulties were encountered in a major cross-national study of health care utilization conducted in 1968–1969. Field surveys on ambulatory medical care encounters were made in Canada, the United States, England, Finland, Poland, Yugoslavia, and Argentina. Identical study methods were used—seeking household information on physician contacts in the previous 2 weeks—with resultant data presented on such contacts per 1,000 persons (standardized for age and sex). The rates varied from 158 contacts per 1,000 in Finland to 306 such contacts in Argentina, but there was no detectable relationship between these rates and the characteristics of the national health systems in the six countries.

Trends over time are no easier to explain. The rate of ambulatory physician services in France rose from 4.7 per person per year in the early 1980s to 7.8 in 1987; in the United States it rose over this period from 4.6 to 5.4 encounters per person per year. On the other hand, the rate of these services in Denmark declined between 1982 and 1985 from 8.4 to 5.2 and in Japan from 14.2 to 12.8. The causes of these variations are obviously complex. One can only say that in all these countries the ambulatory physician services include a great deal of the therapeutic component of primary health care.

Settings for Organized Ambulatory Care

Since the first dispensaries for the poor in seventeenth-century Europe, organized arrangements for ambulatory health care developed throughout the world in many settings. The construction and use of health centers to serve the general population have been most important, especially in developing countries. In large countries, regionalized patterns are the norm, with main health centers, subcenters, and small health posts. Main centers often have a few short-stay beds, with medical staff full-time or part-time. Subcenters and health posts are nearly always staffed by health auxiliaries of several types. Preventively oriented maternal and child health services are usually a major function, handled by assistant nurses, whereas various types of community health workers treat the sick with drugs available.

In the nineteenth century, hospitals developed rapidly in Europe and America, and their out patient departments (OPDs) gradually replaced the free-standing dispensaries. In the older hospitals space for the OPD had to be improvised, but by the twentieth century the OPD quarters became standard. For emergency care, the OPD is open to everyone, although for nonurgent care it may be limited, as in North America, to the poor. The OPD is typically more highly developed in large city hospitals, where scheduled clinics are held according to medical specialties—that is, for medical cases, surgical cases, maternity care, pediatrics, ophthalmology, and so on. The OPD is also the place where patients, on referral from community practitioners, are examined to determine if they should be admitted to a hospital bed.

In the industrialized countries, where general medical care has been financed by social insurance and provided by private doctors, Ministries of Health play a smaller role in ambulatory care. These ministries then typically sponsor clinics for preventive services, not so readily available from private practitioners. Commonest are the MCH clinics for expectant mothers and infants, where immunizations are given along with advice on child rearing. Public health agencies also operate special clinics for sexually transmitted diseases, tuberculosis, dental care of children, and other focused purposes. In developing countries, without social insurance for general medical care, these specialized clinic sessions are scheduled at certain

times in the overall program of a health center or subcenter.

Schools and colleges provide another setting for organized ambulatory health services for children and youth. Educational authorities often organize such clinics in the industrialized countries, appointing special school nurses and part-time physicians. In developing countries, if school children get any special attention, it is usually from the government health agency. These services typically include examinations to identify physical defects, to monitor immunization status, and any necessary referrals to physicians or to hospital OPDs. Attention is given to any illness or injury occurring during school hours. In secondary schools, the health services must deal with the need for contraceptive services and prevention of drug abuse. At the university level, the scope of health services is usually wide, since many or most students are living away from home.

Large industrial or other enterprises throughout the world, whether private or public, have organized health services for their workers, in the interests of heightening productivity. In the affluent industrialized countries, where general medical care is financed through social insurance, the industrial health unit typically limits its services to preemployment examinations and first-aid care of injuries or acute illnesses. For definitive treatment, the worker is referred to outside resources. In developing countries, where the general level of medical care is not considered adequate, large enterprises often organize comprehensive services for both prevention and treatment. In isolated locations, the industrial clinic may serve the worker's dependents as well. In small plants (with fewer than 100 employees) of all types of country, health services are usually limited to first-aid for accidental injuries.

Another type of clinic is one organized by groups of private physicians who wish to work together. *Group medical practice* is usually defined as three or more physicians who may be of different specialties or of a single specialty. Such arrangements can achieve economies in the use of space, engagement of allied health personnel, and acquisition of diagnostic and therapeutic equipment. Private group medical practice is highly developed in the United States and Canada, where specialists are not mainly attached to salaried hospital staffs. It is expanding, however, in the large cities of all countries as a way to demonstrate high technology and to attract patients.

Voluntary health agencies, devoted to fighting certain diseases or to helping certain types of patients, may also sponsor special clinics. Clinics for crippled children, for the detection of cancer, or for the treatment of mental/emotional problems have been organized by various charitable groups. Persons suffering from addiction to alcohol have organized special groups (Alcoholics Anonymous) to overcome their harmful habit, through a type of spiritual self-help.

The offices, the private clinics, the surgeries, or the "rooms" of individual physicians or traditional practitioners may still be the commonest settings for providing ambulatory medical care in many countries. Historical trends, however, are clearly in the direction of organized facilities becoming the customary arrangement, because of the efficiencies achieved by the division of labor and teamwork.

There are numerous types of specialized clinic facilities for certain population groups or special disorders under public or private sponsorship. In most developing countries, at either transitional or very poor income levels, the general *health center* serves several thousand people living within its reach.

In the developing countries of all ideological types in Asia, Africa, and Latin America, the health center is rapidly becoming the standard facility through which government agencies (usually Ministries of Health, but sometimes other entities) provide the population with modern primary health care. The staffing and equipment of these health centers vary markedly with the economic level and health manpower supply. In countries of the lowest per capita GNP, it is customary for health centers to be staffed entirely by auxiliary or mid-level health personnel; perhaps one doctor will be present full-time or part-time—a general practitioner. There are often two levels of health center: *main centers* and *sub centers,* classified

according to their staffing. Even a lower level or more peripheral facility may be the *health post* or *health station,* staffed by a single auxiliary health worker. In the more moderate income developing countries health centers are usually staffed by one or perhaps two or three physicians, along with nurses and midwives, and sometimes a dentist. Health centers are built both in cities and in rural areas, but in the latter their role tends to be more crucial.

The exclusively preventive focus of health centers in some Latin American and other developing countries did not continue for many years after World War II. If only to attract patients for the preventive services, it was soon learned that the treatment of common ailments in the ambulatory person had to be offered each day—generally in the mornings.

In several affluent industrialized countries, however, health centers are still often restricted to the provision of preventive services. In the United States, the health centers authorized for federal construction grants to the states are essentially for the housing of local Health Departments and their prevention-oriented clinics. Prevention is also the function of a large network of health centers in Japan and the approach of many of the health centers of France and virtually all such facilities in Belgium.

As noted, the hospital outpatient clinic, outside of North America, eventually became a resource for ambulatory service to the general population—not solely for the poor. Since hospitals have been staffed by specialists throughout the twentieth century, outpatient care has also been provided by medical, surgical, and other specialists. Nearly everywhere hospital outpatient departments (OPDs) offer three types of services: (1) organized specialty sessions (medical, surgical, pediatric, etc.) at designated hours of the week, (2) the casualty or emergency service, to which patients may come for urgent conditions at any time of the day or night, and (3) clinics to examine referred patients for possible admission. A nonhospital community doctor may refer a patient to this unit, but the decision on admission to a bed customarily depends on a hospital doctor. In most developing countries, the hospital

OPD clinic is the major channel for specialist care to moderate and low income patients.

Thus, organized health services to the ambulatory person or patient have been launched under a variety of sponsorships in a diversity of settings. The objective has always been to extend the service more efficiently and effectively than has been possible as an individual endeavor. When the concept of primary health care matured in the last decades of the twentieth century, the importance of ambulatory service to the overall functioning of national health systems became better appreciated. Along with environmental protection and hospital care of serious illness, organized ambulatory health service could complete the achievement of an integrated system structure to serve national populations.

REFERENCES

Anon., "Primary Health Care is Not Curing Africa's Ills." *The Economist,* 299:91–94, 31 May 1986.

Attinger, E. O., "High Technology: The Pendulum Must Swing Back." *World Health Forum,* 8:305–338, 1987.

Banerji, Debabar, "Primary Health Care: Selective or Comprehensive." *World Health Forum,* 5:312–315, 1984.

Braveman, Paula, "Primary Health Care Takes Root in Nicaragua." *World Health Forum,* 6:368–372, 1985.

Bryant, John H., "Ten Years After Alma Ata." *World Health,* 10–15, August/September 1988.

Burrell, Craig D., and Cecil G. Sheps (Editors), *Primary Health Care in Industrialized Nations.* New York: New York Academy of Sciences, 1978.

Clute, K. F., *The General Practitioner.* Toronto: University of Toronto Press, 1963.

Corwin, E.H.L., *The American Hospital.* New York: Commonwealth Fund, 1946.

Deodhar, N. S., "Primary Health Care in India." *Journal of Public Health Policy,* 3(1):76–99, March 1982.

Djukanovic, V., and E. Mach (Editors), *Alternative Approaches to Meeting Basic Health Needs in Developing Countries* (A Joint UNICEF/WHO Study). Geneva: WHO, 1975.

Fendall, N.R.E., *Auxiliaries in Health Care: Programs in Developing Countries.* Baltimore, MD: Johns Hopkins University Press, 1972.

Fisek, N. H., and R. Erdal, "Primary Health Care: A Continuous Effort" (Turkey). *World Health Forum,* 6:230–231, 1985.

Fonaroff, Arlene, *Community Involvement in Health Systems for Primary Health Care.* Geneva: World Health Organization (SHS/83.6), 1983.

Freidson, Eliot, *Professional Dominance: The Social Structure of Medical Care.* New York: Aldine-Atherton Press, 1970.

Fulop, T., and M. I. Roemer, *International Development of Health Manpower Policy.* Geneva: World Health Organization (Offset Pub. No. 61), 1982.

Gagnon, Anita J., "The Training and Integration of Village Health Workers." *Bulletin of the Pan American Health Organization,* 25(2):127–138, 1991.

Kohn, Robert, and Kerr L. White (Editors), *Health Care: An International Study.* London: Oxford University Press, 1976.

Lee, K., and A. Mills, (Editors), *The Economics of Health in Developing Countries.* Oxford: Oxford University Press, 1983.

Ming, Ho Tak, "The Present Problems and Future Needs of Primary Health Care in Malaysia." *International Journal of Health Services,* 18(2):281–291, 1988.

Mongelsdorf, K. L., J. Luna, and H. L. Smith, "Primary Health Care and Public Policy" (Ecuador). *World Health Forum,* 9:509–513, 1988.

Newell, Kenneth W. (Editor), *Health by the People.* Geneva: World Health Organization, 1975.

Ofosu-Amaah, Virginia, *National Experience in the Use of Community Health Workers.* Geneva: World Health Organization (Offset Publication No. 71), 1983.

Pan American Health Organization (with UNICEF, UNFPA, and Cuban Ministry of Health), *Cuba's Family Doctor Programme.* Washington, D.C.: PAHO, 1991.

Panikar, P.G.K., "Intersectoral Action for Health—the Kerala Case." *World Health Forum,* 5:46–48, 1984.

Peterson, Osler L., L. P. Andrews, R. S. Spain, and B. G. Greenberg, "An Analytical Study of North Carolina General Practice." *Journal of Medical Education,* 31:Part 2, December 1956.

Reinke, W. A., and M. Wolff, "The Lampong Health Development Project: The Road to Health for All?" *World Health Forum,* 4:114–120, 1983.

Rifkin, Susan B., *Health Planning and Community Participation: Case Studies in Studies in South-East Asia.* London: Croom Helm, 1985.

Roemer, Milton I., "On Paying the Doctor and the Implication of Different Methods." *Journal of Health and Human Behavior,* 3:4–14, Spring 1962.

Roemer, Milton I., Carl E. Hopkins, Lockwood Carr, and Foline Gartside, "Copayments for Ambulatory Care: Penny-wise and Pound-foolish." *Medical Care,* 13(6):457–466, June 1975.

Roemer, Milton I., "Primary Health Care and Physician Extenders in Affluent Countries." *International Journal of Health Services,* 7:545–555, Fall 1977.

Salkever, David S., "Economic Class and Differential Access to Care: Comparisons Among Health Care Systems." *International Journal of Health Services,* 5(3):373–395, 1975.

Shryock, R. H., *The Development of Modern Medicine.* New York: Alfred A. Knopf, 1936.

Sidel, V. W., and R. Sidel, *Serve the People: Observations on Medicine in the People's Republic of China.* New York: Josiah Macy, Jr. Foundation, 1973.

Starr, P., *The Social Transformation of American Medicine.* New York: Basic Books, 1982.

Stern, B. J., *American Medical Practice in the Perspectives of a Century.* New York: The Commonwealth Fund, 1945.

Tarimo, E., and F.G.R. Fowkes, "District Health Systems: Strengthening the Backbone of Primary Health Care." *World Health Forum,* 10:74–79, 1989.

Tarimo, E., and A. Creese (Editors), *Achieving Health All by the Year 2000: Midway Reports of Country Experiences.* Geneva: World Health Organization, 1990.

Unger, Jean-Pierre, and James R. Killingsworth, "Selective Primary Health Care: A Critical Review of Methods and Results." *Social Science and Medicine,* 22(10):1001–1013, 1986.

United Nations Development Programme, *Human Resource Development for Primary Health Care* (Evaluation Study No. 9). New York: UNDP, December 1983.

Vadek, Martin To, "Primary Health Care in Papua-New Guinea." *World Health Forum,* 4:313–314, 1983.

Vuori, Hannu, and John Hastings, *Patterns of Community Participation in Primary Health Care.* Copenhagen: WHO Regional Office for Europe, 1985.

World Health Organization, *The First Ten Years of the World Health Organization.* Geneva: WHO, 1958.

World Health Organization, *The Primary Health Worker.* Geneva: WHO, 1974.

World Health Organization, *Primary Health Care* (Report of the International Conference on Primary Health Care, Alma Ata, USSR, 6–12 September 1978). Geneva: WHO, 1978.

World Health Organization, *Sixth Report on the World Health Situation 1973–1977* (Part I: Global Analysis). Geneva: WHO, 1980.

World Health Organization, *Organization of Primary Health Care in Communities.* Geneva: WHO (SHS/1AH 84.1), 1984.

World Health Organization, *Intersectoral Action for Health: The Role of Intersectoral Cooperation in National Strategies for Health for All.* Geneva: WHO, 1986.

World Health Organization, "Primary Health Care in Practice." *World Health Forum,* 8:56–66, 1987.

World Health Organization and UNICEF, *Primary Health Care: The Community Health Worker* (Report of a UNICEF/WHO Interregional Study and Workshop - PHC/80.2). Geneva: WHO, February 1980.

CHAPTER THIRTEEN

Hospital Services

In every national health system there are structures to accommodate in bed seriously ill patients who require medical or surgical treatment. Hospitals are constructed to hold varying numbers of patients (with various types of illness). As shown in Chapter 3, the supply of hospital beds in relation to the population of a country generally varies with the national income level—from 65 beds per 100,000 in Indonesia, for example, to 2,000 beds per 100,000 in Sweden. The size of a hospital building, furthermore, may vary from accomodations of 10 or 20 up to 1,000 beds or more.

ORGANIZATION AND MANAGEMENT

As scientific and medical technology developed, the structure of modern hospitals has become increasingly complex. The maintenance of services for numerous patients requires nurses, technicians, custodial, and other personnel working together in some systematic way. Typically these personnel are supervised by others, all of whom come under the control of a hospital director, who is usually a physician. In all but the smallest hospitals, there is usually a chief nurse who supervises nurses as well as laboratory technicians and others. In large hospitals, with numerous departments, various assistant administrators may oversee technical services (laboratory and X-ray), business matters, hotel-type services, and so on.

The functions of the modern hospital of moderate size are far broader than a century ago. They may be summarized as follows:

1. Inpatient diagnosis and treatment, with increasingly complex technology.

2. Outpatient care, for the ambulatory patient and the emergency case.
3. Education of health personnel, both through formal courses and continuing education.
4. Research, principally through study of the clinical care of patients.
5. Prevention, through screening for case detection and health education.
6. Organized home care, after discharge of patients, both acute and chronic.
7. Rehabilitation through direct services or referral to other resources.
8. Administration or supervision of satellite health facilities.

To keep hospital services functioning efficiently, the hospital management must arrange for food and medication, laundry, waste disposal, and maintenance of medical records. Arrangements must also be made for the discharge of patients whose treatment is completed and the admission of new patients. When surgical operations are to be performed, there are many requirements for the operating room. The X-ray department and pathology laboratory have special needs that must be met. Rehabilitation equipment is another resource located in a modern hospital. In addition, hospital management is responsible for supervising and monitoring the performance of every member of the hospital team.

The general management of small hospitals (with perhaps 20 beds or less) is ordinarily entrusted to one or two individuals each of whom has multiple functions. As hospital size increases, the administrative structure becomes more elaborate. Frequently the top management is assigned to a *board of directors,* each member of which reflects certain interests. Both public and private hospitals may have such supervisory boards, although their composition would differ.

The sponsorship of a hospital is the major determinant of the composition of a supervisory board of directors. As noted in Chapter 3, in the majority of countries governmental sponsorship predominates. In practice, however, the boards of public hospitals meet quite infrequently, and the normal management of the facility is left in the hands of the hospital director and his or her staff.

In theory, the board of directors of a hospital is expected to provide accountability. Complaints about hospital performance can be addressed by anyone to the board. Acceptance of grievances, however, depends on the composition of the board. In public hospitals, board members are theoretically dependent on the electorate who vote. In private hospitals, boards are self-selected, and are dominated by donors and leading citizens. Representatives of workers or farmers are scarce.

The collection of funds from various sources is a requirement of almost every hospital. This means an office of *business affairs* or of finance in the administrative structure. Even if a government-supported hospital is financed entirely by a Ministry of Health, the money must be handled according to certain conventions. When the Hospital Director is an administrative physician, the second-in-command is often an economist or similar person who is qualified to handle financial accounts.

It is often necessary to calculate the cost of certain specific services in a hospital's operation. This might be required by an insurance program or for a patient whose care is exceptional. The hospital business office would have the expertise to make such calculations. This office must also monitor all forms of spending to be certain that accounts are solvent throughout the year.

The technical equipment and staffing of a hospital vary generally with its bed capacity. Small hospitals may have little more than a laboratory microscope and a supply of drugs. Larger hospitals usually have complex X-ray and electronic equipment and instruments for performing several types of endoscopic examination. Record systems may be elaborate, and there are channels for rapid communication between hospital departments.

Payments for hospital service may be based on a variety of mechanisms. At the end of the nineteenth century, charges were made somewhat arbitrarily for each item of service. In the early twentieth century, charges were replaced by overall *per diem* amounts. With the great expansions of population coverage for health care financing in Europe, several countries developed methods of supporting hospitals by monthly budgetary payments. In France and Germany, this was done for all public hospitals and per diem payments were used for the rest. In the Scandinavian countries prospective global budgets were implemented to pay for all hospitals. Adjustments for shortfalls might be made at the end of the year.

Financial support for hospitals in the developing countries is generally indirect. The personnel are usually paid by the Ministry of Health or similar agency out of some provincial or district fund set up to finance all health services. Separate allotments for food, drugs, and other expenses are then made to each hospital. For special emergencies, supplementary grants may be sought. Equivalent support would come for hospitals owned by social security programs or other agencies. Mission hospitals in developing countries are typically subsidized by Ministries of Health, to help in the purchase of drugs and supplies.

Amenities for patient care are highly variable. In affluent industrialized countries, the prevailing style has beds in small rooms, accommodating a handful of patients (perhaps two to six), with ample bedside comforts. In less developed countries, wards of 12 to 30 beds are still common, and amenities for patient comfort are minimal. In very poor countries, beds may even lack pillows and linens. Toilet facilities are usually limited, and there may be no provisions for patient privacy.

In both industrialized and developing countries, as shown in Chapter 9, hospitals absorb a substantial share of national health expenditures. Based on experience from the 1970s, in Europe and North America the hospital share runs 50 to 70 percent. In developing countries of Africa and Asia, the hospital share is more likely to run 25 to 50 percent. The major factor in hospitalization costs is the complement of personnel, which increases with hospital capacity. In a developed country, a hospital of 500 beds is likely to have three or four personnel per bed, whereas a 100-bed hospital would have one or two personnel per bed. Expressed as hospital personnel per occupied bed, the staffing ratios for all-sized hospitals in selected industrialized countries in 1985 were as follows:

Country	Personnel per Occupied Bed
United States	2.75
Great Britain	2.40
Canada	2.40
Sweden	1.85
Switzerland	1.67
Netherlands	1.55
France	1.37

In developing countries, these personnel-to-bed ratios are typically less than 1.0.

MEDICAL STAFF ORGANIZATION

In almost all countries, the complement of hospital personnel is dominated by physicians, who are employed within the hospital the same way as nurses or technicians. The pattern of medical staffing seen throughout the United States—where numerous private physicians, based in their private offices, visit the hospital part time—is seldom seen elsewhere, except for Canada. Only in private proprietary hospitals—usually constituting a minor fraction of total beds—is open staffing common in both industrialized and developing countries.

The pattern of medical staffing with full-time hospital physicians, in various specialties, permanently attached to each hospital is the prevailing one throughout the world. In industrialized countries, there is competition for these hospital appointments, since the hospital physician has high prestige, is well paid by salary, and may also have freedom to treat certain patients privately. These physicians are responsible for both bed patients and outpatients.

Outside the hospital staff, physicians in the

community are typically general practitioners. For continuity of patient care, hospital specialists are expected to send reports on discharged patients back to the primary practitioner. In many countries, hospital medical staffs carry on programs of continuing education for all out-of-hospital physicians.

The high costs of hospital care have stimulated many strategies designed to ensure prudent policies in hospital management and service. In the organization of the medical staff, this is expressed through various committees. These committees review surgical tissues, examine prescribed drugs, check on the completeness of medical records, and control costs by reviewing bed utilization and monitoring the length of inpatient stay. To cope with difficult issues of "life and death," many medical staffs have established ethics committees. In large hospitals, medical staff discipline is applied to each department—surgery, obstetrics, pediatrics, orthopedics, and so on.

As the use of hospitals has increased throughout the world, the scope of hospital functions has broadened. Each of the eight functions listed earlier develops along several lines. The outpatient clinics, for example, may encompass special services for the mentally ill and for other disorders. Emergency services entail connections with ambulances and first-aid responses. Clinics for children provide a setting for routine immunizations.

The medical staff organization in hospitals is associated with the whole issue of quality assessment and promotion. A paradigm proposed by Avedis Donabedian in the 1960s and further developed by several others called for information on the "structure, process, and outcome" of medical care. Structure is the input of resources, process is the service provided, and outcome is the result in terms of morbidity, recovery, or mortality. Most of these evaluations are applied in hospitals, although quality promotion entails actions in the whole health system.

As a practical matter, the most useful and readily available data for quality evaluation relate to the process of medical care. In hospitals, this is ordinarily available from patient records. Reviews of records have been called *medical audits,* and when these are undertaken by medical colleagues on the hospital staff they are regarded as a form of *peer review*. Record reviews are often carried out by an external expert, engaged specifically to evaluate quality of care. This person may employ explicit criteria (prepared in advance for each diagnostic category) or simply go by the overall judgment of the record reviewer. A correct process in the treatment of a patient is assumed to yield a good outcome.

There is much debate, however, on the relationship of process to outcome of medical care. Outcome might be considered a more definitive measure of quality, except that it might be largely influenced by factors other than the medical care process—for example, genetic traits or environmental conditions. Process combined with outcome data might seem the most robust basis for quality evaluation, except that outcomes require a long time to determine.

The general trend of quality evaluation in hospitals is toward a goal of explicit criteria for the process of diagnosis and treatment. Algorithms and decision trees are being formulated for an increasing range of conditions. With such objective guidelines, quality evaluations may be carried out in hospitals, even where expert evaluators are not at hand. The very act of process evaluation may heighten medical staff consciousness of the importance of quality assessment.

The promotion of improved quality of service in any hospital or other health facility depends on a very broad scope of policies. It begins with the appointment to the staff of well-qualified personnel. The organization of clinical departments, with their special modalities and reasonable peer review, is essential. Quality standards in ancillary services, such as laboratories, X-ray departments, pharmacies, and so on, are important. Patient records must be prepared and maintained scrupulously. Medical staff meetings are important, along with clinical conferences. Various surveillance committees on prescribed drugs, medical records, and bed utilization have been noted. In addition to regular clinical conferences, formal courses may be held to meet legal requirements for continuing education. Special educational conferences may be offered on new

medical tasks, such as the diagnosis and treatment of HIV infection and AIDS or the principles of psychopharmacology.

REGIONALIZATION

To facilitate hospital services in large geographic regions, many countries have planned their hospitals according to a rational network. At the periphery of the region, the local hospital would handle simple conditions. The next level would accommodate cases requiring special skills in surgery and medicine. At the regional center would be a large hospital with resources for tertiary-level care. Everyone would have access to the small peripheral hospital for uncomplicated conditions. More complicated cases would go to the second-level hospital in a district or to a tertiary-level hospital in the main city.

Such regionalized hospital schemes have been developed as roads and vehicles for transportation have become available. The full implementation of the regionalization concept depends on the operation of economic support programs. Without such support, the patient's care might be provided in the facility that was nearby (regardless of patient need). With regionalization, patients go to the hospital with resources most appropriate for their condition.

The earliest explicit formulation of hospital regionalization was developed in Denmark in 1912. Patients were transported from rural towns to Copenhagen rather than trying to establish a complete hospital at every cross-road. In the United States, since the 1930s, several specific programs have implemented the regionalization concept. The Bingham Associates Fund supported linkage of 24 small hospitals with 3 larger district hospitals in Maine and a major medical center in Boston. In the early 1940s, the Rochester (New York) Regional Hospital Council developed cooperative services with hospitals in seven surrounding counties. In the late 1940s, the National Hospital Survey and Construction Act required regionalized *master plans* as a condition for federal hospital grants to the states. In 1965, the Regional Medical Programs for Heart Disease, Cancer, and Stroke encouraged regional ties between medical schools and surrounding hospitals. In 1974 the National Health Planning and Resources Development Act gave a further boost to regionalization, involving both hospitals and ambulatory care facilities.

The customary classification of hospitals in a regional scheme defines three types of facility. In Norway, for example, there are 19 provinces grouped into 5 regions. Each province has one provincial hospital and perhaps one or two local hospitals. Each of the five regions has one regional hospital. To implement the scheme, every hospital budget must be reviewed by the central Ministry of Health. The criteria for review depend on the level of the hospital in the regional scheme. Certain personnel for high-technology equipment would be approved in a regional-level hospital but not in a provincial hospital. Other staffing in a provincial hospital might be approved, but not in a local hospital. Thus each hospital is financed according to its theoretical place in the regionalized network.

Cooperative relationships may also be developed among several hospitals in a region. In France, hospitals of the level of *département* may jointly provide outpatient ambulatory service or conduct educational programs. Services for rehabilitation may be offered in several hospitals by physical therapists who travel around a region. Unusual laboratory tests might be done by one hospital on behalf of several other hospitals in a region.

In Great Britain regionalization has been a guiding health policy. The original administrative scheme in 1948 divided England and Wales into 15 *hospital regions* for management of all hospitals and specialist services. In the 1974 reorganization, these became *health regions*—subdivided into districts. The global budget for each hospital depends on its place in the framework of the health region. In this way hospital technology is kept under control and helps to account for the relatively low costs of the British National Health Service. Recent policy moves to create an internal competitive market in the NHS are likely to elevate expenditures.

Full regionalization depends on the coordination of all hospitals under some central authority. In Latin America, where most countries have several separate sets of hospitals under Ministries of Health, Social Security programs, charitable welfare societies, and private ownership, each group tends to have its own regional scheme. In Chile and in Cuba, where several sponsorships have been unified, effective regionalization is feasible.

The benefits of hospital regionalization are both qualitative and economical. Performance of procedures in the hospital properly equipped and staffed obviously contributes to quality. Personnel appropriate for each hospital's type of case achieves economies.

Relationships among health facilities in a region need not be restricted to hospitals. Exchanges should occur also with health centers devoted to ambulatory care. Such centers are extensive in the Scandinavian countries, in the several formerly socialist countries, and in most of the developing countries on all the continents. Since the staffing of health centers in many of these countries is relatively weak, the back-up of hospital personnel in the same region is especially valuable.

Hospitals may be regarded as back-up facilities for primary health care. This is especially true for the *district hospital,* serving a population of about 100,000 people. In Africa, however, this figure reaches about 160,000 people, and in Thailand only 40,000. The catchment population of a district hospital usually defines the boundaries of a health district for overall health care purposes.

HOSPITAL UTILIZATION

The great majority of hospitals are intended to accommodate patients with a wide range of disorders—that is, they are general hospitals. The length of stay of different patients is highly variable, from a few days for a simple surgical case to several weeks for an elderly patient with cancer or heart disease. The average length of stay for all general hospitals in Western Europe is about 20 days; in the United States and Canada it is about 10 days.

Among industrialized countries, the rate of use of hospitals by the population varies substantially. For 1985, the rates of hospitalization are reported in Table 13.1. It is evident

Table 13.1. Hospitalization in Industrialized Countries: Hospital Days Per 1,000 Per Year, 1985

Country	Days	Country	Days
Turkey	700	Switzerland	3100
Portugal	1100	Australia	3200
Spain	1200	Austria	3300
Greece	1400	France	3400
Ireland	1500	Germany	3500
Italy	1700	Iceland	3500
United States	1700	Luxembourg	3700
Canada	2000	Japan	3800
Denmark	2100	Netherlands	3900
Great Britain	2200	Finland	4400
New Zealand	2700	Sweden	4500
Belgium	2800	Norway	5200

Source: Organization for Economic Development and Cooperation, *Health Care Systems in Transition.* Paris: OEDC, 1990.

that hospital use in the Scandinavian countries is several times the rate experienced in countries of the Mediterranean region.

The sponsorship of hospitals has an inevitable influence on their rate of use. Public hospitals, for which there is an established scheme of economic support, are kept more fully occupied than hospitals under private sponsorship, even if nonprofit. As shown in Chapter 3, government sponsorship predominates in both industrialized and developing countries.

A day of hospital care implies a rich mixture of diagnostic, treatment, and social services. Elaborate diagnostic work-ups of complex cases are done in hospitals, of course, largely because of the difficulty of carrying out such procedures on the ambulatory patient. The range of possible therapies that can be done only in hospitals has steadily widened—organ transplants, open-heart surgery, kidney dialyses, rehabilitation of severely disabled patients, or short-term treatment of acute mental disorders.

The general hospital serves patients with any type of illness or injury, as well as maternity cases. The great majority of general hospitals are intended to serve short-term or acutely ill patients with a duration of illness lasting under 30 days. Sometimes there are separate hospitals for maternity care, communicable disease, and sick children. Every country has special hospitals for the mentally ill.

This discussion has focused on the delivery of service in hospitals, and the expansion of the hospital's many functions. Still—as observed in Chapters 3 and 12—the very complexity and high costs of hospital care have given rise to various strategies for reducing hospital use. Home care programs, operated by the hospitals themselves as well as by other agencies, have been noted. Hospital outpatient departments may treat patients adequately without admission to a bed. In several industrialized countries, there are outpatient *surgicenters* for simple operative procedures, such as lens replacements for cataracts, hernial repairs, treatment of varicosities, splinting of fractures, and abortions. Most important is the community health center that is playing an increasing role in both developing and industrialized countries. The multipurpose functions and teamwork characteristic of hospitals are coming to apply to the larger health centers or polyclinics. For long-stay cases, usually in the elderly, nursing homes and custodial facilities are developing everywhere to reduce the utilization of expensive hospital care.

LONG-TERM CARE

Another aspect of hospital services that is associated with several types of institutional care is the care of the long-term patient. With the survival of greater numbers of elderly patients who need care—but not elaborate hospital service—many other forms of long-term care are being developed. In the industrialized countries, these problems have long been recognized, and they are now becoming evident in numerous developing countries as well.

Long-term care may be defined as a continuum of programs, starting with the most intensive and moving to the simplest. These include

1. The care of long-stay patients in general hospitals
2. Nursing homes, providing skilled nursing and other services to long-stay patients
3. Custodial care in old people's homes
4. Residential living for the elderly
5. Organized home care to elderly patients in their own homes

It is difficult to give a time of onset of long-term care and even more difficult to give a time of termination.

The exact meaning of each of these stages of long-term care differs somewhat between countries, and sometimes terminology differs completely, so that cross-country comparisons must be made with great caution. In general the first two of these basic types of long-term care are sponsored and financed by health authorities and the last three by social welfare authorities. Exact sources of financing are very complex. Our focus therefore is the patterns of delivery, rather than the source of economic support.

Long-term care in general hospitals is very expensive, so that every effort is made to discharge patients. Where nursing home beds are relatively few, however, as in Japan, this extravagance is tolerated under national health insurance financing. In the United States some outstanding hospitals that specialize in long-term patient care have been developed. The Montefiore Hospital in New York, which evolved into a great medical center, is one of the most creative of such long-term hospitals. In many hospitals, the long-term patient population stimulated the entire field of hospital-based rehabilitation.

In most industrialized countries long-term care patients occupy an increasing proportion of hospital beds. This is feasible because of the support of national health insurance programs. At the same time this has probably been the major force promoting the development of nursing homes. These have been under both public and private sponsorship, varying with the character of the national health system. Thus in the United States, with its entrepreneurial health system, private sponsorship of nursing homes is strongly predominant.

The organization and financing of nursing homes and their supervision by government have come to dominate discussion in the entire field of long-term care. The policies are so variable between countries and bewildering even within countries that it is impossible to generalize. It will be most helpful for understanding long-term care if we examine nursing homes in selected countries: Great Britain, Norway, Japan, Canada, New Zealand, and the United States.

Our focus, of course, is on the organization of long-term care in national health systems and not on the clinical aspects of such care. One aspect of clinical medicine, however, should be noted—the development in several countries of a specialty of geriatrics. (This has been especially prominent in England.) With such leadership in the medical profession, all aspects of long-term care have acquired greater dignity, especially in the medical centers for teaching and research.

In Great Britain, nursing homes providing skilled nursing service under public sponsorship are rare. Growing numbers of such nursing homes under private sponsorship, however, are being organized. Since they are outside the National Health Service, they must be privately financed by affluent families.

The British *Old People's Home* is administered by local health and welfare authorities, but it does not provide skilled nursing care. It is essentially a custodial facility for frail patients who need help in activities of daily living. These old peoples homes are financed by local government, but the individual is asked to contribute if possible. Other services for persons entirely outside of institutions in Britain are discussed below.

In Norway, there is a strong development of public nursing homes, financed and controlled by the county governments. About 50 percent of their support comes from national health insurance funds. The demand for nursing home beds, however, is much higher than the supply, and there are long waiting lists. The trained personnel and the quality of services in Norwegian nursing homes are usually very high.

For the elderly who are frail but still ambulatory, there are public old people's homes in Norway. The shortage of nursing home beds has also forced these facilities to accept sick elderly in nursing home sections. These units are financed entirely by local municipalities without any support from national health insurance. They have become combinations of custodial and nursing home programs.

In Japan, where the aging of the population is more recent, the development of nursing homes has been relatively weak. As noted earlier, general hospitals furnish most of the long-term care. Policy now is to promote the development of private nursing homes as in the

United States. The local welfare office pays for low-income residents (equivalent to Medicaid support in the United States).

Canada supports a great deal of nursing home care. Since 1977, when the federal government gave block grants to the provinces for *extended care*, such services have been a regular benefit in nearly all provinces under the provincial-national health insurance program. Each province decides exactly how these grants should be used, within the long-term care spectrum of services. The chief problem is an inadequate number of nursing home beds. For the majority of long-stay patients, costs are covered by the national health insurance program; for welfare recipients there is financial assistance from the Canada Assistance Plan.

Proximity to the United States, with its large supply of skilled nursing home beds, has encouraged the construction of skilled nursing homes in Canada. Private groups, both nonprofit and for-profit, are being encouraged to play a part. Canada has a good supply of trained personnel to staff these facilities.

In the affluent Canadian setting, as in the United States, there is another type of protected living for the elderly—in residential living projects. These are simply small settlements of private homes, with provision for meals, recreation, entertainment, and community life. There may be a local medical care program that is entirely private. In Western Europe in public housing projects, some residential units may be reserved for the elderly. The Netherlands has been encouraging such arrangements.

New Zealand illustrates a comprehensive health system, in which skilled nursing homes have not developed. Instead, long-term care is simply provided in general hospitals. For the frail elderly, who are still ambulatory, there are old people's homes; these are principally controlled by private nonprofit organizations. The New Zealand Ministry of Health sets minimum standards for the old people's homes.

Finally we may examine the United States, where nursing homes play a very large role in the provision of long-stay care. The field is dominated by privately owned for-profit facilities. Many of these are owned by corporate chains. Financial support of patients comes from different sources. The oldest source is the private individual or family, sustained in a limited share of cases by private insurance. Since 1965, when the federal Medicare insurance program was enacted, it has included Medicaid for public assistance recipients of several categories. The costs under Medicaid are shared with the states. A small percentage of patients is supported by local *general assistance*.

As private businesses, there is a great deal of competition among U.S. nursing homes, especially in large cities. This results in many cost-cutting practices that may seriously affect the quality of care. Patients are deeply sedated, because this simplifies their care although it is not good for them. Some patients with mental deterioration may be physically restrained instead of being provided proper nursing care. To reduce abuses, government regulations under Medicaid have been tightened by the state authorities. Even the federal government requires nursing home administrators to be trained and licensed. Enforcement of regulations rests with the states, and there are often difficult choices between upholding standards and closing down a nursing home completely.

The whole issue of skilled nursing home care in the United States is tied up with the larger question of national health insurance. In the many debates about national health insurance, the inclusion of benefits for long-stay care in nursing homes is being urged. This is especially prominent in the 1988 policy recommendations of the Pepper Commission on National Health Insurance and Long-Term Care. Senior citizen groups are naturally very active in the whole debate about long-stay care under national health insurance. Such care is, of course, expensive, but its exclusion raises ethical questions about the rights of the elderly.

This completes our discussion of nursing home care in the general field of long-stay care of selected countries. We proceed to a more general discussion of custodial care, based on the experience of the same countries. Custodial care, as here discussed, consists of two types: services provided in facilities and services provided in the patient's home.

In virtually all industrialized countries, programs have been organized to help elderly people to live more comfortably. In Norway, as noted, there are old people's homes, which have become blended with nursing homes. In addition, there are separate arrangements for residential living and community service. These are controlled by the Social Welfare Board of the local municipality. Although some pay a share of the costs, the great majority of residents are welfare recipients who make no payments. Most important is organized service for the patient living in a personal or family home. Home nursing services are financed 25 percent by the municipalities and 75 percent of the national health insurance. In addition there are homemaker services provided in all of Norway's 444 municipalities, at small charges. National welfare authorities reimburse the municipalities for 50 percent of these expenses.

Japan has had a stronger development of custodial programs than of its nursing homes. In 1980 there were about 1,000 old people's homes, with about 70,000 beds. The resident must bear part of the cost, according to a sliding scale. In addition there are community services brought to elderly people in family homes. Nurses or physical therapists may visit personal homes periodically. Homemaker services are offered by the municipalities through the local social welfare agencies.

The policy in many countries is to shift care as much as possible out of institutions—nursing homes, old people's homes, and even residential homes—to community-based services, supportive of life in the home of the individual or family. This is well illustrated in Great Britain, where, since the nineteenth century, home nursing services were designed to keep people out of hospitals. In the twentieth century, it has been formulated as home care programs of wider scope. It includes organized homemaker services, friendly visitors, and *meals on wheels.* It also includes opportunities for elderly people to keep busy with visits to day centers.

In countries of Western Europe—Germany, France, Netherlands, Belgium, and Switzerland—long-term care has been financed from several sources. Statutory health insurance pays for certain benefits. Pension funds have provided retired persons with money that can be used for long-term care. For the elderly with little personal income, social welfare programs of municipalities are often the principal source to pay for nursing home care or organized

home care. Since so many elderly people are very poor, municipal government carries the major responsibility for long-term care.

Organized home care has become a worldwide movement in the industrialized countries. The sponsoring agencies differ among countries, but they operate principally at the local level. In welfare-oriented and comprehensive health systems, sponsorship is mainly by public bodies—hospitals and public health agencies. In entrepreneurial health systems, sponsorship is often by voluntary Visiting Nurse Associations or entirely by private enterprises. In the United States, where home health agencies are financed by the 1965 Medicare law, there are 5700 home health agencies, of which 33 are sponsored by proprietary corporations.

In the United States community-based services, designed to enable elderly people to stay in their own homes, are also being explored through dozens of experimental projects. Social workers use several modalities noted above, with financial support provided by Medicaid and the federal Older Americans Act. This typically requires partial support from state governments as well.

Social services—both in facilities and in family homes—are obviously very diverse. Terminology across countries is quite confusing. The organization and financing are more frequently under social welfare agencies than under health agencies; both of these tend to involve responsibilities for local government.

The entire field of long-term care throughout the industrialized world is in great ferment. This is true of all five major components: (1) hospital services, (2) nursing home services, (3) custodial services, (4) residential living, and (5) organized home care.

Services in nursing homes—in response to epidemiological trends—require the most attention. Yet to stem this tide, custodial services are being developed in facilities, along with home care at home. As an overriding policy goal, the objective of long-stay care is to maximize life in the patient's own home. This is linked with other movements of the World Health Organization on self-care and primary care.

This entire discussion has focused on national health systems in industrialized and affluent countries, where long-stay care has been a prominent issue. In the less developed countries, however, equivalent issues are just coming to the foreground. This is clear in large countries, such as India, China, or Indonesia, or moderate sized ones, such as Brazil or Nigeria. Even though the percentage of elderly people in these countries is relatively low, the number of such people is very large. As the incidence of infectious diseases caused by poverty declines, and the elderly live longer, the requirements for organized programs of long-term care for the elderly will rapidly increase. Many have pointed out the double burden in developing countries, requiring continued programs of primary health care and the new assault required in long-term care.

REFERENCES

Hospital Organization and Management

Bridgman, R. F., and M. I. Roemer, *Hospital Legislation and Hospital Systems.* Geneva: World Health Organization, 1973.

Faxon, Nathaniel W. (Editor), *The Hospital in Contemporary Life.* 1949.

Georgopoulos, B. S., and A. Matejko, "The American General Hospital as a Complex Social System." *Health Services Research,* 2:76–112, 1967.

MacEachern, Malcolm T., *Hospital Organization and Management.* Berwyn, IL: Physician Record, 1962.

Mills, Anne, "The Economics of Hospitals in Developing Countries." *Health Policy and Planning,* 5:107–117, 1990.

Paine, L.H.W., and F. Siem Tjam, *Hospitals and the Health Care Revolution.* Geneva: World Health Organization, 1988.

Pan American Health Organization, *Bulletin—Special Issue on Bio-Ethics.* (4), 1990.

Perrow, C., "Hospitals: Technology, Structure and Goals." In J. March (Editor), *Handbook of Organizations.* Chicago: Rand McNally, 1965. pp. 142–169.

Regionalization

Koff, Sandra Z., "Regionalization and Hospital Reform in Italy." *Journal of Public Health Policy,* 3:205–228, 1982.

Macagba, Rufino L., "Hospitals and Primary Health Care." *World Health Forum,* 6:223–229, 1985.

Palec, Rudolf, "The Regional System and Postgraduate Medical Training in Czechoslovakia." *Milbank Memorial Fund Quarterly,* 44(4):414–424, 1966.

Roemer, Milton I., "Regionalized Health Services in Seven Countries." *Hospitals,* 53:72–82, 1979.

Saward, Ernest W. (Editor), *The Regionalization of Personal Health Services (Revised Edition).* New York: Milbank Memorial Fund, 1976.

Somers, Anne R., "The Rationalization of Health Services: A Universal Priority." *Inquiry,* 8(1):48–60, 1971.

Van Lergerghe, W., and Y. Lafort, *The Role of the Hospital in the District: Delivering or Supporting Primary Health Care?* Geneva: World Health Organization (Division of Strengthening of Health Services), 1991.

World Health Organization Expert Committee, *Hospitals and Health for All.* Geneva: WHO, 1987.

Medical Staff Organization in Hospitals

Glaser, William A., *Social Settings and Medical Organization.* New York: Atherton, 1970.

Lembcke, Paul A., "Hospital Efficiency: A Lesson from Sweden." *Hospitals,* 1 April 1959.

Roemer, Milton I., "General Hospitals in Europe." In J. K. Owen (Editor), *Modern Concepts of Hospital Administration.* Philadelphia: W. B. Saunders, 1962.

Roemer, Milton I., and Jay W. Friedman, *Doctors in Hospitals: Medical Staff Organization and Hospital Performance.* Baltimore, MD: Johns Hopkins University Press, 1971.

Shortell, Stephen M., *Effective Hospital-Physician Relationships.* Ann Arbor, MI: Health Administration Press, 1991.

Smith, H. L., "Two Lines of Authority Are One Too Many." *Modern Hospital,* March 1984.

Hospital Utilization

Brook, R. H., *Quality of Care Assessment: A Comparison of Five Methods of Peer Review.* Washington, D.C.: National Center for Health Services Research and Development, 1973.

Coyne, Joseph S., and Milton I. Roemer, "Paying for Hospital Care: Evolution and Implications." *Journal of Public Health Policy,* 8:65–83, 1987.

Donabedian, A., *Explorations in Quality Assessment and Monitoring.* Ann Arbor, MI: Health Administration Press, 1980.

Ellwood, Paul M., et al., *Assuring the Quality of Health Care.* Minneapolis: InterStudy, 1973.

Organization for Economic Cooperation and Development, *Health Care Systems in Transition.* Paris: OECD, 1990.

Roemer, Milton I., "Political Ideology and Health Care: Hospital Patterns in the Phillippines and Cuba." *International Journal of Health Services,* 3:487–492, 1973.

Rosenfeld, L. S., "Quality of Medical Care in Hospitals." *American Journal of Public Health,* 47:856–865, July 1957.

Shapiro, S., "End Result Measurement of the Quality of Medical Care." *Milbank Memorial Fund Quarterly,* 45(2):7–30, 1967.

Sheps, M. C., "Approaches to the Quality of Hospital Care." *Public Health Reports,* 70:877–886, September 1955,

Long-Term Care

Bererfelt, Eva, "Norway." In Erdman Palmore (Editor), *International Handbook on Aging: Contemporary Developments and Research.* Westport CT: Greenwood Press, 1980.

Campbell, A. John. "Implications of Policy and Management Decisions on Access, Quality and Type of Services for the Elderly in New Zealand." In Marshall W. Raffel and Norma K. Raffel (Editors), *Perspectives on Health Policy: Australia, New Zealand, United States.* University Park: Pennsylvania State University Press, 1987.

Davies, Michael A., "Older Populations, Aging Individuals and Health for All." *World Health Forum,* 10:299–321, 1989.

Glaser, William A., *Health Insurance in Practice,* San Francisco: Jossey Bass, 1991.

Kalve, Trygve, "Help for Old People: Private Care and Public Responsibility." *World Health Forum,* 7:178–180, 1986.

Kane, Robert L., and Rosalie A. Kane, *Long-term Care in Six Countries: Implications for the United States.* Washington, D.C.: Fogarty International Center for Advanced Studies in Health Sciences, 1976.

Kane, Robert L., and Rosalie A. Kane, *A Will and a Way: What Americans Can Learn about Long-Term Care from Canada.* Santa Monica, CA: Rand, 1985.

Kane, Robert L., and Rosalie A. Kane, "Special Needs of Dependent Elderly Persons." In *Oxford Textbook of Public Health,* Vol. 3, Chapter 30. New York: Oxford University Press, 1991, pp. 509–521.

Kane, Robert L., J. G. Evans, and D. Macfadyen (Editors), *Improving the Health of Older People: A World View.* New York: Oxford University Press for the World Health Organization, 1990.

Koo, Jason, and Donald O. Cowgill, "Health Care of the Aged in Korea." *Social Science and Medicine,* 23(12):1347–1352, 1986.

Levey, Samuel, and N. Paul Loomba (Editors), *Long-term Care Administration: A Managerial Perspective.* New York: Spectrum, 1977.

Levinson, Dorothy, *Montefiore: The Hospital as Social Instrument 1884–1984.* New York: Farrar, Straus & Giroux, 1984.

Maeda, Nobuo, "Long-Term Care for the Elderly in Japan." In Teresa Schwab (Editor), *Caring for An Aging World: International Models for Long-Term Care, Financing, and Delivery.* New York: McGraw-Hill, 1988.

Nusberg, Charlotte, "Community Services: Social Care." In *Innovative Aging Programs Abroad: Implications for the United States.* Westport, CT: Greenwood Press, 1984.

Nusberg, C. H., *Improving Health Care of the Elderly: Examples from Around the World.* Washington, D.C.: Pan American Health Organization, 1985.

Palmore, Erdman (Editor), *International Handbook on Aging: Contemporary Developments and Research.* Westport CT: Greenwood Press, 1980.

Palmore, Erdman B., and Disaku Maeda, *The Honorable Elders Revisited.* Durham, NC: Duke University Press, 1985.

Shanas, Ethel, and M. E. Sussman (Editors), *Family, Bureaucracy and the Elderly.* Durham, NC: Duke University Press, 1977.

Shanas, Ethel, *Old People in Three Industrial Societies.* London: Routledge and Kegan Paul, 1968.

Zwick, Daniel I., "Home Health Services for the Elderly: The English Way." *Home Health Care Services Quarterly,* 5:13–65, 1985.

CHAPTER FOURTEEN

Health Programs for Certain Populations

In all countries there are special-purpose health programs that may be classified into three types: those serving certain types of person, those focused on certain types of disease or disorder, and those providing certain types of health service. In this chapter we examine health programs for certain types of population groups. In Chapters 15 and 16 we consider special programs for certain types of disorder and programs providing certain types of health service.

The main population groups on which certain programs are focused include mothers and children, industrial workers, and rural people, each of which has several subdivisions. Other groups include military personnel, prisoners, aboriginal people, and the poor. The manner of providing health services to these populations depends on the national health system, of which the special program is a part.

MOTHERS AND CHILDREN

In virtually every national health system, expectant mothers, infants, and small children have been served with special attention. The welfare of newborn babies, and therefore of their mothers, has an emotional appeal in all societies. The maternal and child health (MCH) services have come to include a whole spectrum of organized programs for subdivisions of this population. We may examine these according to conventional categories of organized efforts: pregnant women, infants and children, students in school, family planning, and abortion.

Pregnant Women

Special public health clinics for the antenatal care of pregnant women operate throughout the world. They were first started in western Europe. In the early nineteenth century, officials of local government in France and Great Britain organized dispensaries to instruct low-income mothers about proper infant feeding. The doctors staffing these units stressed the benefits of breast-feeding and that, if cow's milk was used, it should be boiled.

Antenatal—and also postpartum—clinics were soon adopted in the Ministry of Health programs throughout Europe. In the early twentieth century, they were organized in North America, not in hospital out-patient departments, but as free-standing structures. Initially these were in New York and a few other large cities, but in 1921 the Sheppard–Towner Act established a Board of Maternal and Infant Hygiene in the U. S. Department of Labor. This led to grants-in-aid to the State Health Departments for organizing antenatal as well as child health clinics. In the conservative atmosphere of the 1920s, however, opposition from the medical profession forced a termination of this federal support in 1929.

With the U.S. Social Security Act of 1935, in the depths of a great economic Depression, federal grants for MCH services were resumed, and they greatly strengthened prenatal clinic services in the states. These became a standard component of local Health Department programs in America, as they had become in Europe. The clinics were staffed by physicians and nurses and, unlike Europe, they were limited to women of low income. In larger towns and cities, where there were numerous private practitioners, medical opposition often forced the termination of prenatal clinics, on the ground that they were usurping the role of private medicine. With World War II (1939–1945), a special maternity and infant care program was organized for services by private physicians, paid by fees. This was the Emergency Maternal and Infant Care (EMIC) insurance for the dependents of noncommissioned military personnel.

In Western Europe, during the first half of the twentieth century, antenatal clinics were extensively developed. They were operated by Ministries of Health and staffed by physicians and midwives. All expectant mothers, of any income level, were encouraged to attend these clinics as early as possible in pregnancy. Incentives were even provided, through a requirement of prenatal care as a condition for receipt of a financial maternity bonus. In France, the requirements were quite specific, with three prenatal visits necessary for entitlement to the bonus.

These antenatal clinic services were developed earlier than the great extension of social insurance in Europe. As health insurance or national health services broadened to cover virtually everyone, mothers were free to consult private physicians for preventive services. Patients in France and Germany customarily saw a private doctor, while a substantial minority visited the clinics of public health authorities. In Great Britain, where general practitioners were paid by capitation, clinic services were more heavily used. In Scandinavian countries, with the greater use of health centers, public health nurses were routinely on hand to check infants and to counsel the mothers.

As social insurance coverage has been extended, enabling every woman to consult a private physician, the use of public health clinics has naturally declined. Some local health authorities tried to maintain prenatal or well-baby clinics, to be helpful to women of lower socioecomonic status (who might not be comfortable with a private practitioner). Prenatal services in most European countries are rendered by midwives or nurse-midwives, backed up occasionally by an obstetrician. In Germany, legislation of the 1960s mandated the provision of a full range of preventive services to be available from *sickness fund* doctors, so that public clinics declined further.

Since World War II, therefore, maternity-related services in Western Europe have been provided mainly by private medical practitioners, paid by social insurance. In Belgium,

France, Germany, Norway, and Switzerland the pregnant woman normally seeks prenatal care from the general practitioner or obstetrician of her choice. In Great Britain and most of Denmark, everyone is registered with a generalist (paid by capitation), who ordinarily refers the woman to a hospital for the childbirth.

In several countries—Germany, France, Denmark, the Netherlands, and Switzerland—prenatal clinics have been deliberately phased out. In Norway, Great Britain, Belgium, Spain, and Ireland, organized clinics have been kept available as an alternative to private physicians. Clinics tend to serve low-income people who do not seek immunizations and other preventive services from the physicians in the sickness funds. Most of the local public health authorities have social workers who provide outreach into the community.

Regarding services to pregnant women, the local public health authorities in Germany continue to provide selected services, not to be expected from private physicians. These include counseling on mental health problems, general health education, and family planning. Public health agencies also provide social work services in the fields of drug abuse and AIDS. In Ireland and Spain, where the social insurance program for medical care is not so politically powerful, special public health clinics for pregnant women are numerous and well attended.

Midwives are extensively used for overall maternity care in all Western European countries. They provide not only the antenatal care, but also perform most of the deliveries in hospitals. Only if the childbirth has complications, is an obstetrician called in. The record of perinatal mortality, which may be attributed to the childbirth process, is slightly lower in the European countries using midwives than in the United States, where obstetricians perform most deliveries.

Childbirth is, or course, the crucial goal of all efforts to advance maternal and child health. This has become a hospital event almost everywhere in the industrialized countries. (Home deliveries are retained for one-third of the childbirths in the Netherlands.) In most such countries, the birth of a child in a hospital is routinely reported to the public health authorities, so that a public health nurse can visit the mother at home. The mother is then encouraged to visit a *well-baby clinic* promptly or to consult her regular physician.

Cesarian sections, to cope with complicated deliveries, have been increasing in almost all industrialized countries. For 1983, the rates ranged from 6.5 percent in Spain to 13.2 percent in Germany. No European rate, however, was as high as that in the United States, which in 1985 was 23 percent. Inside the U. S. the cesarian rate was higher for women with health insurance to ensure the payment of medical fees.

Maternal deaths are caused by many clinical complications in the childbirth process. One of these is clearly preventable—hemorrhage or infection due to mishandled abortion. Such mishandling is found to some extent in all countries. It is estimated that throughout the world, about 40 percent of maternal deaths are due to complications of improper abortions. These may have been performed by an incompetent "back alley" person or by the desperate woman herself. Solutions are widely debated, with respect to legislation as well as provision of resources for the proper interruption of pregnancy.

Adolescent pregnancy is a major difficulty contributing to both legal and illegal abortions. The young woman is unable to raise a child properly. The rates are high in almost all European countries, but none is as high as in the United States. These problems call for greater education about contraception in high schools.

Another important aspect of maternity in all countries is policy toward breast-feeding. In Europe, from about 1940 to 1970, the prevalence and duration of breast-feeding declined; as women entered employment and became generally more liberated in social relations, breast-feeding became regarded as an inconvenience. Infant formula manufacturers sold scores of products for bottle-feeding. The breast-feeding rate fell to about 30 percent of mothers. In the United States, the rate declined to 26 percent in 1973.

Then a reaction set in, and public health policy, supported by private physicians, stressed the benefits of breast-feeding. This was not only better for the infant's health, but it was simpler and more economical. As a result, the prevalence of breast-feeding rose everywhere in Europe; in Sweden it reached 90 percent. In the United States, it more than doubled to 54 percent in 1980. It is noteworthy that the cultural norm in almost all countries is for women to nurse their babies in public.

The entire picture of maternity care in the developing countries is quite different from that in Europe and North America. The extremity of the comparison is dramatically shown by maternal mortality rates. In the United States for the 1980s, maternity-related deaths occurred at the rate of 8 per 100,000; in Sweden the rate was 2 per 100,000. In India, such deaths occurred in different states at the rates of 500 to 800 per 100,000. In Egypt it was 200 to 300 per 100,000 and in Indonesia about 700. The World Health Organization estimates that about 500,000 maternal deaths occur globally each year; of these 99 percent occur in the developing countries.

There are differences in maternity care, of course, among Africa, Asia, and Latin America, and also differences among countries within these regions. Africa has the most deficient conditions, and several Latin American countries (e.g., Argentina, Chile, Costa Rica, Cuba) have the least deficient. On the whole, however, the great majority of childbirths in these regions take place in the home, attended principally by traditional birth attendants (TBAs). Unlike the professional midwife, the TBA has had little or no formal education, although a growing share of them has received limited hygienic training from field personnel of the Ministry of Health. In India, a study in 1982 compared perinatal mortality rates of deliveries performed by completely untrained women with those handled by hygienically trained TBAs, and found the latter to be half the former.

Formal recognition of the TBAs, through registration with the Ministry of Health, is sometimes linked to brief training. A WHO study in 1972 found 36 percent of countries, where TBAs are thought to attend a high proportion of births, offering such recognition. By 1982, this had risen to 82 percent. Among developing countries throughout the world, 80 percent now have TBA training programs. Deficiencies in supervision are continuing to impede progress in the quality of TBA performance.

The TBA in developing countries rarely provides antenatal care. Often a trained government midwife in rural areas attempts to provide such care, even though the expectant mother engages the TBA for the actual delivery. In the hospitals of developing countries, especially those under government control, the trained midwife performs most deliveries, as in Europe.

Cesarian sections are relatively rare in developing countries. In some major cities, however, the rates are as high as in the United States. Moreover, as in affluent countries, the rates vary with the method of remuneration. In São Paulo, Brazil, a highly industrialized city, the cesarian rate in 1982 was 14 percent among indigent patients, 35 percent among patients covered by social security, 53 percent in commercially insured patients, and 73 percent in patients paying privately. Although this study did not report clinical conditions, the fiscal influences are obvious.

Ambulatory care of pregnant women by professionally trained personnel in Asia, Africa, and Latin America is provided predominantly in government health centers. In the large health centers of developing countries, especially within cities, this facility is usually staffed by a general physician and several other professionally trained personnel, including nurses and medical assistants. In the rural areas the staffing seldom includes a doctor. The prenatal care of women is usually a major function of health center nurses. After the baby is born, mothers are advised on good nutrition, personal hygiene, and child-rearing practices.

Only rarely does a prenatal patient in these countries seek care from a private physician, as in Europe and North America. Aside from the expense, the private practitioner is not considered as skilled at prenatal care as the health center nurse. Most health centers are sponsored by Ministries of Health, but many in India and Pakistan are operated by religious missions or other nongovernmental bodies.

In Latin America, where social security programs, unlike Europe, have their own polyclinics, these provide prenatal care by physicians.

Breast-feeding in the developing countries is generally more highly prevalent than in the industrialized countries. In Africa, for obvious economic reasons, it is practically universal for a protracted time. It is practiced among urban and rural people, privileged and poor. In rural populations, the duration is not 3–6 months, as in Europe, but about 20 months. In middle and south Asia, it is almost universal for about 6 months duration. In eastern Asia, the rate is also high—80 percent in Malaysia and 90 percent in the Philippines. In Latin America, breast-feeding is also generally high, but the average duration is quite variable.

In some large cities of these developing countries, the rate of breast-feeding in the mid-1970s showed slight declines. These were believed to be mainly among elite professional women. A major influence was attributed to the advertising and general promotion of breast-milk substitutes by multinational corporations. This became a hot issue in the WHO World Health Assembly, leading to enactment of the "International Code of Marketing of Breast-Milk Substitutes" in 1981. Although the code is not mandatory, it calls for action by Ministries of Health to discourage marketing of these products.

The World Health Organization has distinguished three phases in the dynamics of breast-feeding; these apply in different degrees to both affluent and developing countries:

1. Traditional phase, with high prevalence and duration of breast-feeding.
2. Transformation phase, with prevalence of breast-feeding declining and duration becoming shorter.
3. Resurgence phase, with rising prevalence and shorter duration.

The addition of solid infant foods early in the first year of life may be the major cause of robust child growth in the affluent countries and in the upper social classes of developing countries.

Infants and Preschool Children

Just as clinics to advise expectant mothers were started in nineteenth century France, so were "infant welfare stations." At Nancy, several such stations were organized to counsel mothers on infant feeding. In the 1890s, a large network of infant consultation centers was developed in Paris. In the early twentieth century, the infant welfare station became a standard part of local public health programs in France and Great Britain. It was emulated in America in the relatively few large cities with stable Health Departments. In the 1920s "well-baby clinics" were promoted by federal grants to the states for eight years.

In modern France, infant and child health services are especially well developed. There are more than 6,800 clinics for advising mothers on infant care, plus another 2,000 clinics for children of 3–6 years of age. There are also 445 clinics for expectant mothers and 25 for fertility problems. To staff these maternal and child health (MCH) clinics some 7,000 physicians are appointed—mostly part-time but some on a full-time basis—plus hundreds of social workers and nurses. The French "social assistant" really combines the training of a nurse and social worker.

The maternal and child health services in France are organized to have significant linkage to various social security benefits. The prenatal care requirements for a maternity bonus have been noted. Likewise the newborn baby must be registered, for the family to be entitled to the children's allowance. Thus, MCH clinics in France are available to everyone for preventive services only—screening and immunizations. The physicians are not allowed to prescribe. Private practitioners—both generalists and pediatricians—deliver the same type of service, including immunizations.

Funding of the MCH services in France is especially strong through a separate flow of money from the top, and out to each department. These funds are identified as PMI or "Protection of Mothers and Infants" support. The mother must keep a record *(Carnet de Santé)* on her child's health examinations to

continue
lowance
aminat
cian, t
less re

If
nati
Fra
me
Pl
to
exchange
tending physician or
on nutrition and child-rearing, not
all the necessary immunizations.

In Great Britain, all patients may choose whether to have their maternal and child health development monitored by their general practitioner or by the organized health services provided by the District Health Authority. Under their 1990 contract, GPs may claim a new capitation supplement for all preventive services provided to child patients under age 5, if such services are part of the District Health Authority's program of child health care. The 1990 contract with the GPs makes clear that health promotion and illness prevention are within the definition of general medical services for which they receive an overall capitation fee, and the contract spells out specific kinds of services that may be provided.

In the developing countries, organized health services for infants and preschool children are extensive. Unlike the industrialized countries, however, these services are seldom separately identified, but are simply a major component of primary health care (PHC) offered throughout the country. The setting for provision of PHC services is typically a health center or subcenter for service to the ambulatory patient. In welfare-oriented health systems, such as in India and Malaysia, there are thousands of health centers, staffed with doctors, and subcenters, staffed with medical assistants, nurses, and other auxiliary personnel. Egypt has a relatively large supply of doctors, so that all urban and rural health centers are medically staffed.

In an entrepreneurial health system, such as that in Indonesia, health centers are abundant,

staffed. Regarding in-
...xaminations and counsel-
... generally done by assistant
... child requires treatment, this
...n by a male medical assistant. In
...th centers or smaller health stations
...lly staffed entirely by auxiliary per-
... Physicians are so few that they work
...n hospitals or in private practice. Almost
... of these PHC programs are sponsored by
...he Ministry of Health (at various jurisdictional levels), but in Africa and Asia some religious missions have broadened their work
from hospitals to ambulatory services.

Most of the welfare-oriented health systems
in Latin American countries have two major
sources of organized health service for infants
and children. The Ministries of Health provide
PHC services through health centers and subcenters, in which child health services are always a prominent part. In many of these
health facilities, preventive as well as therapeutic services for children are so conspicuous that
other persons, such as adult males, hesitate to
come for care.

The second source of infant and child service in Latin American countries is the Social
Security program for employed workers and
usually their dependents. These are most often
provided in large polyclinics, which usually include a medically staffed Department of Pediatrics. Although social security programs emphasize treatment of the sick, for small
children they designate certain days for preventive services.

The clinical content of preventive services
for children in developing countries has been
widely discussed. Counselling the mother on
nutrition and hygiene is universal. Babies are
usually weighed, so that their growth and development may be followed, and basic immunizations are routinely given. An extremely
common problem is infant diarrhea, for which
mothers are taught *oral rehydration therapy*
(ORT). Widespread ORT implementation,
promoted by UNICEF, has contributed to the
reduction of infant mortality rates. Combining
growth monitoring, oral rehydration, breast-
feeding, and immunization yields an acronym,
GOBI, which has been broadcast by UNICEF.
These health targets for "Child Survival"

have given rise to some contention between
UNICEF and WHO. A comprehensive program of primary health care, it is maintained
by WHO, and is necessary to ensure continuity
of a health infrastructure in communities after
enthusiastic campaigns are over. Yet, UNICEF
contends, a dramatic victory in one selected
program can pave the way for future broad
PHC policies. Child health service, in itself, is
always a socially appreciated point of entry to
comprehensive and enduring primary health
care.

Thus in the health systems of virtually all developing countries, a general pattern for delivery of health services to children has taken
shape. Unlike Europe and North America, relatively few families outside the large cities can
afford to consult private physicians. Even
though a high proportion of doctors may engage in private practice full-time or part-time,
their market of patients is relatively small. Traditional healing constitutes a varying share of
the private market. For provision of scientific
service to children throughout the developing
world, health centers of various levels and
small health stations, staffed mainly with auxiliary personnel, constitute the prevailing pattern. These services are seldom regarded as the
output of MCH clinics, but rather as an element—and usually a large one—within primary health care.

School Children

When children become old enough to attend
school, their health protection assumes forms
quite different from those for the preschool
child. In the industrialized countries, responsibilities are generally taken by educational authorities that operate the whole school system.

The idea that school children should be
medically examined was advocated by Johann
Peter Frank in central Europe around 1780. In
1840, Sweden appointed *school doctors* to do
these examinations. Later in the nineteenth
century, France, Germany, and Russia started
school health services; these included also inspection of the schools for sanitary conditions.
In Great Britain, school health services were
provided by certain local authorities in advance of legislation.

Early school health services were concerned mainly with detection of communicable disease, that might spread rapidly. In France a Royal Ordinance of 1837 required school authorities to supervise the health of school children and to provide sanitary conditions in school buildings, but this order was seldom followed. Not until 1879 was an effective program for the protection of school child health actually implemented in Paris.

French legislation in the 1880s required action throughout the country. It mandated medical examinations of children at the onset of school, to be repeated two or three times along the way until public schooling was completed. When any physical or mental disorder was discovered, the child's parent or guardian was to be notified and advised to seek medical attention. By the 1980s in France, for protecting the health of school children, there were some 1,000 physicians (one quarter being full-time), along with 1,200 nurses and 1,100 social workers.

Germany was the second country to develop health supervision of school children. An investigation of children's eyesight in 1866 led to further initiatives at the local level. In Great Britain also, the first school health services were developed by local units of government. There were great local variations; aside from concern for the spread of infection, special attention was directed to the needs of handicapped children.

The first British legislation of national scope, therefore, applied to school children with epilepsy or other serious disorders; for them appropriate types of school were necessary. This law was permissive, however, and was not implemented in many areas. The impetus for mandatory examinations came from popular concern about the large number of army recruits for the Boer War (1899–1902) in South Africa who were found to be physically unfit. As a result, legislation in 1907 required local school authorities to provide medical examinations immediately before and soon after admission to a public elementary school. Each child was also to be examined three times during the school years.

In 1918, as a sequel to World War I, another Education Act strengthened school health services in Great Britain even more. It required school authorities to ensure *treatment* for medical and dental defects found in the physical examinations. This could be done through referral to hospital outpatient departments or to a private physician remunerated by the school. For dental disease—extremely common in school children—special school clinics were operated in Britain.

In the first 25 years of the British National Health Service, 1948–1973, it is noteworthy that the school health services remained administratively under school authorities and separate from the NHS. Only with the Reorganization of 1974 were these services fully integrated into the NHS, with management by the local District Health Authorities. Under this management, periodic examinations of school children are still performed, but necessary treatment is given the same way as for anyone else.

School child health services were first organized in the United States in the 1890s. Boston set up a program for medical examination of children to control contagion in 1894. Chicago, New York, Philadelphia, and other major cities soon followed. After a while it was realized that screening for infections was not enough, and that education of parent and child was necessary to combat the conditions that spawned disease. Gradually the scope of school health services has broadened even further.

The agency responsible for these programs in Western Europe has almost always been the Ministry of Education at all levels. (The exception was the socialist countries of eastern Europe, with their comprehensive services under a Ministry of Health.) The same was true in the programs of large American cities, as they took shape. Local autonomy, however, was the guiding principle in the United States, and in smaller towns and rural counties school health responsibilities were often vested in public health agencies. There is an on-going debate in America about which of these two patterns is best for the child, for quality and for efficiency. In Japan school health services have been brought under the jurisdiction of public health authorities.

Whatever the administrative arrangements, the content of school health programs in the industrialized countries has achieved a general consensus. It includes: (1) maintenance of a safe and sanitary school environment, (2) instructing children in the classroom about health and healthful living, and (3) personal health services. The latter always include examinations for case detection and may include deliberate preventive services (e.g., immunizations) and medical/dental treatment. Schools in many countries arrange for the basic education of teachers in the identification of childhood communicable diseases. Personal health counselling is also included in the later school years, to cope with mental and emotional problems, the hazards of drug abuse, and prevention of teen-age pregnancy.

In modern school health services, the school nurse is a key operator. She serves in the school full-time or part-time, depending on the school size, and is available for sickness episodes that occur during the school day. She occupies and maintains a small clinic in the school building. She makes arrangements for various medical services, and she visits the homes of children with health problems. She counsels secondary school students and she makes referrals for medical care. Special training is ideally provided for school nurses under the general rubric of "public health nursing." In American and some European schools, furthermore, there may be school lunch programs, which advance the nutritional status of low-income children. (These involve the Department of Agriculture as well as the school authorities.) Nutritional education is also embodied in the instructional program.

In the developing countries, it is rare for school authorities to organize any special health services. Relative to their instructional role, these would be regarded as a luxury. Instead, nursing personnel of the Ministry of Health may visit the schools to carry out immunizations or to give educational talks on health subjects. In practice, personal health services for school children, if provided at all, are limited to schools in the large cities. In rural schools, the commonest service from a Ministry of Health is the inspection of school sanitary facilities and advice on proper water supply and waste disposal.

The Ministry of Health in developing countries often makes use of the public schools as convenient settings for mass screening to detect intestinal parasites, malaria, or disorders such as tuberculosis. In Bangkok, Thailand, for example, a small team of health auxiliaries from the Ministry of Health examined thousands of children in elementary schools. They focused on the eyes, and some 11 percent of children were found to have trachoma or other eye infections. Such screening examinations are typically authorized by the school authority, but carried out by public health personnel.

As more students attend secondary schools in developing countries, the hazards of drug abuse and teen-age pregnancy are usually increased. At the same time, opportunities for discussion and education about these problems are enhanced. Large schools in the main cities of Asia and Latin America are offering such health education with rising frequency.

An important extension of school health services is programs for university students. These are highly developed in both public and private universities of the industrialized countries, and usually financed out of the general university budget. Sometimes the university health service is limited to ambulatory care, and hospitalization is provided in the community. University health services in most developing countries are rudimentary, although at major universities in the national capital they are sometimes well established.

Family Planning Services and Abortion

Along with the maternity component of MCH services, most national health systems offer services to help women control their reproductive lives. Originally defined as *birth control,* the task is now usually described as *family planning* (FP). The practice is highly relevant to the health and welfare of women as well as to the larger social question of population policy.

The origins of family planning programs from the courageous initiative of Margaret Sanger in Brooklyn, New York have been discussed in Chapter 11. This was in 1916, and by 1937 most U. S. states had enacted laws permitting contraceptive education and practices.

The motive was entirely oriented to the welfare of the individual family and preventing the birth of more children than could be properly raised. Many countries with large Catholic populations, however, opposed contraception on religious grounds. A French law of 1920, for example, barred any advertising or distribution of contraceptives. Such policies were also adopted by French colonies in Africa and Asia. For similar reasons, contraceptive practices were prohibited in most Latin American countries.

After World War II, the main objective of family planning, especially in developing countries, acquired a different orientation. With the emancipation of colonies in Asia and Africa, many developing countries became keenly aware of their rate of population growth. They realized that advances in economic productivity could be lost by increase in family size, unless some controls were put on human reproduction. The obvious channel for such controls was in connection with the provision of services to pregnant women. The decision on limiting further childbirths could naturally be made by the mother, after the birth of a baby. As a purely private service, contraceptive techniques had been disseminated by doctors to higher income women for many years.

Even in the liberal democratic atmosphere after World War II, international action on family planning was inhibited for several years. The World Health Organization established a research unit on human reproduction, but did not promote FP services. On the other hand, the World Bank—aware of the negative effect of excessive population on economic development—promoted family planning in its health projects. The same was done by the U.S. Agency for International Development (USAID) bilateral program.

Around 1960, the political leadership in India recognized the great importance of contraception for the nation's entire socioeconomic development. Incentives were given to people—both women and men—to undergo sterilization. The majority of women, however, chose to use other methods, such as the contraceptive pill or the intrauterine device (IUD). In later years, vasectomies in men were

strongly encouraged, with major political repercussions. Eventually almost all developing countries implemented family planning programs in close connection with maternal and child health services. Sometimes nongovernmental organizations were deliberately chosen to spread the message on contraception.

The effectiveness of family planning education is dependent on larger questions of national culture and the place of women in it. When women are expected to have six to eight pregnancies, as in Africa, one can hardly expect FP strategies to have an impact. Social policy can give rewards to the one-child family, as is done in China. Economic development tends to bring greater urbanization, where small families are appropriate. If infant lives are saved, there is less need for replacement with new infants. Maternal mortality is tragically high in the developing countries, so that FP programs are launched as a strategy for women's health, as well as population policy.

Despite all FP efforts, studies in Africa have shown that less than 15 percent of married couples are regular "acceptors" of contraceptive advice. Nevertheless, when faced with unwanted pregnancies in almost any country, women frequently resort to an abortion. This is done, however, in many countries where a woman's access to a safe induced abortion is restricted. As a result, women throughout the world undergo illegal and often badly mismanaged abortions. These patients end up as cases of uterine hemorrhage in the wards of public hospitals. Maternal mortality is highest wherever abortion is illegal.

As the legal rights of women have become increasingly recognized, several large countries have liberalized their laws on access to abortion. In the 1980s, among countries permitting abortion essentially on the demand of a woman were three of the world's largest countries—China, the Soviet Union, and the United States. Also India was among the countries permitting abortion for a social reason. Indonesia, Iran, and Iraq were among the numerous countries that restrict abortions only to cases in which the woman's life is endangered by a pregnancy. In the 1990s, legal access to abortion in the United States was being debated politically and in the courts.

All the evidence suggests that the rate of abortions in a country largely depends on the availability of effective methods of family planning. Abortions can be reduced much more by good family planning than by laws making them illegal. Progress in the technology for terminating pregnancy has made abortion, under proper conditions, a very simple and safe procedure. The greatest challenge is to extend economical and effective methods of family planning to all developing countries, so that unwanted pregnancies are reduced to a very low level.

INDUSTRIAL WORKERS

The development of industry has inevitably created conditions that are hazardous to the health of working people. Since the pioneer studies of Ramazzini in 1700, enormous progress has been made over the years in identification of toxic substances and harmful practices. Our approach is to examine official regulations for protecting workers from harm, in-plant health services, and worker's compensation.

Government Regulation

As noted in Chapter 11, early laws were passed in France, then Great Britain, not directly on worker's health but on child labor. This was in the early nineteenth century, and then around 1860 protection was extended to women, and later to adult workers of both sexes.

With the Industrial Revolution, working conditions in the factories became congested and dangerous. Machinery was not shielded and accidents were frequent. Ventilation was lacking and factory air was filled with dust and fumes. Governmental factory inspection to enforce correction of these conditions increased its rigor only slowly; the concept of inspection by a knowledgeable physician—a medical inspector—originated in Belgium in 1895. Administrative responsibility for inspections was quite naturally assigned to Ministries or Departments of Labor. Sometimes an industrial hygiene unit in the Ministry of Health was developed to do studies and offer consultation.

Standards for factory inspection have advanced appreciably in the industrialized countries. Technological advances have disclosed the presence of toxic substances in very small amounts. In Great Britain factory inspection is one of the few health functions maintained outside the National Health Service. British research in the 1950s, for example, disclosed the pathology of coal-miner's pneumoconiosis, and American research revealed the tragic extent of asbestosis.

Factory inspection by Ministries of Labor became the major strategy for protecting workers in almost all countries. Among the industrialized countries, these programs were especially strong in those with comprehensive health systems, such as Sweden or Great Britain. In many welfare-oriented and even entrepreneurial health systems in industrialized countries, Ministries of Labor also tend to apply relatively broad occupational health and safety standards.

After World War II, Scandinavian countries passed laws to protect workers in clear relationship to their political labor parties. In France, glowing from victory over Fascism, a very broad set of in-plant services was required; the Minister of Labor was a Communist and every plant was required to have one full-time physician for each 1000 workers. In Australia during the 1970s it was a growing labor union movement that led to legislation on higher workplace standards. This was the situation also in Japan. In Italy, the trade union movement, combined with a generally heightened appreciation of the environment in society, has strengthened workplace standards.

There are many gaps, however, between official standards for occupational safety and health and their proper enforcement. In the western European countries, in Japan, Australia, and Canada, it is generally recognized that, despite reductions in the rate of industrial injuries, enforcement of the standards is deficient. In the United States, where the important federal Occupational Safety and Health Act (OSHA) law was enacted in 1970, severe cutbacks in funding and regulations in the 1980s emasculated this program. In almost all countries, factory inspection personnel are typically inadequate in numbers and training; only a fraction of workplaces can be visited, usually the larger ones. Moreover, if orders are given to correct hazards, they may not be followed, and penalties are weak.

A major factor in achieving enforcement of standards has been found to be the influence of workers in the entire process. If the workers are provided information about the materials they are working with and the hazards, they can exercise considerable influence on the formulation of standards and their enforcement. This issue has given rise to the slogan about the worker's "right to know." Workers in the Netherlands, France, Belgium, Germany, and all the Scandinavian countries hold at least half the places on occupational health and safety committees. In Canada, several *occupational health centers* have been established to do physical examinations of workers from any firm.

A study was made in the 1980s to explore the relationship between organizational arrangements for occupational health and safety and the strength of the labor movements. Labor strength was reflected in political labor parties, large and effective unions, high employment levels, and other conditions. It was found that where the labor movement was strong, workers participated more fully in planning the whole process of production and in ensuring its safety. The rank order of labor strength in the countries investigated was Sweden, East Germany, Finland, West Germany, Great Britain, and the United States.

To cite just one measurement, in Sweden some 85 percent of workers are in unions, compared with under 15 percent in the United States; occupational health and safety policy is roughly parallel. The Swedish program implements effective controls concerning accident hazards, chemicals, ergonomics, effects of piece work, shift work problems, and psychosomatic difficulties. Every place of work with 50 or more workers must have a joint labor–management committee to operate the program. A National Board of Occupational Safety and Health gives specialized training for physicians, occupational health nurses, safety engineers, and others. Financing for the entire program is derived half from employers

and half from Sweden's National Health Service.

In developing countries, the entire field of occupational health service to protect workers is generally rudimentary. In the countries of transitional economic level, where there are usually a few larger cities with major industrial plants, factory inspections may be performed. As in Europe, the Ministry of Labor is typically responsible, but its medical staffing is usually so weak that the Ministry of Health often becomes involved.

São Paulo, Brazil illustrates a situation found in many large cities of these countries. There were 94 electroplating plants, in which a survey found 87 percent of the workers to have chromium-induced lesions. Even in the unionized plants, 60 percent had poor working conditions; only 50 percent of employers had installed exhaust systems. Personal protective equipment supplied to workers was of very limited value. Conditions in nonunionized firms were probably even worse. Yet the São Paulo Department of Labor was very weakly staffed to cope with these problems. Industrial hygienists could visit only 50 percent or fewer of the large plants in a year and hardly any of the small plants. Their technical skills are limited and their power of enforcement is weak.

As summarized in a recent USAID report:

> Some stringent regulations are in place, (but) the Brazil Ministry of Labor has maintained virtually no workplace inspection capacity, and little enforcement has occurred. If a violation is discovered, a labor justice may impose a fine, but the maximum amount prescribed by law is only 10 times the minimum wage for a month. Large firms must have Internal Committees for Accident Prevention with labor–management composition. The chairman, however, is always from management, and corrective measures are rare.

In a very poor country, even with a welfare-oriented health system, such as India, the gap between occupational health legislation and its implementation is even wider. Even before independence, India had such legislation, and after liberation in 1947, it was strengthened.

There are provisions for inspection of large factories and enforcement of physical standards, such as water and sanitation for the workers. Occupational health is equated with labor welfare, but without any reference to occupational diseases. There are separate laws for miners and also agricultural workers, but hardly any means of enforcement.

As summarized by a WHO report in 1980:

> despite the existence of laws and regulations (in India), there is no effective monitoring machinery to detect flaws in the implementation of the various acts. Implementation of labor laws cannot succeed because of the availability of cheap labor. Employers can flout laws with impunity when workmen acquiesce to any indignity or ill-treatment for the sake of sheer survival. Legislation becomes useless in such circumstances.

In the very poor countries of Africa, there is seldom even legislation to protect the health of workers. The major exception applies to mining, which is usually controlled by foreign corporations. Standards call for the control of dust to prevent silicosis, but these are typically not enforced. Requirements for on-site medical services, to treat sick workers and their families, are more often implemented, if only to preserve working productivity. South Africa is a transitional level country, with entrepreneurial health policies, where management-operated medical services for workers (not dependents) are well developed. On the other hand, the problem of asbestosis, with its long incubation period, has been seriously neglected. Because of the generally weak structure of government in Africa, occupational health functions are most often assigned to the Ministry of Health; a Ministry of Labor ordinarily does not exist.

In Socialist China, the working conditions in factories are very congested, the machinery is unprotected, and atmospheric exhaust is very poor. Provincial and county branches of the Ministry of Health are attempting to enforce standards, but progress is slow. Much effort is being put into the training of industrial hygienists.

In-Plant Medical Services

As industry has developed thoughout the world, enterprises have realized the value of promptly available medical care. Having one or more doctors and other health personnel at the workplace could ensure immediate care of industrial injuries, and other health services for prevention and continuing treatment.

The first general medical service for industrial workers was initiated in the textile mills of Manchester, England, in 1796. Other such doctors were appointed in England, and they soon developed interest in preventing occupational diseases and accidents, as well as giving general medical care. In 1830, enlightened entrepreneurs recommended medical inspectors to visit large factories daily, and explore the effects of work on the worker's health. In 1898, the post of Medical Inspector was established in the municipality. One of the functions of these doctors was to certify individuals as physically fit for employment.

The first industrial nurse engaged by a company was also in England in 1872. She was expected to look after the nursing and social needs of the workers. The use of industrial nurses, with special training, spread generally throughout Europe, especially in moderately large plants. In large enterprises full-time or part-time industrial physicians were appointed to provide on-site treatment of injuries and acute illnesses.

In Germany full-time factory doctors were appointed in the chemical industry as early as 1866, long before this was required by law. For identification of occupational diseases, however, workers did not trust these "company doctors." The workers feared that they would simply be told to stop working, which they could not afford to do. Nevertheless, management-controlled in-plant medical services were increasingly organized in Europe, and later in America, to provide both preventive and treatment services.

In the very large plants of industrialized countries, there are usually well staffed and equipped clinics and even small hospitals. In France and a few other countries, legislation requires all companies to have a certain ratio of physicians and nurses; for large firms these must be full-time, but even for small firms part-time services must be provided through cooperative multiplant arrangements. In most countries, such in-plant medical services are not mandated by law, but they are organized for productive efficiency.

In many countries, there is a range of in-plant services according to the size of firm. In the smallest firms, there may be little more than first-aid equipment, with a few workers taught how to use it. Larger plants would have a part-time or full-time industrial nurse. Still larger plants might supplement the industrial nurse with a part-time physician. The largest plants would have full-time medical and nursing staffs, working in well-equipped facilities.

The national health systems of the former socialist countries of Eastern Europe may be mainly of historical interest, but they provided worksite health services of exceptionally broad scope. Comprehensive health care was available to workers at their place of employment to the same extent as it was in a community polyclinic. Since the socialist health systems have not yet been completely dismantled, many such workplace-related health care programs are still in operation.

After liberation from colonial status in the 1950s and 1960s, many developing countries enacted legislation to require in-plant medical services in firms above a certain size (e.g., 500 workers or more). Sometimes such legislation had existed before liberation, but was not enforced. These large firms were usually under foreign multinational corporations, and the new regulations were intended to emphasize the newly won national sovereignty. Standards generally stipulated the resources in physicians, nurses, and even hospital beds that were required for each 100 workers or thereabouts. Most of these large enterprises were located in the outskirts of cities, but some were at isolated locations. From the viewpoint of the large corporation, these health services contributed to worker productivity and promoted the loyalty of workers to the company.

At isolated locations in both industrialized and developing countries, large enterprises often provide comprehensive health services for workers and their families as well. In the United States, with its great geographic size, such isolated firms are found in mining, lumbering, and power. The Tennessee Valley Authority (TVA) for electric power generation has organized comprehensive health care for its personnel. Mines for coal and metals have routinely provided physicians for general medical care. The same applies at isolated enterprises in developing countries, such as copper mines in Peru, tea estates in Sri Lanka, or rubber plantations in Liberia.

Even in large cities, certain giant companies have organized comprehensive health care programs for their employees and dependents. In the Netherlands, for example, there is the Philip's Company, in France the Renault Company, in Italy the Fiat Company, and in the United States the Consolidated Edison Company. Under national health insurance (NHI) programs in a country, these company-based programs usually continue to operate as efficient modes of delivering service. In India, the comprehensive health program in Tata Industries has special value for thousands of workers and their families.

In the developing countries, whether of transitional or very poor economic level, small plants have virtually no organized arrangements for protecting the health of workers. If a worker is injured, he is simply sent to the nearest private physician or hospital outpatient department for care. There may be a small clinic nearby, where private physicians specialize in prompt treatment of industrial injuries. These clinic doctors realize that payment will be forthcoming from worker's compensation funds.

In all in-plant health programs with physicians on hand, the functions since the 1950s have broadened beyond medical care. Prevention has come to include preemployment and even preplacement examinations. If done fairly, such matching of the worker to the demands of each job is beneficial to the worker as well as the production process. There are naturally arguments about the implementation of policy with regard to the demands of each job. The requirements of a job can also be adjusted to human capabilities, rather than expecting workers to adjust to any job conditions.

After employment and reasonable placement of the worker in a job, prevention calls for periodic reexaminations. These may detect the onset of chronic disease, whether occupationally caused or not. Continuing prevention may include immunizations and worker education about health promotion. Education may be provided on the hazards of tobacco, along with smoking cessation classes. Problems of drug abuse and alcoholism may be discussed. The entire issue of sound nutritional education and, better yet, demonstration through industrial lunch programs, is being increasingly recognized.

Training programs for industrial physicians and nurses are increasing in the most affluent countries. These may be in schools of public health or in special sections of a Ministry of Labor. Where specialization in medicine is well developed, as in the United States or Great Britain, "industrial medicine" may be a formal subspecialty.

Worker's Compensation

Another important aspect of protecting workers is the issue of financial compensation for losses caused by work injuries. Known originally as "workmen's compensation," social insurance for this problem was first established in Germany in 1884. This legislation came soon after the first law for general sickness insurance, the cost of which was shared between employer and worker. The injury compensation, by contrast, was financed solely by the employer.

For decades before work-injury compensation, the adjudication of work accidents in Europe was governed by "Employers' Liability" Acts. These, in brief, made employers theoretically responsible for safety in the workplace. An injured worker who took legal action against the employer, however, seldom won. The employer's defense included the "contributory negligence" of the worker, the fault being due to a "fellow worker," and the worker's "assumption of ordinary trade risk" when taking

the job. It was to cut through these unfair litigations in court that the worker's compensation laws were passed, first in Germany and soon in almost all other industrialized countries. These social insurance laws established essentially a "no fault" policy that yielded rewards if accidents occurred at the workplace.

Under worker's compensation, financial awards are generally more modest than might be decided in a courtroom litigation. These are virtually assured, however, and the worker basically gives up the right to sue, in exchange for this assurance. Despite the simplicity of the concept, there have been countless political and legal arguments about the meaning of the laws—for example, the difinition of "accident" or the boundaries of the "workplace." Awards in almost all countries consist of (1) financial, for loss of wages, and (2) medical, for treatment of the injury. Financial awards are usually specified for each type of bodily injury, such as loss of one finger, loss of an arm, loss of an eye, and so on.

The medical services in compensation cases correspond to the type of national health system in the country. In the British National Health Service and other NHS systems (New Zealand, Scandinavian countries), medical care is simply provided in the NHS facilities. This was true also in the former socialist health systems of Eastern Europe. In some welfare-oriented health systems, such as Canada and Chile, compensation medical care may be provided in special facilities. Canadian compensation programs in some provinces operate their own rehabilitation centers. In entrepreneurial countries, such as the United States, the Philippines, or Kenya, medical care of injured workers is simply given by private physicians in the open market.

Insurance carriers for both the financial and the medical benefits under worker's compensation differ also in the various types of health system. In most states of the United States, South Korea, and Ghana, where entrepreneurial policies prevail, worker's compensation insurance for both financial and medical benefits is carried by commercial insurance companies. Their administrative expenses tend to be quite high. Even in some welfare-oriented systems, as in Switzerland or Brazil, commercial carriers provide insurance to companies for compensable work injuries.

In most welfare-oriented and comprehensive health systems, worker's compensation insurance is carried by special branches of the Ministry of Labor or its equivalent. This is the practice in France, Austria, and Japan. In Australia there are Workmen's Compensation Boards in each of the states, but an employer may get insurance through a private commercial carrier. In the comprehensive health systems of Great Britain, Norway, and Sweden, compensation insurance is handled in two ways. For monetary benefits, it is carried by the general social security program, along with unemployment and other monetary awards. For the medical benefits, there is no special insurance and the injured worker simply gets treatment within the general NHS.

Administration of compensation insurance in the United States shows how complex this can be in an entrepreneurial system, with jurisdictions distributed among 50 federated states. In only 6 states is there an exclusive fund, with which every employer must be insured. In 12 states, employers may choose to be insured either by a state fund or a private carrier. In the remaining 32 states, insurance is carried by scores of private companies. In practically all states, moreover, large employers may organize self-insurance.

Looking at the entire world, work injuries are the most extensive type of risk buffered by social security. Of 145 countries with any type of social security legislation, 136 have work-injury protection. The general trend of these programs has been toward placing responsibility in public insurance bodies, rather than private commercial carriers. About two-thirds of the 136 countries manage their work-injury benefits through a central public fund. The remaining countries may also have public funds, but private insurance carriers may be chosen as well, and they play a large role.

Although the premium costs of private carriers are generally higher than those of public funds, one theoretical advantage is their level being adjusted to accident experience. (Public funds charge the same to all enterprises, in order to spread the risk between high-hazard and low-hazard industries.) This experience rating of premiums is expected to give incentives to management to improve safety in the production process. It may also encourage firms to develop in-plant medical and nursing services. Where this "adjustment" of insurance premiums is not implemented, as in some public programs, other incentives must be used to encourage safe working conditions. One country, New Zealand, has extended the concept of *no fault* compensation to *all* accidents in any situation. An Accident Compensation Corporation gives thousands of financial awards without litigation, at very low administrative costs, leaving medical service to the national health system.

COMMENT

There are obvious interrelationships among the various programs, intended to protect the worker's health. Government regulation through factory inspection affects the environmental safety standards, as well as the adequacy of in-plant health services. Worker's compensation can influence the standards of in-plant programs. Among these is progress in the field of rehabilitation and in health promotion.

The detection of and compensation for occupational diseases present problems very different from accidents. The exposure to toxic substances ordinarily has a long history at different places of employment. Compensation responsibility must be borne by many different employers. The strong linkage of asbestosis to one large corporation in the United States is exceptional. Coal-miner's pneumoconiosis and occupationally caused cancers are due generally to employment with many different companies. Some countries, therefore, have set up separate social insurance funds, to which numerous employers contribute, to compensate victims of occupational disease.

The general development of industry in the affluent free-market countries, as well as in several transitional countries, gives some ground for optimism about in-plant medical services. The average size of the firms in most industries is increasing, so that workplace health care becomes more feasible. Even though small shops with meager health and safety programs are still predominant, especially in developing countries, the workforce in large establishments is an increasing proportion of the total. The organization of workers in unions usually enables them to have a stronger voice in health policy. Likewise, the generally forward development of national health systems has a positive impact on occupational health programs within them.

There is still another type of work, in public transportation, for which many countries have developed separately organized health programs. The railroads, merchant ships, and airlines, in both affluent and low-income developing countries, often have health personnel and facilities to serve their special needs. The earliest actions applied to men at sea. For merchant mariners, clinics or contract-physicians may be arranged at major ports domestically and also in foreign countries. Norway—a small country with a relatively large merchant fleet—has organized health programs for its merchant seamen at ports in California and elsewhere.

Great Britain organized health services of its merchant seamen at domestic ports in the mid-nineteenth century. The idea spread to the American colonies, which in 1798 passed an "Act for the Relief of Sick and Disabled Seamen." This led to organization of the U.S. Marine Hospital Service, which evolved into the U.S. Public Health Service. Most of these marine hospitals have now been converted to other purposes, but a few survive.

The most highly developed services for transportation workers in most countries—both industrialized and developing—are in the railroads. Special clinics are built and operated at major junctions. Health services are part of general social protection. In the United States, even before the enactment of federal old-age insurance (1935), there were extensive private pension programs for railway workers and a Railroad Retirement Act for social insurance became law in 1934. Any worker with 10 or more years of railroad work becomes entitled to benefits beyond those under the general Social Security Act.

The health services for railway workers are typically provided by salaried medical and allied personnel. A certain pride and esprit de corps often develops in these health care teams that try to excel in the performance of their functions. There is even an International Union of Railway Medical Services, founded in 1948 and based in Brussels; it has representation from 37 countries.

RURAL PEOPLE

In both industrialized and developing countries, people living in rural areas are the subjects of special-purpose health programs. *Rural* is usually defined as a complex of living conditions, rather than by strictly statistical criteria. It has social, economic, geographic, and psychological meanings. Even as the world is becoming urbanized disproportionately, the sheer numbers of rural people remain great, because of the growth of the general population. This is especially true in developing countries, where overall population growth rates exceed those in industrialized countries. The strategies for strengthening health services in rural areas permeate all components of health systems, among which the enlargement of human resources is especially important.

Health Personnel for Rural Areas

Several methods have been used for increasing the supply of health personnel to serve rural populations: (1) mandatory requirements, (2) provision of incentives, and (3) regulations on location.

Physicians. Mandatory rural service may be made a condition of licensure for physicians. Since its first Five-Year Plan in the 1920s, the Soviet Union required 3 years of rural service from all medical, dental, and nursing graduates. In the 1930s, Mexico became the first nonsocialist country to require a period of "social service" (6 months) as a condition of earning the medical degree and licensure. Since then many other Latin American countries have adopted similar requirements. In various forms the same practice has been adopted in several nations of the Middle East and Asia.

Egypt has hundreds of rural health centers, which are staffed mainly by new medical graduates. Iran requires a period of military services as its mandatory strategy. Malaysia requires duty in its Rural Health Services Scheme. Lebanon requires two years in service from all new graduates. It may be noted that in India, one of the Five-year Plans contemplated a period of rural medical service, but it was rejected on the grounds that it invaded the doctor's personal freedom and that doctors were needed everywhere.

In all these mandatory programs, exceptions are made for outstanding medical graduates, who may be permitted to enter specialty training in an urban hospital directly. There are also problems in the guidance and supervision of new graduates in their rural posts. Ministries of Health attempt to make rural service more agreeable by provision of adequate housing and transportation for the new graduate.

Professional licensure may also strengthen rural health manpower, with respect to cross-national migration. A physician wishing to enter Canada, for example, was granted licensure on condition of his settlement in a rural area for 5 years. Peru set similar conditions for physicians from Europe. The entire rigor of licensure laws in the United States, with respect to foreign medical graduates, was modified in connection with national needs for skilled immigrants.

In most industrialized countries, especially with welfare-oriented health systems, medical education is financed by government, with no tuition costs for the student. Obligatory rural service after graduation, therefore, is accepted as morally justified (paying back a "debt" to society). In the United States, however, medical school training is costly; even though 58 percent of schools are publicly sponsored and 42 percent are private, tuitions in all schools are relatively high. In 1970, therefore, an Emergency Health Personnel Act was passed, providing for a "National Health-Service Corps." This program financed medical education for students, who then became obligated to serve in a rural or other "underserved" area for the same duration as the subsidy of his schooling. (Before the federal law, several states had operated similar pro-grams, but with mixed results.) Although some graduates escaped from this commitment by repaying the education loan, the principle of mandatory rural health service has been accepted on a limited scale in the United States. In implementation, the rural assignments have not involved private practice, but usually posts in organized programs, such as the Indian Health Service, public clinics for migratory farm workers, or variously sponsored community health centers.

Much commoner than these mandatory health manpower strategies have been various policies to attract physicians voluntarily to rural areas. Incentives have been offered to private practitioners in the open medical care market, as well as to medical officers within a government health service. In western Canada, for example, in the 1920s private general practitioners were offered salaries to settle in a rural municipality; for the salary they would provide primary care to everyone, and fees could be charged for certain services. Also in the 1920s, small towns in the northeastern United States offered rent-free homes to attract private physicians. In Australia, certain states have guaranteed a minimum annual income to private physicians choosing rural settlement; the financial assurance came from the state government. Some Canadian provinces have done likewise.

Within organized governmental health programs, incentives are also employed throughout the world to achieve coverage in rural areas. One might expect that medical personnel in public programs could be easily moved around by a central authority, but this is seldom done outside of national emergencies. To maintain morale and a stable health system, all sorts of incentives are furnished to keep personnel satisfied in rural posts. The most frequent incentive is a higher salary for rural service than the same work would yield in a city. This is done in the governmental health programs of Brazil, Mexico, Costa Rica, and Panama. Sometimes the incentive is called a "hardship allowance." Adequate housing that is often rent free is also provided.

In Africa, where the physicians shortage is so great that almost any place of settlement is reasonable, few countries offer incentives. In Kenya and Mauritania, however, there are financial attractions for serving in small rural hospitals. Egypt and Saudi Arabia, with their relatively large output of doctors, offer premium salaries for service in a rural health center. This is done also in Thailand, South Korea, and New Zealand. In Europe, few countries have found incentives necessary to achieve rural coverage, but salary increments are applied in Greece and Turkey.

Beyond compulsory policies and incentives, an improved rural supply of physicians may be achieved by various regulations. The policy in Great Britain (from 1948 until the recent free market changes) has been a model. For general practitioners, the country was divided into areas that were reasonably supplied, "underdoctored," and "overdoctored." New GPs could theoretically settle wherever they wished, but if they chose an "overdoctored area," they could not acquire a capitation list of patients under the NHS. (They could engage only in private practice, which would be difficult.) This policy soon led to a relatively even distribution of GPs throughout the country.

A somewhat similar strategy was applied in some developing countries, illustrated by Tunisia. Here new medical graduates were barred from settlement in Tunis, the national capital, for 5 years after qualification. Such a policy has been advocated in Thailand regarding Bangkok, and in Peru regarding Lima, but it has not yet been implemented.

Another nonmandatory method of achieving coverage of physicians in rural areas is illustrated in Norway. There are 444 municipalities, most of them rural. In the post-World War II years, when local governments were weak, Municipal Health Officers were appointed by the central Directorate of Health Services, with local approval; in the 1980s this was decentralized. General practitioners are now appointed by municipal governments, with some guidance from the provincial (often called "county") Health Officers, representing the central Directorate.

Municipal Health Officers (also called *district doctors*) are officially responsible for all preventive services—sanitation, child health, communicable disease control, and so on. For treatment services, fees are paid by the national health service program. Two nurses—one for the office and one for field work—assist the district doctor, who serves also as chairman of the local Board of Health. This whole program has acquired a rich tradition, and through it virtually all rural people in Norway have access to primary health care.

Finally, with regard to physicians, the total national output is expected to have an influence on the numbers that will settle in rural areas. Even though settlement in cities may be the first preference, more physicians are available for rural work when the cities have become saturated. This has been evident in the United States, where the physician ratio to population has improved over the years, especially in very small towns. With greater physician resources, various incentives can be more effective. Such dynamics are over and above the increased access of rural people to medical care due to improved transportation.

In some affluent countries, where private medical practice predominates, the medical association may have a committee to study problems of medical care. These committees sometimes work with Agricultural Extension Services to prepare educational material on nutrition and hygiene. Some offer information to new medical graduates about rural localities, with promising opportunities for private practice.

Auxiliary Personnel. The above programs for strengthening rural health resources have focused on physicians, since this was the prominent approach throughout the world up to the end of World War II. With postwar liberation of the colonies and the birth of so many new independent nations, the manpower focus has shifted to various medical assistants and community health workers. This general movement has been reviewed in Chapter 2, but here it may be noted that the issue is largely rural.

Most of these auxiliary personnel are trained in relatively brief courses to provide both preventive and curative services. Perhaps the main historical precedent occurred in Czarist Russia, where the *feldsher* was drawn from discharged military auxiliaries in the mid-nineteenth century. For civilian work, the feldsher was given further training and posted mainly in the large rural areas of the country.

Many other forms of "middle medical" or auxiliary personnel were trained and used in rural areas of various countries. In the late nineteenth century, *dispensers* were formally trained in Jamaica, *assistant medical officers* were trained in Fiji, and in India *assistant surgeons* were designated from medical school graduates with low academic performance.

In the early twentieth century, even under colonial governments of Asia and Africa, many types of medical assistants were used; they were often called *dressers* or hospital assistants. In India medical assistants were trained and in Ceylon (later Sri Lanka) at the health centers there were *apothecaries.* In Ethiopia, a paramedical *health officer* was trained in a special school at Gondar for 3 years. In Venezuela, the program was developed after 1960 and was called *medicina simplificada;* it entailed much contention with the medical profession. In French Indo-China 4 years of training was given to *assistant doctors* to serve in the rural areas.

With experience, the interest turned to persons with only a few months of training, built on a primary school education. The sensational achievements of China with its huge supply of *barefoot doctors* made a worldwide impression after 1971. It was noteworthy that barefoot doctors were selected for training by the local people; the only prerequisite was literacy, and they continued to work part-time in farming.

This strategy for achieving rural health care coverage spread rapidly. In different forms, it was adopted in Iran, India, Latin America, and a few countries of Africa. In Latin America personnel were designated as *promoters of health,* and emphasized education of rural people to make use of established health centers and health stations. These *community health workers,* as they came to be called generically, were usually volunteers at the outset, but to achieve continuity, various methods were found to pay them. (One method was earnings from the sale of contraceptive pills.) Community health workers in Asia have usually been taught how to treat minor ailments and give preventive service. Evaluations have

been made of community health workers in rural areas, as discussed in Chapter 12, and these have unfortunately shown uneven performance. Difficulties are usually traced to inadequate initial training and weak supervision. With maturation of the whole public health infrastructure in rural areas, the effectiveness of both community health workers and medical assistants may be expected to improve.

It should be realized that medical assistants and community health workers are scientifically trained personnel. These are not to be confused with traditional healers, found throughout the developing world, especially in rural areas. This large multicultural subject has been explored in Chapter 1. Here we may simply note that in a few countries there is a policy of integrating traditional healers into the national health system. This is most impressive in China, where the integration of traditional doctors is with fully qualified physicians, even in government health facilities. In India, the Ayurvedic practitioner is not integrated, but constitutes a vast separate manpower resource essentially in a private market. Where traditional healers do not have a formal educational background, as in Africa and Latin America, they may sometimes be given limited training to serve as community health workers.

Organization and Financing

The organization of Ministries of Health in overall national health systems is heavily influenced by the requirements of rural people. These ministries are largely regionalized to provide health services for the rural population. Their typical pyramidal frameworks have three, four, or even five levels from center to periphery, and are intended to ensure some health services for people at the remotest locations. All too often, of course, the end result is less effective than suggested by the lines and boxes on the organization chart. Still, the very existence of an organizational framework provides a basis for planning the allocation of both physical and human resources throughout a country.

Outside the national headquarters, almost all Ministries of Health have planned a network of large, intermediate, and small hospitals, health centers, and health posts. These facilities, in turn, help to determine the geographic location of health personnel. In welfare-oriented health systems, this applies to medical and surgical specialists who are typically employed by the facility on salary. In entrepreneurial systems, where most hospital beds are in nongovernmental facilities, doctors are less often employed by hospitals; even so, the location of a rural facility helps to attract physicians as well as other personnel. Hospitals also need professional nurses, and ambulatory care facilities provide positions for assistant nurses and medical assistants.

Other agencies besides Ministries of Health can make special contributions to rural health services. Ministries of Agriculture in developing countries sponsor "community development programs" that include health activities—particularly programs of environmental sanitation and nutrition. Social security agencies, providing medical care directly (that is, not merely financing it) in developing countries, can serve workers on large agricultural estates as well as their families. This is seen especially in Latin America and the Middle East. Large agricultural enterprises, such as the United Fruit Company in Central America, provide relatively comprehensive services for their workers, usually independent of social security.

Perhaps the most fundamental strategy for strengthening rural health is to provide economic support. Rural populations are almost always poorer than urban. In the cities, a purely private market can finance a good deal of modern medical care, but in rural areas private family funds can support little. In welfare-oriented systems, such as in France and Germany, special legislation has applied social insurance to farmers and agricultural workers. In comprehensive systems, such as in Scandinavia, Great Britain, Italy, and Spain, agricultural workers and farmers are covered and financed along with everyone else.

Long before social insurance was extended to rural populations, small insurance schemes have been organized in certain rural areas. This was done, under voluntary agency sponsorship, in selected villages of India. Rural health cooperatives were prominent in Chi-

nese communes, before their dismantling in the 1980s. In Yugoslavia, long before its socialist years, health cooperatives were organized in rural villages.

When developing countries have extended their social security coverage for health service to rural populations, they must usually make special arrangements to be sure that the services can be delivered. This applied to Brazil, when it extended coverage to 83 percent of the population. Departing from its usual delivery pattern in polyclinics, Brazil social security had to make contracts with individual doctors and others to serve beneficiaries. (In fact, not everyone in rural regions who is entitled to coverage can actually get care.) Financing has been derived partly from taxes on agricultural products at the point of marketing, and partly from urban revenues, in a spirit of "social solidarity."

Everywhere in the world, both in cities and in rural regions, the provision of scientific health services depends largely on organized social financing of some sort. There are many arguments, however, between the advocates of social security financing and those favoring general revenues. As discussed in Chapter 6, revenues are believed to be derived more equitably and to be usable more flexibly. On the other hand, general revenues are competing with the claims of many other government programs, including military affairs. They are easily decreased. Social security, with its separate trust fund, has much greater long-term stability. Furthermore, whatever theoretical inequity may apply to the financial contributions, entitlement to services is the same for all covered persons. Since initial social insurance coverage usually applies only to regularly employed urban workers, Ministry of Health efforts can be more concentrated on meeting rural health needs.

In the United States, special financing by the federal and state governments has long been provided for migratory farm workers. This was done in the 1930s, as part of a general assistance program for low-income farm people—under the Farm Security Administration. When this was terminated after World War II, separate federal grants to the states for migratory worker clinics were authorized. In Mexico in the 1980s, national grants were made for "the extension of social protection to marginal groups in rural zones"—the COPLAMAR health care program.

Still another population, largely rural, has attracted special financial support—refugees from one country to another. The reasons for people fleeing from their native lands are always complex, involving extreme economic, political, ethnic, or wartime difficulties. Whatever the reason, there are many hundreds of thousands of refugees, occupying very crude camps in Asia and Africa. The U.N. High Commissioner for Refugees attempts to coordinate efforts to help refugees, but funding is never adequate. For health services, voluntary international agencies provide much support, and health personnel often serve without pay.

Delivery of Health Services

Because of the special conditions of rural life, health services require patterns of delivery quite different from those in the cities. Most of the problems arise from the dispersion of the population and the difficulties of transportation.

Environmental sanitation, with regard to both water supplies and waste disposal, demands special techniques for small villages or isolated homes. In place of public water pipelines, there are wells, and in place of public sewerage, there are latrines. Ministries of Health usually carry out major programs for helping families construct these units. Vector control to reduce mosquitoes, flies, or snails requires appropriate strategies, according to climate, terrain, and other factors. Developing proper water and sanitation facilities in the cities is usually a responsibility of Ministries of Public Works or other agencies, employing sanitary engineers. The rural sanitation programs of Health Ministries require not only simple construction skills, but also ability in education and persuasion to ensure that families make use of the facilities created.

Delivery of personal health service to rural people demands special stragegies in almost all countries. If the private market is relied on, little can be expected in developing countries, aside from traditional healers, drug sellers, and

a handful of modern practitioners to serve the affluent few. The typical solution in nearly all countries of Africa, Asia, and Latin America has been to organize tax-supported networks of facilities, as noted above. If a country devotes substantial resources to rural health, in the manner of Cuba or Malaysia, doctors may also be on the teams of major health centers.

In some developing countries with entrepreneurial health systems—such as Thailand, South Korea, and the Philippines—patients are asked to pay certain charges for care in both rural health centers and hospitals. (Although very poor patients may not be turned away, pride may inhibit their coming in the first place.) In most developing countries, however, the services of rural health care networks are simply supported by the Ministry of Health. A common problem, however, is vacancies in the medical positions.

Mobile clinics are a special modality for serving rural people who are extremely isolated. Vehicles with supplies of drugs and vaccines are based at rural health centers from which they travel outward periodically. These are especially relevant for maternal and child health services. Staffing is variable, but usually requires auxiliary personnel.

On a more sophisticated level, there are transportation strategies to help the seriously sick in rural areas. Organized ambulance services bring the patient from a distant point to an urban hospital. The Red Cross has operating responsibilities for these in many countries. In large territories like Canada or the Soviet Union there are airplane ambulance programs. Australia, with its huge territory, has developed a unique program known as the "flying doctor service"; it is sponsored by a voluntary agency, but financed mainly by government.

Health services, rural or urban, financed by social security are often regarded as being limited to curative medical care. Although treatment is undoubtedly emphasized, many such programs give special attention to preventive services. The Preventive Medicine Law of Chile's social security in 1938 was a conspicuous example. Preventive maternal and child health services are widely offered. Immunizations, case-detection screening tests, and Pap smears in women are offered. Social work services may be provided to help the elderly and disabled. Although such special services are more likely to be offered in the industrialized countries, they are done in both the rural areas and the cities of such countries.

Altogether, rural health services have made great improvements, with numerous strategies emanating from national governments. Most important has been human resource distribution along many lines. Organizational structure involves Ministries of Health in regionalized activities. Finally, special strategies for delivery of rural services have emphasized teamwork and designed imaginative forms of transportation. Nevertheless, the great handicaps of rural life remain in the more entrepreneurial developing countries. A WHO conference in 1989 reported that in Jakarta the infant mortality rate (IMR) was 33 per 1,000 live births, compared with 84 in the rest of Indonesia. In Manila it was 32 compared with 45 in the rest of the Philippines. In Bangkok it was 17, compared with 41 in the rest of Thailand. In Egypt, where a welfare-oriented health system seems to have had an equalizing effect, the IMR was 41 in Cairo and 47 in the rest of the country. In Pakistan, the IMR is generally high, with 79 in Karachi and 116 in the rest of the country. In Lagos, the IMR has been reduced to 21, compared with 90 in the rest of Nigeria.

Rural living conditions are doubtless more important than health services in explaining infant mortality. But health services can counteract some of the worst impacts of the physical and social environment, if there is political will. This has been shown in the State of Kerala in Southern India and in rural Costa Rica. Other developing countries have a long way to go to match these achievements.

OTHER SPECIAL POPULATIONS

Certain populations in nearly all countries live in highly organized circumstances, part of which include health services. Four main types of programs may be identified:

1. Most extensive are active military person-

nel, with very structured health service programs.
2. Groups associated with the military as dependents and later as military veterans are relevant.
3. On a much smaller scale there are services for prisoners.
4. In certain countries, there are special health programs for aboriginal populations.

Active Military Personnel

Medical arrangements for armies can be traced back to ancient Greece as early as 1200 B.C. Later in the Roman Empire military hospitals were established, called "valetudinaria." By 250 A.D., however, the military structure of the Roman army had deteriorated. In Byzantium (527 A.D.), a modern medical corps was established—not to be found in the west until the fifteenth century, when national military hospitals were built. The eighteenth century was a major turning point in military medicine. In 1752, a British textbook appeared on *Observations on Diseases of the Army.* This emphasized the importance of maintaining sanitation, nutrition, and so on, as well as coping with battle wounds.

In the nineteenth century at Solferino (Italy) there occurred a tragic battle, which led to the organization of the Red Cross and the formulation of international conventions on rules of war. Florence Nightingale did her pioneer work on military nursing around 1855. By World War I (1914–1918), medical administration in the military forces was well established. Special leadership came from the British, who set up hospitals close to the front lines, backed up by base hospitals in the rear. With World War II, the numbers of men in military service grew substantially. In 1945, the British military had 1,180 medical service units, the Germans had 1,200, the Russians had 1,500, and the United States had 2,200.

With such a history, we might expect that the contemporary structure of military health services in countries would be highly varied. In fact, there is a high degree of uniformity between countries of the same general economic level. The political orientation of the health system (whether entrepreneurial, welfare oriented, or comprehensive) seems to make no difference.

The essential characteristics of military health services are their high degree of organization in all countries. All personnel are engaged on full-time salaries. There is a hierarchy of command from a national center outward to various base hospitals and then to medical stations under them. The elements within this hierarchy reflect the whole range of health services. They are shown in a listing of British Army medical service units published in 1968:

1. Regimental medical establishments
2. Field ambulance
3. Casualty clearing station
4. Field hygiene section
5. Ambulance train
6. General hospital
7. Convalescent training depot
8. Hospital ship
9. Advanced depot of medical stores
10. Base depot of medical stores
11. Mobile hygiene laboratory
12. Mobile bacteriological laboratory
13. Motor ambulance company
15. Base malaria field laboratory
16. Base transfusion unit
17. Beach medical unit
18. Burns team
19. Central pathological laboratory
20. Chest surgery team
21. Field dressing station
22. Field hygiene company
23. Field medical company
24. Field surgical team
25. Field transfusion team
26. Malaria control company
27. Maxillofacial surgical team
28. Medical forward treatment unit
29. Mobile ear, nose, and throat team
30. Mobile malaria field laboratory
31. Mobile neurosurgical team
32. Mobile ophthalmic team
33. Special treatment team

This lengthy list of units in military health service may reflect the degree of organization in a comprehensive program. Although prepared in Great Britain, the account is based on practices in Canada, Australia, New Zealand, and India, as well as in Britain.

Further insight on military services in the modern world may be gathered from an account of policies in the United States published in 1980. Each military branch—army, navy, and air force—has its own medical department, but a policy of reciprocity among resources in various geographic regions is applied. The structure of the Army Medical Department, for example, is highly authoritative. Top authority is vested in the Surgeon-General of the Army and his staff located in Washington, D.C. There is central determination of all policy matters—both administrative and technical.

Great stress is put on professional dignity, and this is sought through the operation of a separate corps for each occupational group—the medical corps, dental corps, nurse corps, and so on. At each post, the chief of health service is always a member of the medical corps, even if a member of another corps is of higher military rank. The medical chief reports to the general commanding officer of the post on all administrative but not technical matters. Technically, the medical chief is responsible to his counterpart at the next higher health service echelon.

The entire network of Army medical services is a regionalized hierarchy, related to physical facilities. At the local level are various medical stations or clinics. For anything beyond immediate care, the patient is sent to a military hospital class I. (There are about 150 of these within the continental United States.) Difficult cases are relayed to a larger class II facility of 500 to 1,500 beds. These are known as Army General Hospitals, of which there are 6 in the United States.

The range of health services provided by the military establishments is comprehensive. Great emphasis is put on prevention through periodic health examinations, all feasible environmental controls, and so on. There is one limitation, however: the treatment of chronic illness from which the individual is not likely to recover. Persons with such illness are of no further military use, and they are discharged.

Under battle conditions, modern military establishments must be highly flexible. The

United States Army has shown special ingenuity in setting up surgical stations close to the field of battle; then later, injured soldiers are sent to the rear. Modern warfare, with its emphasis on aerial attack, has medical requirements quite different from infantry hostilities.

The cost of military medical services are met wholly from the general revenues of the federal government. Since national defense is generally accorded the highest priority in federal budgeting, this entire program rarely faces financial restrictions. On the larger political scene, of course, there are many reasons to regard United States military expenditures as excessive.

The quality of U.S. military health services is undoubtedly high, in comparison with care in the general health system. Top officials of the federal government, from the President down, are treated for serious conditions in central facilities such as the Army's Walter Reed Hospital and the U.S. Naval Medical Center. The weaknesses of the military medical establishment are obvious enough. As in any large bureaucratic structure, there is inhibition of innovations, without approval up the line. The morale of personnel may be poor, and the decisions of high officers may be faulty. The overall effects of teamwork and organization, however, protect against deficiencies. This account has been based on the United States, but it would doubtless apply to the dynamics of military health services in other industrialized countries. Services for active military personnel are being constantly developed throughout the world.

In developing countries, the remarkable feature of military medical services is their frequent exceptionally high development. In transitional and even very poor countries, where health care of the general population is usually beset with problems, the military program may be efficient, well staffed, and well equipped. This reflects, of course, the high priority politically assigned to military strength, although it is usually called "national defense." Developing countries that spent more than 10 percent of their GNP on military affairs in the 1980s included Guyana, Nicaragua, Iran, Iraq, Israel, Jordan, Oman, Saudi Arabia, Syria, Yemen Democratic Republic, Mongo-

lia, Angola, and Libya. No industrial country spent such a high share of GNP for military purposes, except the former Soviet Union. The absolute military expenditures of the industrialized countries, of course, are much higher than those of developing countries.

The military forces of affluent countries often assist developing countries in strengthening their own military capabilities. Great Britain has assisted its colonies and ex-colonies. France has done likewise. The United States has helped developing countries that were faced with domestic hostilites, such as El Salvador and the Philippines. Training may take place in the foreign country or in the United States.

Groups Associated with Military Personnel

During peacetime in most countries, the family dependents of active military personnel are entitled to health services at military installations. There may be various restrictions, but the basic idea is to promote the morale of the soldier or sailor. This policy prevails in both industrialized and developing countries, and it usually means the use of services at regular health stations and hospitals by military wives and children. In some developing countries, these benefits are provided only for the dependents of officers, not enlisted men. Sometimes it may be implemented only in cities, but not at isolated military camps, where there is no housing for families.

In the United States, a special variation of this entitlement occurred during World War II. Since large numbers of dependents were entitled to service, it was not considered reasonable to restrict them to military posts. A law was passed to permit dependents to use any private physician, who would then be paid by the federal government. In the entrepreneurial health system of the United States, the payment of fees was not direct, but mediated through private insurance companies. This relatively complex arrangement for military dependents is known as the Civilian Health and Medical Program for the Uniformed Services (CHAMPUS).

A much more extensive type of health program linked to active military personnel provides services to these men and women after they are discharged from active duty. The military veteran attracts strong political support in many countries, especially in the case of disabilities acquired during military service. Even for other disorders, if they are very serious, veterans may receive governmental (not military) medical care. Many countries maintain special facilities for disabled veterans. France, Italy, and other Western European countries have developed rehabilitation facilities for the seriously disabled and institutions for the elderly, some of which are reserved for disabled military veterans. There are also purely custodial facilities for elderly veterans, which are often called "old soldier's homes."

In the United States, the political strength of veterans after World War I led to a remarkable development. The Veterans Act of 1924 provided for a national network of general hospitals to serve veterans both with "service-connected disabilities" (that is, connected with military duty) and with other "non-service-connected disabilities." The latter persons had only to declare that it would be an economic hardship to obtain this care in the general health system. Periodic concern over the quality of medical care in veteran's hospitals has led to several reorganizations of their clinical services. Most important has been the establishment of affiliations between about half of the 175 hospitals and medical schools nearby.

Such a highly developed medical care program for veterans could be expected only in a country whose health system lacked national health care financing for the general population. In 1924, when the Veterans Administration (V.A.) started, health insurance protection in America was almost totally lacking, but even after voluntary insurance became extensive, many veterans were not covered.

In Canada in the 1930s, special veterans hospitals were also built. This was long before the first provincial initiative on hospital insurance. The capital and operating costs were met entirely by the federal government, so that later insurance programs by the provinces could exclude responsibility for these federal hospitals. Even after Canada was entirely covered with economic protection for hospital and physician's care, the costs of veterans hospitals remained a federal obligation.

By the 1980s, the proportion of V.A. Hospital patients with non-service-connected conditions in the United States came to occupy two-thirds of the beds. As the U.S. Veterans of World War II and other hostilities (Korea, Vietnam, etc.) grow older, the composition of patients naturally contains higher proportions of the chronically ill. It also contains higher proportions of homeless or lonely men, since those with stable family lives tend to have insured access to local community hospitals. Average lengths of stay are naturally very long. The Veterans Administration, which manages this entire program, is an independent federal agency. Its budget is separate from the U.S. military budget, but there are natural political alliances between the two.

Prisoners

Quite different from active military personnel, but living also under very regimented conditions, are prisoners. The first formal attention to prisoner medical care came in England, with the establishment of a Prison Medical Service in 1779. This specified that each local prison must have a surgeon or apothecary to preserve the health of inmates. Since then to the present, the law requires that each new prisoner be medically examined on admission.

The British Prison Medical Service is a separate agency under the Home Office, and does not come under the National Health Service. It employs 200 full-time or part-time medical officers and 600 nurses and other health personnel. Medical officers coordinate the services of the prison health care staff and outside consultants. They work also with prison administrative personnel to provide treatment in a "nonjudgmental setting." When the NHS was reorganized in 1974, the Prison Medical Service was still kept separate.

France also developed a national prison health program with its own prison hospitals. At least one physician is assigned to each prison. Sick inmates are treated by the prison physician or referred to one of the prison hospitals in the region. There is even a large prison hospital for chronic disease cases. Physicians intending to make a career of this field may undertake a year of training. The centralized management of the French prison health services reflects the policies of the overall national health system.

In Canada, in spite of the usual responsibilities of the provinces, the Canadian Prison Health Service, established in 1962, is a federal activity. Some 200 doctors and other health personnel are able to handle most problems in the prison and, for hospitalization, cases are sent to federal veterans hospitals nearby. It is noteworthy that health decisions are made by the federal program, rather than the administration of each prison. Policies have been similar in Australia for a longer time. With that country's founding from a population of convicts in the early nineteenth century, there is a natural interest in having humane treatment of prisoners.

Poland in its socialist period organized prison health services through special hospitals serving prisons in a region, as in France. Each Polish prison had a small clinic, staffed by the same doctors as those serving prison employees.

These selected national accounts offer perspective on the prison health services in the United States. By contrast with all the countries reviewed, there is simply no national program in this field. There are about 4,000 jails and prisons in the country and each takes care of itself. A study made by the American Medical Association in 1980 found that only 59 of the 4,000 jails met minimal standards in their health operations. These were mainly at large prisons or penitentiaries operated by the federal government, under the U.S. Department of Justice. In these large federal facilities, there are full-time medical officers and auxiliary *physician's assistants.*

In the United States there are diverse ways that local jails provide medical coverage. They may have their own health care providers and share them with neighboring jails. A jail may contract for health services with a local private group practice or an HMO; it may make similar contracts with individual physicians or hospitals. It can obtain services through local health departments of the state, county, or city. A contract typically calls for provision of primary care at the jail, surgical care in an area hospital, and dental care in a dentist's office. Any arrangement, of course, calls for close surveillance of convicted prisoners. The utilization rate of prison health services tends to be high—about 10 percent each day. For angry men behind bars, this is easy to understand.

In developing countries, health care of prisoners has a very low priority. Unless some critical problem arises, nothing is done and the sick inmate may be ignored. In a large national prison, there may be some arrangement with a local physician, paid a part-time salary. On the whole in most developing countries, deficient health care of the prisoner is part of his punishment. There are exceptions, of course, in countries undergoing rapid economic development. In all countries there are some attempts to utilize the prison experience as a strategy for rehabilitation rather than punishment.

Aboriginal People

There is nothing pejorative about the term "aboriginal," which simply means the original inhabitants of a land, before some sort of invasion by outsiders. When the newcomers came in great numbers and acquired power, the original inhabitants have often become a segregated population. They generally suffer from a lower social status, but at the same time may become entitled to special programs in health care. These may arise simply from a central government decision, paternalistic in its motives, or from agreements (even treaties) between the national authorities and the aboriginal people.

The largest population of aboriginal people, dominated by an invading population of foreigners during the last 500 years, were the prior inhabitants. This gave rise to the world's most highly developed program of this type. It concerned American Indians or Native Americans, and for the provision of health care was organized in the U.S. federal government as the Indian Health Service.

In 1832, a United States Supreme Court decision created obligations of the U.S. Government to work with scores of Indian tribes. After several decades in the U.S. Department of the Interior, the health service was transferred to the U.S. Public Health Service in 1954. The United States is divided into 12 administrative regions, and under these are 123 health units; with a policy of encouraging local self-determination, administrative controls in 44 of these have been turned over to the tribes. Each health unit consists of a hospital (51 of these) or a health center (99 of these). Beyond these are 400 health service units for delivery of primary health care. Much emphasis is put on preventive services, including environmental sanitation. The program trains many of its own medical assistants and community health workers, although this has been reduced with federal funding cutbacks in recent years.

Financial support of the U.S. Indian Health Service (IHS) is almost entirely from the federal government. This is true even under the supervision by the tribes, which receive all their operating and capital funds from government. The IHS health budget amounts to 20 percent of the total Indian Affairs budget. This reflects a high priority, and can be credited at least partially with a reduction of infant mortality between 1955 and 1979 from 63 to 15 per 1,000 live births.

Another country with well developed services for original inhabitants is Canada. These people are mostly Eskimos, Inuits, and other ethnic groups in the far north. The entire program is directed by the central Department of National Health and Welfare and 9 regional offices. These administer a network of hospitals (8 general and 6 cottage type), 150 health centers, and more than 300 health stations. Dental services are provided mainly by contracts with private practitioners.

The Australian service for aboriginal people is much smaller and has a very different character. Instead of maintaining a network of facilities, it concentrates on training the aborigines themselves to give primary health care. At a few places, the federal government has built small health centers, but the great majority of services are simply rendered in the villages without having a health station.

Among developing countries there are special arrangements in Panama (which are sometimes found in other Latin American countries). In Panama there are three major Indian groups with distinct languages, constituting about 5 percent of the national population. These live in three widely separated localities. There are no special services, however, beyond the usual program of the Ministry of Health. In the national MOH office there is a medical officer for overseeing services in the three localities, in light of the special ethnic relationships.

In Malaysia there is a well-developed network of general hospitals under the Ministry of Health. Quite separate is an Aboriginal Hospital operated by the Ministry of Land and Mines. There are radio connections with some 45 health stations in scattered and isolated settlements. A seriously ill patient will sometimes be brought to the hospital by a military airplane. Patients come often with their families, who prepare food and help to take care of the nursing needs. The Aboriginal Hospital has no connection with the Malaysian Ministry of Health, except for occasional assistance in procuring drugs and supplies. Its medical staffing has been mainly by foreign physicians.

A different policy has been applied to the Maoris, who were the original inhabitants of New Zealand. For years the Maori people tried to live in separate settlements, without any contact with the general population. Government, however, opposed this and has tried to integrate the Maoris with everyone else, including the use of regular public medical care.

This review of health services for aboriginal people shows that there are two general approaches in health systems—the development of separate programs versus a policy of assimilation and integration. Countries with large aboriginal populations tend to adopt the first policy and with relatively small populations the second. It must be realized that in all six countries discussed here, the aboriginal population lives at much lower standards than the national average. In view of this, the choice between the two general options must depend on many social and economic factors.

The Poor: A Note

In the United States, where—except for the elderly and totally disabled—social insurance for health care does not protect the general population, a conspicuous group entitled to special governmental health services is the poor. Prior to 1965, the states and counties operated diverse programs for treating the sick poor; many of these programs had salaried physicians and designated health facilities. With the important Social Security Act amendments in 1965, the financial support for care of many (not all) of the poor was brought under a joint federal–state program, known generally as Medicaid. The largest category of public asisstance recipients entitled to Medicaid is "aid to families with dependent children" (AFDC). The intent was to bring care of the poor into the "mainstream" of private American health service. The states determined eligibility, fees paid, and many other features, but a minimum range of services was laid down by federal law.

In 1990, about 27,000,000 persons were covered by Medicaid; another 34,000,000 people were covered by Medicare insurance for the elderly and disabled, who are also mainly of low income. This amounted to 61,000,000 or 24 percent of a national population of 250,000,000 people. With serious economic difficulties in most states, the fees payable for services under Medicaid are relatively low, and many physicians and hospitals refuse to accept these patients. Furthermore millions of low-income people are not covered by either Medicaid or Medicare and do not have private insurance. As a last resort for care of serious illness, these poor people—numbering at any one time around 30,000,000 or 40,000,000—seek care at large public hospitals. These were built to serve the poor in large cities, long before enactment of the federal insurance and public assistance laws. The funding of large public hospitals, however, is grossly deficient almost everywhere, because it depends on inadequate local and state tax support. A saving grace of several public hospitals is their well-qualified medical staffs, due to linkage with medical schools. The circumstances of personal patient care unfortunately are typically congested and often inhumane.

Categorical programs of medical care for the poor, equivalent to U.S. Medicaid, are not found in the industrialized countries of Western Europe. In France, for example, there are Public Assistance Hospitals constructed long before social insurance (1928), which were intended to serve the poor. They have now been converted into first-class general hospitals for everyone, with small patient rooms replacing the large communal wards. They are still patronized by the poor, because no copayment is required of them as in private hospitals. With salaried medical staffs, there is no free choice of doctor, but frequent ties to medical schools assure high quality service. Low-income patients, who have a good reason to use private hospitals, may even have the copayment paid for them by Public Assistance. For basic coverage under French social insurance, the poor are simply enrolled in a sickness fund at the expense of the Public Assistance authorities.

In Germany, the financial support of health care of the poor is handled at the local government level. Public assistance may pay private medical practitioners by fees or may pay the premium for enrollment in a local sickness fund. This choice rests with the local government. Hospitalization is provided in a public hospital, supported by local and provincial tax revenues.

Medical care of the poor in Canada is a responsibility of the provincial Department of Social Welfare. For the hospital and physician care benefits of Canadian social insurance, the indigent are simply enrolled in the provincial programs. Since these are mainly supported by general revenues, no special premiums need be paid on their behalf. For service not included in the provincial insurance scheme, such as dental care or prescribed drugs, the costs are often assumed directly by provincial welfare authorities.

In national health systems with universal coverage and comprehensive benefits, such as the British National Health Service or the systems in any of the Scandinavian countries, the care of the poor presents no special problem. They are simply entitled to service like anyone else. In fact, the administration takes pains not to identify the indigent, lest it affect the attitude of the providers.

In developing countries, where the masses of people are typically of low income, there is hardly any programmatic recognition of the poor. It is assumed that almost all governmental health programs for ambulatory or hospital care are mainly serving the poor. The more conspicuous issue in some developing countries is to rule out services for the well-to-do who, it is assumed, could purchase medical care in the private market. In developing countries with entrepreneurial health systems, personal charges may be levied in public hospitals and health centers, from which only the very poor are excused.

REFERENCES

Mothers and Children

Bader, Michael B., "Breast-Feeding: The Role of Multi-National Corporations in Latin America." *International Journal of Health Services,* 6(47):609–626, 1976.

Banerji, D., "Population Planning in India: National Foreign Priorities." *International Journal of Health Services,* 3(4):773–777, 1973.

Bankowski, Z., J. Barzellato, and A. M. Capron, (Editors), *Ethics and Human Values in Family Planning.* Geneva: Council of International Organizations of the Medical Sciences (CIOMS), 1989.

Berelson, Bernard (Editor), *Family-Planning Programs: An International Survey.* New York: Basic Books, 1969.

Birdsall, Nancy, *Population and Poverty in the Developing World.* Washington, D.C.: World Bank (Staff Working Paper No. 404), July 1980.

Bosch, Samuel J., and Jaime Arias (Editors), *Evaluation of Child Health Services: The Interface between Research and Medical Practice.* Washington, D.C.: U.S. Dept. Of Health, Education, and Welfare, 1978.

Chase, H. C., "A Study of Risks, Medical Care, and Infant Mortality." *American Journal of Public Health,* 63(Supplement):1–56, September 1973.

Conable, Barber B., "Safe Motherhood." *World Health Forum,* 8:155–160, 1987.

Cook, Rebecca J., "Abortion Laws and Policies: Challenges and Opportunities." *International Journal of Gynecology and Obstetrics,* Supplement 3:61–87, 1989.

Dixon-Mueller, Ruth, "Abortion Policy and Women's Health in Developing Countries." *International Journal of Health Services,* 20(2):297–314, 1990.

Dunning, James M., and Nora Dunning, "An International Look at School-Based Children's Dental Services." *American Journal of Public Health,* 68(7):664–668, 1978.

Forum Interview, "Prevention of Maternal Mortality." *World Health Forum,* 7:50–55, 1986.

Grant, James P., *The State of the World's Children 1989.* New York: UNICEF, Oxford University Press, 1989.

Hanlon, John J., "School Health" in *Public Health Administration and Practice.* St. Louis, MO: Mosby, 1974, pp. 335–343.

Henshaw, Stanley K., "Induced Abortion: A World Review." *Family Planning Perspectives,* 22(2):76–89, March–April 1990.

Hernandez, Donald J., "Fertility Reduction Policies and Poverty in Third World Countries: Ethical Issues." *Studies in Family Planning,* March–April, 1985.

Institute of Medicine, *Legalized Abortion and the Public Health.* Washington, D.C.: National Academy of Science, 1975.

International Congress of School and University Health and Medicine, *Proceedings of Congress VII.* Mexico, November 1975.

International Union of School and University Health and Medicine, *School Health Symposium in Stockholm 1974.* Stockholm, 1975.

Janowitz, Barbara, et al., "Method of Payment and the Cesarian Birth Rate in a Hospital in Northeast Brazil." *Journal of Health Politics, Policy, and Law,* 9(3):515–526, 1984.

Jelliffe, D. B., and E.F.P. Jelliffe, *Advances in Maternal and Child Health,* Vol. 5. Oxford: Clarendon Press, 1985.

Jones, Elise (Study Director), *Teenage Pregnancies in Industrialized Countries.* New Haven, CT: Yale University Press, 1986.

Jones, Elise F. (Study Director), "Unintended Pregnancy, Contraceptive Practice and Family Planning Services in Developed Countries." *Family Planning Perspectives,* 20(2):53–67, March—April 1988.

Kaminski, M., et al. (Editors), *Perinatal Care Delivery Systems: Description and Evaluation in European Community Countries.* Oxford: Oxford University Press, 1987.

Maglacas, Amelia, and Helen Pizurki, *The Traditional Birth Attendant in Seven Countries: Case Studies in Utilization and Training.* Geneva: WHO (Public Health Papers 75), 1981.

Malloy, James M., and Silvia Borzutsky, "Politics, Social Welfare Policy, and the Population Problem in Latin America." *International Journal of Health Services,* 12(1)77–98, 1982.

Miller, C. Arden, "A Review of Maternity Care Programs in Western Europe." *Family Planning Perspectives,* 19(5):207–211, 1987.

Miller, C. Arden, *Maternal Health and Infant Survival.* Washington, D.C.: National Center for Clinical Infant Programs, 1987.

Mitchell, Ross G. (Editor), *Child Health in the Community.* See especially Frank N. Bamford, "The School Health Service: Organization." London: Churchill Livingston, 1980.

Mosley, W. Henry, "Child Survival: Research and Policy." *World Health Forum,* 6:352–360, 1985.

National Board of Health and Welfare, *The Swedish Health Services in the 1990s.* Stockholm: Liber Trycle Stockholm, 1985.

Pan American Health Organization, *Maternal Health: The Perennial Challenge.* Washington, D.C.: PAHO, 1991.

Population Information Program (Johns Hopkins University), "Mothers' Lives Matter: Maternal Health in the Community." *Population Reports,* Series L (7), September 1988.

Pratinidhi, A. K., et al., "Birth Attendants and Perinatal Mortality." *World Health Forum,* 6:115–117, 1985.

Rosen, George, "The Health of the School Child." In *A History of Public Health.* New York: MD Publications, 1958, pp. 365–374.

Royston, Erica, and Sue Armstrong (Editors), *Preventing Maternal Deaths.* Geneva: World Health Organization, 1989.

Sai, Fred T., "Family Planning and Maternal Health Care: A Common Goal." *World Health Forum,* 7:315–324, 1986.

Savage, Wendy, "Taking Liberties with Women: Abortion, Sterilization, and Contraception." *International Journal of Health Services,* 12(2):293–308, 1982.

Silver, George, *Child Health: America's Future.* Germantown, MD: Aspen, 1978.

Stickle, Y., and P. Ma, "Some Social and Medical Correlates of Pregnancy Outcome." *American Journal of Obstetrics and Gynecology,* 127(2):162–166, 1977.

Task Force for Child Survival, *Protecting the World's Children* (Conference Report "Bellagio II" at Cartagena, Columbia). Decatur, Georgia, March 1986.

Torres, Alberto, and Michal R. Reick, "The Shift from Home to Institutional Childbirth: A Comparative Study of the United Kingdom and the Netherlands." *International Journal of Health Services,* 19(3):405–414, 1989.

UNICEF, *Assignment Children: A Child Survival and Development Revolution.* Geneva: UNICEF, 1983.

Wallace, Helen M., MCH Responsibilities and Opportunities under National Health Insurance." *Public Health Reports,* 89(5):433–439, 1974.

Wallace, Helen M., and Kanti Giri, *Health Care of Women and Children in Developing Countries.* Oakland, CA: Third Party Publishing Co., 1990.

Willett, Margaret K., "Midwifery in Seven European Countries." *Journal of Nurse-Midwifery,* 26(4):28–33, 1981.

Williams, Cicely D., and Derrick B. Jelliffe, *Mother and Child Health: Delivering the Services.* London: Oxford University Press, 1972.

Williams, Glen, "Save the Babies." *World Health Forum,* 7:391–398, 1986.

World Health Organization, *New Trends and Approaches in the Delivery of Maternal and Child Care in Health Services.* (Sixth Report of the WHO Expert Committee on Maternal and Child Health). Geneva: WHO, 1976.

World Health Organization, *International Code of Marketing of Breast-Milk Substitutes.* Geneva: WHO, 1981.

World Health Organization, "The Extensions of Health Service Coverage with Traditional Birth Attendants: A Decade of Progress." *WHO Chronicle, 36(3):92–96, 1982.*

World Health Organization, "The Prevalence and Duration of Breast-Feeding: A Critical Review of Available Information." *World Health Statistics Quarterly, No. 2:92–116, 1982.*

World Health Organization, "The Dynamics of Breastfeeding." *WHO Chronicle,* 37(1):6–10, 1983.

Industrial Workers

Berlinguer, Giovanni, and Marco Biocca, "Recent Developments in Occupational Health Policy in Italy." *International Journal of Health Services,* 17(3):455–474, 1987.

Berman, Daniel M., "Why Work Kills: A Brief History of Occupational Safety and Health in the United States." *International Journal of Health Services,* 7(1):63–87, 1977.

Bull, D., *A Growing Problem: Pesticides and the Third World Poor.* London: OXFAM, 1982.

Cassou, Bernard, and Bernard Pissarro, "Workers Participation and Occupational Health: The French Experience." *International Journal of Health Services,* 18:139–152, 1988.

Elling, Ray H., *The Struggle for Worker's Health.* Farmingdale, NY: Baywood Pub. Co., 1986.

Frumkin, Howard, and V. de M. Camara, "Occupational Health and Safety in Brazil." *American Journal of Public Health,* 81(12):1619–1624, 1991.

Garbarino, Joseph W., *Health Plans and Collective Bargaining.* Berkeley, CA: University of California Press, 1960.

Gevers, J.K.M., "Worker Control Over Occupational Health Services: The Development of Legal Rights in the EEC (European Economic Community)." *International Journal of Health Services,* 15(2):217–229, 1985.

Landrigan, Philip J., and Dean B. Baker, "Workers." In *Oxford Textbook of Public Health.* Volume 3, Chapter 27. Oxford: Oxford University Press, 1991, pp. 449–465.

Laurell, A., "Mortality and Working Conditions in Agriculture in Underdeveloped Countries." *International Journal of Health Services,* 11:3–20, 1981.

Levenstein, C., and S. Eller, "Occupational Safety and Health Regulation: An International Labor Perspective." *International Journal of Health Services,* 11:303–309, 1981.

MacSheoin, Tomas, "The Dismantling of U.S.

Health and Safety Regulations under the First Reagan Administration: A Bibliography." *International Journal of Health Services,* 15(4):585–608, 1985.

Michaels, David et al., "Economic Development and Occupational Health in Latin America: New Directions for Public Health in Less Developed Countries." *American Journal of Public Health,* 75:536–542, 1985.

Millis, Harry A., and Royal E. Montgomery, *Labor's Risks and Social Insurance.* New York: McGraw-Hill, 1938.

Mullan, Fitzhugh, *Plague and Politics: The Story of the U.S. Public Health Service.* New York: Basic Books, 1989.

Myers, J.E., et al., "Asbestos and Asbestos-related Disease: The South African Case." *International Journal of Health Services,* 17(4):651–666, 1987.

Myers, Jonathan E., and Ian Macun, "The Sociological Context of Occupational Health in South Africa." *American Journal of Public Health,* 79(2):216–224, 1989.

Navarro, Vicente, "The Determinants of Health Policy: Regulating Safety and Health at the Workplace in Sweden." *Journal of Health Politics, Policy, and Law,* 9(1):137–156, Spring 1984.

Palmer, G., *Compensation for Incapacity.* Wellington, NZ: Oxford University Press, 1979.

Pearse, Warwick, and Chloe Refshauge, "Workers Health and Safety in Australia: An Overview." *International Journal of Health Services,* 17:635:650, 1987.

Phoon, W. O., "Occupational Health in Developing Countries: A Simple Case of Neglect." *World Health Forum,* 4:340–343, 1983.

Phoon, W. O., and C. N. Ong (Editors), *Occupational Health in Developing Countries in Asia.* Tokyo: Southeast Asian Medical Information Center, 1985.

Reich, Michael R., and Howard Frumkin, "An Overview of Japanese Occupational Health." *American Journal of Public Health,* 78:809–816, 1988.

Roemer, Milton I., "From Factory Inspection to Adult Health Service." *British Journal of Industrial Medicine,* 10(July):179–194, 1953.

Roemer, Milton I., "Workmen's Compensation and National Health Insurance Programs Abroad." *American Journal of Public Health,* 55(2):209–214, 1965.

Shor, G.M., "Worker's Compensation: Subsidies for Occupational Disease." *Journal of Public Health Policy,* 1:328–341, 1980.

Sigerist, Henry E., "Historical Background of Industrial and Occupational Diseases." *Bulletin of the New York Academy of Medicine,* 12:597–609, November 1936.

Somers, Herman M., and Anne Ramsey Somers, *"Workmen's Compensation: Prevention, Insurance, and Rehabilitation of Occupational Disability.* New York: John Wiley, 1954.

Stern, Bernhard J., *Medicine in Industry.* New York: Commonwealth Fund, 1946.

Straus, Robert, *Medical Care for Seamen: The Origin of Public Medical Service in the United States.* New Haven: Yale University Press, 1950.

Teleky, Ludwig, *History of Factory and Mine Hygiene.* New York: Columbia University Press, 1948.

U.S. Department of Health, Education and Welfare, *Social Security Programs in the United States.* Washington, D.C.: 1968.

U.S. Department of Health and Human Services, *Social Security Programs Throughout the World—1989.* Washington, D.C.: DHHS, 1989.

Vilanilam, J.V., "A Historical and Socioeconmic Analysis of Occupational Safety and Health in India." *International Journal of Health Services.* 10:233–249, 1980.

Weindling, P., *The Social History of Occupational Health.* London: Croon Helm, 1985.

Wolfe, Samuel, "Worker Conflicts in the Health Field: An Overview." *International Journal of Health Services,* 5(1):5–8, 1975.

Yassi, Annalee, "The Development of Worker-Controlled Occupational Health Centers in Canada." *American Journal of Public Health,* 78(6):689–693, June 1988.

Rural People

Airhihenbuwa, Collins O., "Nigerian Heads of Households Attitudes Toward Modern and Traditional Medicines." *Journal of Rural Health,* 3(1):21–30, 1987.

Australian Information Service, *The Flying Doctor.* Canberra 1974.

Bannerman, Robert H., John Burton, and Ch'en Wen-chieh (Editors), *Traditional Medicine and Health Care Coverage.* Geneva: World Health Organization, 1983.

Bodenheimer, T. S., "Mobile Units: A Solution to the Rural Health Problem?" *Medical Care,* 7:144–154, 1969.

Chandra, Shiv, and G. M. Mathur, "Health Care Through Mobile Camps." *World Health Forum,* 6:153–154, 1985.

Drobny, Abraham, "Latin American Experience Related to the Solution of Rural Health Problems in the United States." *New England Journal of Medicine,* 285:124–127, July 1974.

Fendall, N.R.E., *Auxiliaries in Health Care: Programs in Developing Countries.* Baltimore: Johns Hopkins University Press, 1972.

Gish, O., and G. J. Walker, *Mobile Health Services: Study in Cost-Effectiveness.* London: Tri-med, 1977.

Halstead, Scott B., Julio A. Walsh, and Kenneth S.

Warren (Editors), *Good Health at Low Cost.* New York: Rockefeller Foundation, 1985.

Hu, Teh-Wei, "The Financing and the Economic Efficiency of Rural Health Services in the People's Republic of China." *International Journal of Health Services,* 6(2):239–242, 1976.

Israel, E., *Incentives Offered to Civil Servants in the Medical Field for Services in Remote, Semi-Rural, and Rural Areas.* Geneva: World Health Organization (Processed document, WHO/SHS/76.1), 1976.

Jajoo, U.N., V.P. Gupta, and A.P. Jain, "Rural Health Services: Towards a New Strategy." *World Health Forum,* 6:150–152, 1985.

Mejia, Alfonso, Helena Pizurki, and Erica Royston, *Physician and Nurse Migrations: Analysis and Policy Implications.* Geneva: World Health Organization, 1979.

Mott, F. D., and M. I. Roemer, *Rural Health and Medical Care.* New York: McGraw-Hill, 1948.

Ofosu-Amaah, V., *National Experience in the Use of Community Health Workers: A Review of Current Issues and Problems.* Geneva: World Health Organization (Offset Pub. No. 71), 1983.

Roemer, Milton I., "Rural Health Programs in Different Nations." *Milbank Memorial Fund Quarterly,* 26:58–89, 1948.

Roemer, Milton I., *Rural Health Care.* St. Louis, MO: Mosby, 1976.

Roemer, Milton I., "Strategies for Increasing Rural Medical Manpower." *Public Health Reports,* 93(2):142–146, 1978.

Rosenthal, Marilynn M., and Deborah Frederick, "Physician Maldistribution in Cross-cultural Perspective: United States, United Kingdon and Sweden." *Inquiry,* 21:60–74, 1984.

Savy, Robt., *Social Security and Agriculture and Rural Areas.* Geneva: International Labour Office, 1972.

World Health Organization, *City Health.* Geneva: WHO (processed), 1990.

Other Special Populations

Armstrong, G. E., "Medical Program of Veterans Administration." *Journal of the American Medical Association,* 171:540–544, 1959.

Berry, Frank B., "A Complimentary Report on the Medical Services of the Armed Forces." *Military Medicine* (Washington, D.C.), 128(10): 951–959, October 1963.

Cohen, Irvin J., "The Veterans Administration Medical Care Program." In Leslie J. DeGroot (Editor), *Medical Care Social and Economic Aspects.* Springfield, IL: Charles C Thomas, 1966, pp. 425–436.

Davis Karen, and Cathy Schoen, *Health and the War on Poverty.* Washington, D.C.: Brookings Institution, 1978.

Dewdney, J., *Health Services in Australia.* Sydney: John Wiley, 1984.

Fitzgerald, M., and J. Sim, *British Prisons.* Oxford: Basil Blackwell, 1982.

Fully, G., "Penitentiary Medicine in France." *Ciba Foundation Symposium on Medical Care of Prisoners and Detainees.* Amsterdam: Associated Scientific Publishers, 1972.

Garrison, F. H., *Notes on the History of Military Medicine.* New York: Hiddesheim, 1970.

Goldsmith, Seth B., "The Status of Prison Health Care." *Public Health Reports.* 89(6):569–575, 1974.

Hetzel, Basil S., et al., *Better Health for Aborigines.* St. Lucia, Queensland: University of Queensland Press, 1974.

Lacronique, Jean-François, "Health Services in France." In Marshall Raffel (Editor), *Comparative Health Systems,* University Park, PA: Pennsylvania State University Press, 1984, pp. 258–285.

Laffin, J., *Surgeons in the Field.* London: J.M. Dent, 1970.

MacNalty, Arthur S., and W. Frank Mellor (Editors), *Medical Services in War: The Principal Medical Lessons of the Second World War.* London: Her Majesty's Stationary Office, 1968.

Marmor, Theodore R., *The Politics of Medicare.* Chicago: Aldine, 1973.

Newport, John, "Review of Health Services in Correctional Facilities in the United States." *Public Health Reports,* 92(6):564–569, 1977.

Nordlicht, Stephen, "Punishment or Rehabilitation?" *New York State Journal of Medicine* 75(6):1085–1087, 1975.

Roemer, Milton I., "History of the Effects of War on Medicine." *Annals of Medical History,* 4:189–198, May 1942.

Roemer, Milton I., *The Organization of Medical Care under Social Security.* Geneva: International Labour Office, 1969.

Roemer, Milton I., "Organized Programs of Medical Care." In John M. Last (Editor), Maxcy-Rosenau, *Public Health and Preventive Medicine,* 11th ed. Chapter 49. New York: Appleton-Century-Crofts, 1980, pp. 1634–1700.

Sandrick, Kazren M., "Health Care in Correctional Institutions in the United States, England, Canada, Poland, and France." *Quality Review Bulletin,* 7(7):28–31, 1981.

Schewe, D., K. Nordhorn, and K. Schenke, *Survey of Social Security in the Federal Republic of Germany.* Bonn: Minister for Labour and Social Affairs, 1972.

Smith, Richard, "History of the Prison Medical Services." *British Medical Journal,* 287:1786–1788, 1983.

Smith, Richard, "Medical Care in the Dutch Penal System." *British Medical Journal,* 288:925–927, 1984.

Soong, F. S., "Aboriginal Health Workers in Austra-lia." *World Health Forum,* 3(2):166–169, 1982.

Spicer, Edward H., *A Short History of the Indians of the United States.* New York: Anvil, 1969.

Spiegel, Allen D., and Simon Podair (Editors), *Medicaid-Lessons for National Health Insurance.* Rockville, MD: Aspen Systems Corp., 1975.

U.S. Army Handbook, *Panama.* Washington: Department of Defense, 1981.

U.S. Public Health Service, *Indian Health Service: A Comprehensive Program for American Indi-ans and Alaska Natives.* Washington, D.C., 1980.

U.S. Public Health Service, *Indian Health Service Chart Series Book.* Washington, D.C.: Government Printing Office, 1985.

World Health Organization, *Health Services in Europe,* 3rd ed. Copenhagen: Regional WHO Office for Europe, 1981.

Zajtchuk, Russ, et al., "Medical Success in El Salvador." *Military Medicine,* 59–61, February 1989.

CHAPTER FIFTEEN

Health Programs for Certain Disorders

In every health system there are organized efforts to cope with special disorders, varying with epidemiological conditions. The oldest of these efforts have concerned the control of communicable diseases, but with the changing picture of morbidity and mortality in countries, other objectives of disease control have become prominent. In this chapter we shall examine the principal strategies of disease control under five major categories: (1) communicable diseases, (2) sexually transmitted diseases, (3) mental disorders, (4) chronic noncommunicable diseases, and (5) dental disease.

COMMUNICABLE DISEASES

The earliest social action to control communicable diseases was taken in Europe of the twelfth and thirteenth centuries to combat leprosy and the plague. Facilities were built outside the towns, to isolate the unfortunate patients so that their disease would not be spread. Isolation and quarantine continue to be strategies in communicable disease control, for selected disorders, up to the present time.

The scope of communicable disease control programs in most health systems is very broad and only the highlights can be reviewed. They concern acute communicable diseases, tuberculosis, vector-borne infections, and other chronic communicable diseases.

Acute Communicable Diseases

The acute communicable infections are largely diseases of childhood. Although many features of life affect their occurrence, the principal strategy of control has been immunization of the child. Such immunizations, of course, have

been given in child health clinics throughout the world for decades. Enforcement often comes from school authorities, who require certain immunizations for entry to public school.

Nevertheless, studies by the World Health Organization and UNICEF around 1970 showed that there were serious deficiencies in the immunity status of children regarding major childhood infections, especially in developing countries. This led in 1974 to the launching of WHO's Expanded Program on Immunization (EPI). The goal was to achieve full immunization of children against six major infections: diphtheria, pertussis, tetanus, poliomyelitis, measles, and tuberculosis. Mass campaigns were carried out through the whole Ministry of Health infrastructure. Problems encountered by the EPI program have included lack of awareness (in government and in the general population) of the scope and seriousness of the target diseases, ineffective program management, and inadequate skills and equipment for vaccine storage and handling.

Nevertheless, progress has been made. When EPI started in 1974, less than 5 percent of children in developing countries were receiving poliomyelitis and full DPT (diphtheria, pertussis, and tetanus) immunization in their first year of life. By 1987, these coverage levels surpassed 50 percent in developing countries. Poliomyelitis immunization efforts have been so successful that the Pan American Health Organization is leading a drive to eradicate this crippling disease from the Americas in the near future. The strategy of EPI calls for major campaigns in nations or regions, followed up by inclusion of immunizations in on-going primary health care programs.

The EPI program was preceded in the World

Health Organization agenda by strategies to combat a single major virus disease. In the 1960s, one of the oldest communicable diseases, smallpox, became the object of a worldwide eradication effort. Through painstaking organization in dozens of countries, especially in Asia and Africa, the disease was reduced and by 1977 was declared to be eradicated from the earth—the first such achievement. This great accomplishment has been recognized as social and organizational, rather than medical. The organization of vaccine transport under proper conditions—an effective "cold chain"—was the indispensable strategy, requiring the full cooperation of countries with WHO regional offices and headquarters.

The control of acute communicable diseases in all health systems begins with the notification of public health authorities about cases. Legislation or regulations usually specify the diseases that must be reported. Public health personnel are then expected to investigate the case and trace contacts who may also be infected. Depending on the disease, the patient may be isolated—at home or in a hospital—to prevent spread. In fact, notification is seldom complete, even in industrialized countries. In periods of epidemics and for the more serious diseases, it tends to be more nearly complete. Some countries still operate contagious disease hospitals, but more often such cases are admitted to isolation wards in general hospitals.

The maximum provision of immunizations in the first year of life is an on-going task of maternal and child health programs. In the industrialized countries, this is most effective when MCH clinics are available; immunizations through private medical practitioners are usually less dependable—if only for cold chain problems. In developing countries almost all immunizations are provided in health centers or health stations offering primary health care. All countries must develop laboratories for examination of specimens from infected patients.

To promote immunizations, health education is very helpful. It is provided by posters, pamphlets, films, and other media. Community health workers have a largely educational role, to persuade people to obtain preventive services. The availability of medical care in a health facility is often the most persuasive reason for seeking preventive immunizations at the same time. WHO studies have shown that contrary to common belief, there is no danger in vaccinating children who have minor illnesses.

Each of the acute communicable diseases has had special problems in the perfection of effective vaccines. Most of the early vaccines came from research in Europe, although methods of large-scale production were developed in America. Poliomyelitis has two types of vaccine, both developed by U.S. scientists. Each of the vaccines is in use by different countries. Numerous vaccines have been developed for prevention of influenza, but with very uncertain benefits. Hepatitis B is a serious liver infection in southeast Asia and parts of Africa, against which immunization has not yet been perfected. Rheumatic fever is a serious infectious disease, related to streptococcal infection, that has declined greatly in affluent countries, but remains high in many developing countries; it often leads to rheumatic heart disease. Although no immunization is available, it can be prevented by basic primary health care.

In every local public health jurisdiction, as part of all political types of health system, the control of acute communicable diseases is a basic function. It is an aspect of the work of all health personnel—public health nurses, sanitarians, auxiliary health workers, health educators, and others. Whatever may be the primary duty of a public health worker, discovery of a communicable infection calls for immediate action. The general effectiveness of communicable disease control programs in industrialized countries is reflected in the steady decline of mortality rates from such diseases over the last 100 years. These declines began even before the era of immunizations, reflecting the influence of improvements in the general physical and social environment. In developing countries, urbanization and improved standards of living have also brought large declines in communicable disease. Improvements in rural areas are probably attributable more to immunizations and other preventive interventions.

Tuberculosis

The control of tuberculosis has been the subject of special efforts in national health systems since the late nineteenth century. Robert Koch of Germany had discovered the tubercle bacillus in 1882, and this gave rise to the movements to prevent its spread. The first initiative was taken by voluntary community groups in Europe. A French League against Tuberculosis was founded in 1891 at Bordeaux, France, and in 1898 the British organized a National Association for the Prevention of Consumption and Other Forms of Tuberculosis.

The first physical facility focused on tuberculosis was the Victoria Dispensary for Consumption, opened in Liverpool, England in 1887. In the early twentieth century, voluntary tuberculosis associations constructed special sanitaria for these patients. In 1904, the National Association for the Study and Prevention of Tuberculosis was formed in the United States, after several similar agencies had been organized at the state level. But the problem was much greater than voluntary agencies could handle; in 1900, pulmonary tuberculosis was the number one cause of death in many industrialized countries. Major responsibility had to be assumed by government.

Ministries of Health at the national or provincial levels in both Europe and North America constructed sanitaria exclusively for tuberculosis patients. Although these facilities treated patients, mostly with bedrest and nutritious food, they also served a crucial preventive function: the isolation of cases. Accordingly the construction and operation of large sanitaria, for treatment and isolation of active cases, were the main strategies of tuberculosis control throughout industrialized countries.

Declines in tuberculosis mortality began to occur soon after 1900. The occupancy rates of the sanitaria therefore decreased. By the 1920s and 1930s, tuberculosis sanitaria began to be converted to other uses. They served often as reasonable facilities for general long-term care of elderly and chronically ill patients. In developing countries, on the other hand, special tuberculosis sanitaria were seldom built. These patients were treated in isolation sections of general hospitals.

After the discovery of streptomycin in 1947, the rate of decline in both incidence and mortality from tuberculosis accelerated further. Tuberculosis sanitaria were closed down almost completely. Instead the global strategy, in both industrialized and developing countries, shifted to the purely preventive goals that had always been advocated.

A strategy for prevention of tuberculosis has achieved wide acceptance, especially in developing countries, where the incidence and prevalence of the disease remain high. Case finding is basic, both by mass screening with miniature chest X-rays and by identification of patients attending health centers and other facilities. Sputum specimens are collected for bacteriological study. This requires laboratory facilities with trained technicians. Case finding can be expanded by interrogation of household heads and community leaders about possible victims of the disease. Routine chest X-rays of all patients admitted to hospitals are done in many transitional (middle income level) developing countries.

Laboratory services that are essential in case finding need not be limited to identification of the tubercle bacillus. They are one component in multipurpose bacteriological, chemical, and other analyses of specimens. In the affluent countries and many moderate income developing countries there are national networks of laboratories, with large central units, intermediate, and small but multipurpose local laboratories. Certain specimens may be sent from peripheral laboratories to the center for more elaborate study.

After tuberculosis cases are identified, the next preventive action is chemotherapy. The patient continues to live at home and takes medication for 3 to 6 months. Streptomycin is now supplemented with isoniazid and several other drugs. The exact regimes of therapy differ among countries, but all of them are quite inexpensive, compared with the previous approach of institutionalization. The procurement of an adequate supply of antituberculosis drugs by most countries requires foreign currency, acceptable to the industrialized countries that produce them. UNICEF and the World Bank have provided loans and grants for this purpose. China and India have developed pharmaceutical industries that produce most of these drugs domestically.

An even more basic preventive approach is immunization of small infants against tuberculosis with bacillus Calmette-Guerin (BCG) vaccine. This French discovery of bacilli with low virulence (BCG) has led to a vaccine that is effective in developing countries, where exposure to tuberculosis is high. BCG is included in the EPI program, even when it is implemented in industrialized countries, and even though further research is needed. In developing countries, examination of the personal contacts of cases is seldom feasible, so that mass prevention through a vaccine holds much greater promise.

Finally, for advanced cases of tuberculosis, it is still necessary to have hospitalization and intensive therapy. Patients are thereby isolated and can often be cured. Despite the gradual decline in tuberculosis sanitaria, in 1975 there were still some 600,000 beds worldwide reserved for the disease. Fortunately the trend in all types of countries has been for further decline of these categorical facilities and beds.

The history of tuberculosis control programs in both industrialized and developing countries has often been one of strong central leadership, with peripheral activities coming under central authority. This "vertical" management had certain short-term benefits, but serious long-term weaknesses. Since the 1970s, as the approach of primary health care became dominant, the task has been to integrate tuberculosis control and all other categorical programs at the local level. If various aspects of control come under separate social security agencies, universities, quasigovernmental corporations, and private medicine, integration is necessary under the leadership of the Ministry of Health.

The most fundamental approach to the prevention of tuberculosis would be sweeping improvement of the physical and social environment, to enhance standards of living. This requires, of course, economic development, higher levels of education, good housing and sanitation, full employment, and world peace. The costs and political will for such a social order are incalculable, even though some progress toward it is being made. In the absence of an ideal society, strategies for the control of tuberculosis—and many other afflictions—can

correct some of the worst outcomes of existing society. By so doing, they strengthen the ability of men and women to move ahead.

Vector-Borne Diseases

In contrast to the acute childhood infections and tuberculosis, several major communicable diseases are spread by insect vectors or other animal forms. The most important in the world is malaria, transmitted by mosquitoes and occurring in some 100 countries. Another vector-borne disease causing great disability from parasites is schistosomiasis, spreadly by snails. There are many others, but the programs to control these two vector-borne disorders are analyzed as major examples of the general field.

Malaria. Social efforts to combat mosquitoes date back to ancient Greece, and marshy lands breeding mosquitoes were believed to emit "miasms" causing fevers. Peruvian Indians discovered the value of cinchona bark (later found to contain quinine) in the treatment of fevers before 1500. By the nineteenth century quinine was being taken as a preventive of malaria. The malaria parasite in human blood was first identified in 1880 and the role of mosquitoes as vectors in 1897. This knowledge, coming from research in France and England, laid the basis for extensive malaria control programs after 1900.

The earliest control efforts were directed to combat the breeding of mosquitoes. This meant the drainage of swamps and the application of pesticides around the water's edge, where mosquito larvae bred. In relatively affluent countries, like Italy or the southern United States, this strategy worked, but it was too expensive to carry out in most developing countries.

The great breakthrough occurred after World War II, when the Swiss synthesis of DDT provided an extremely powerful insecticide. When it was sprayed on the interior walls of houses, the residual chemical could continue to be an effective insecticide for several months. Mosquitoes would simply light on the walls and die. Teams of DDT sprayers visited houses in malarial regions once or twice a year, and great reductions in malaria were achieved.

WHO provided the initial teams in several Asian countries, to demonstrate the technique, and eventually most developing countries with malaria organized spraying programs themselves. Meanwhile improved drugs for personal prophylaxis of malaria had been synthesized, but they were too expensive for widespread use in most malarial countries.

Numerous problems arose in the house-spraying programs—development of insecticide resistance by mosquitoes, inadequate funding, management inefficiencies—that slowed up progress. Nevertheless in the 1960s, the World Health Assembly voted to embark on an international effort to *eradicate* malaria from the earth. With increased funding and political commitment, substantial progress was made, but in the late 1960s the disease burst out epidemically again in areas where eradication had been thought successful.

The policy taking shape in the 1970s was that malaria "control" could be best achieved as part of stable and long-term programs in primary health care. WHO analysis divides the world into four situations with respect to malaria:

Region	Percent of World Population
1. Malaria never existed or disappeared without intervention	27
2. Malaria was endemic, but disappeared after control campaign	32
3. Malaria was much reduced after control measures, but tranmission recurred, and the situation is unstable	32
4. Malaria is endemic and no national control program was ever implemented	9

The type of malaria control program needed must obviously differ among these regions. An upward trend in cases reported has been prom-

inent in certain Latin American and Asian countries. Some 83 percent of the cases reported annually to WHO come from Brazil and Mexico in the Americas and in Asia from China, India, Philippines, Sri Lanka, Thailand, Viet Nam, and Afghanistan (these are absolute numbers, not rates). In Sri Lanka and Afghanistan, the disease has reached epidemic proportions. In Africa, there are probably more malaria cases than anywhere else. About 2 to 7 million are reported each year but extrapolating from fever and parasite surveys, WHO estimates about 90 million cases per year. This prevalence must be seen in the perspective of a worldwide total of malaria cases, estimated to be about 110,000,000 per year. Compared with estimates for 1900, when there were 250,000,000 cases of malaria each year (and 2.5 million deaths), the control programs of the period 1945–1985 brought a spectacular drop in morbidity and mortality, even though a partial reversal has occurred.

To quote from the WHO Division of Control of Tropical Diseases:

> The lack or shortage of trained personnel for the planning, organization, monitoring and evaluation of programs remains one of the major constraints in many countries. The policy advocated is the development of malaria control within the framework of primary health care at the district level. The aim is the prevention and reduction of malaria mortality by providing prompt diagnosis or recognition and adequate treatment of malaria cases through the basic health services and primary health care. This implies also the creation of efficient referral systems for the management of severe and complicated cases, and for treatment failures.

Difficulties complicating control programs are poor housing and sanitation; lack of knowledge about the biology and ecology of the mosquito vectors; the expansion of agriculture, forestry, and mining into new areas, causing migration; and an inefficient or nonexistent health care infrastructure. Aggravating all these difficulties is inadequate financing to support all control efforts.

The biological aspects of malaria transmissions require whole textbooks to explain. It should be noted here that the anopheles mosquito that transmits malaria may be of many species, in different environmental circumstances. The parasite infecting people may also be of several types, the most lethal being *Plasmodium falciparum*. This organism has developed resistance to chloroquine, the most widely available antimalaria drug. Adaptation of control efforts to these two biological variables is difficult but essential.

The best combination of strategies for malaria control differs not only with the general degree of endemicity, but also with the physical environment. In sub-Sahara Africa, with its great arid open plains (savanna), transmission of the parasite is so continuous that virtually every small child is infected. Diagnosis and drug treatment of cases must be the main strategy here. In areas having traditional agriculture in plains and valleys, outside of Africa, house spraying and personal health services are called for. In forest areas, classical vector control methods are not applicable and individual diagnosis and treatment are most feasible. In areas of extensive agricultural development, breeding control techniques should ideally be built into irrigation systems; house spraying, drug prophylaxis, and personal protection against mosquitoes (netting over beds) should be used. Urban malaria should ideally be prevented by proper location of houses, design of buildings, and environmental sanitation. Malaria in coastal and marshland areas calls for drainage and landfills as well as house spraying.

The control of malaria is nearly always a responsibility of Ministries of Health and its geographic subdivisions. The work is largely in rural regions, where there are few other government or voluntary agencies on hand. Managerial efficiency depends on the whole structure of this ministry, at different administrative levels. There is need, of course, to encourage community participation, so that individuals are motivated to cooperate in malaria control efforts. Political support is necessary to acquire proper funding. Because malaria usually persists for many years, community awareness must be of long duration.

Numerous other parasitic diseases are spread by insects—filariasis, onchocerciasis, trypanosomiasis, and even the virus of yellow fever—and their control requires destruction of the insect vectors in different ways. A quite different form of vector is involved in the transmission of schistosomiasis, which is second only to malaria in its public health and socioeconomic importance in tropical areas of the world.

Schistosomiasis. The epidemiology and mode of transmission of this parasitic disease are very complex, but their dependence on polluted water is crucial. The parasite is discharged from infected persons into water, where snails are the intermediate hosts. Freely swimming larvae emerge from the snail and penetrate the skin of persons, usually during agricultural work. In the human body the adult parasite settles in veins, causing serious deformities—elephantiasis in severe cases.

The control of schistosomiasis requires careful planning of water resources to maintain their purity. The land around the waterways should have proper sanitation facilities, so that the water is not contaminated with urine. Decent housing must be provided for migratory agricultural workers, and personal health service for prompt drug therapy of infected persons.

Since prudent planning of water sources has usually been lacking, the practical strategy for schistosomiasis control has usually required various efforts to eliminate the intermediate host—certain species of snail. Aside from drainage of nonproductive swamps, snail-breeding places are treated with various molluscicides. In addition the treatment of infected persons with effective drugs can help to reduce the transmission of the parasites.

People in endemic areas must be educated about the mode of transmission of schistosomes. If agricultural workers have to move about in contaminated water, they should wear protective clothing, although this is seldom feasible in developing countries. Potable water, of course, has to be provided nearby for drinking, bathing, and washing clothes. Because these preventive measures are so difficult to carry out in the lowest income developing countries, schistosomiasis remains endemic in much of Africa and certain sections of southeast Asia and Latin America.

In the late 1980s, WHO reported that schistosomiasis was endemic in 74 countries, with over 200,000,000 persons estimated to be infected. Much larger numbers of people are exposed to infection. Water resource development for irrigation and agricultural purposes is important, and yet such projects often increase the intensity of schistosomiasis transmission. The construction of dams is imperative for economic development, but inevitably they affect the environment and may foster disease.

Certain major impoundment and irrigation projects have dramatized rapid increases in schistosomiasis. In Egypt, the construction of the Aswan Dam in the 1930s brought perennial irrigation to several provinces. This was followed, however, by an increase in schistosomiasis from 2–11 percent up to 44–75 percent of persons. Similar escalation of rates applied after dam construction in Sudan. In west Africa, the damming of Lake Volta was followed by a rise in the infection of children from 5–10 percent to 90 percent. These epidemic levels of schisotomiasis led to the array of control efforts noted above, especially the chemical strategies against the breeding of snails.

The campaign against schistosomiasis in China in the 1950s was a dramatic illustration of control efforts, even without molluscicides. In certain high prevalence areas, the entire rural population was mobilized to carry out a "people's war against snails." Old ditches and ponds had to be filled up and new channels dug. The banks of the waterways, where snails bred, were dug up and smoothed down so that the snails were buried. In addition, the people had to be educated about the handling of human excreta, the provision of safe drinking water, and improved personal hygiene. Outcome data are not available, but the severity of schistosomiasis in the endemic areas seems to have declined.

Other Communicable Diseases

Many other communicable diseases have been the object of organized programs in national health systems, of which a few may be considered.

Leprosy. This ancient disease, against which communities took stern actions to isolate cases, still survives in many developing countries. As noted in Chapter 3, "lazarettos" for leprosy patients were built throughout Europe in the twelfth and thirteenth centuries, and the unfortunate patients were condemned to live in them for life. This brutal form of isolation did reduce the prevalence of leprosy in Europe, and after the fourteenth century, it gradually subsided. In developing countries, however, the disease persists to the present time.

It is estimated that in 1976 there were 10–12 million leprosy cases in the world. The prevalence rates (cases per 1,000 population) were highest in Africa, but to some extent the disease exists in Latin America, southeast Asia, and even Australia. An especially large increase in cases was reported in India during the 1970s and 1980s.

The leprosy bacillus was identified in 1868, and since then the control of the disease shifted radically away from isolation of cases to treatment of infected persons while they live in their own homes. The leprosaria had already been closing down in Europe, but they were operating in developing countries in the nineteenth and twentieth centuries. It became a political task of enlightened public health leaders to persuade governments in developing countries to discontinue use of leprosaria and promote drug therapy of all cases.

The proper therapy with drugs for effective control of the disease took years to work out. Since 1981, WHO has promoted a combination of three drugs that are taken monthly for 6–24 months. The regime has now been adopted by 45 of the 53 countries in which leprosy is endemic, although in another 50 countries some cases are reported. In endemic regions, treatment centers have been established, where drug supplies are maintained and records are kept. In one district of India, for example, the cases dropped from 30,000 to 4,000 over a 4-year period. Drug therapy, in place of forced isolation, is not only much less expensive, but it has removed the dreadful stigma of leprosy, so that cases are more readily reported. Even without drug therapy, the incidence of leprosy has declined in areas with generally improved standards of living, demonstrating the influence of personal hygiene. With this new more hopeful spirit about the disease, it is expected that complete eradication may be possible in a few decades. Elimination of leprosy "as a public health problem" would be achieved by reducing the prevalence of the disease to less than 1 case per 10,000 population.

Diarrheal Diseases. The several infectious diseases of the gastrointestinal tract have long been concerns of public health control, although in much more diversified ways than the communicable diseases so far reviewed. If we begin with the end of World War II, the main problems may be examined.

Because of its severity and its propensity for rapid epidemic spread, *cholera* has received the greatest attention. An outbreak in Egypt in 1947 was the first occasion in 30 years that the disease had spread west of India. In the early 1960s, cholera spread as far westward as Iran, Iraq, and parts of the USSR. The World Health Organization responded with the organization of training courses, creation of cholera combat teams, assistance to countries in setting up laboratories, and general improvement of sanitation. The use of anticholera vaccines was found to be of little value, but the simple ingestion of *oral rehydration salts* (ORS) was found to be effective. Despite the high concern for cholera, increasing attention was also paid to typhoid and paratyphoid fevers. Large field trials in the 1960s showed the limited effectiveness of vaccines and the necessity of control through environmental sanitation.

In 1970, cholera spread to western Africa, where it rapidly invaded 39 countries. Rehydration centers were set up at strategic sites in three WHO regions. Antibiotics were also found to be effective for cholera, and supplies of these had to be acquired. Manufacturers of oral rehydration salts were persuaded to produce small packets for distribution to families. Emphasis was always put on health education, food safety, and other sanitary measures.

Research in the 1970s identified new viral and bacterial agents as causes of diarrhea, such as rotavirus. The most important finding of practical value was that ORS treatment was effective in treating all the diarrheas, including cholera, and in persons of all ages. Although children were the commonest victims, it worked also in adults. ORS packets were delivered by health centers and health stations, and this was done by assistant nurses and various auxiliary health workers—often in connection with dietary education in maternal and child health programs.

Acute diarrheas had always been known to be a greater problem in developing countries than cholera, but in the absence of a specific preventive, there was little enthusiasm in Ministries of Health to undertake control efforts. The demonstrated simplicity and effectiveness of ORS therapy in reducing diarrheal morbidity and mortality convinced authorities to regard this strategy as an essential component of national primary health care programs. In developing countries, it is part of the service offered at every Ministry of Health facility for ambulatory care.

Because of the enormity of the task, the support and collaboration of various international agencies have been necessary. In addition to WHO, in the early 1980s UNICEF became a major contributor in country programs. Some 29 international and bilateral agencies (such as USAID) have given financial support. The use of ORS therapy has clearly increased. By 1987, diarrheal control programs were operative in 96 countries, which included 98 percent of the population of the developing world. A comprehensive program includes not only ORS therapy, but also proper breast-feeding, use of safe water, and hygienic waste disposal.

In many countries, mothers are taught how to prepare ORS solutions at home. Countries are also setting up domestic plants for producing ORS packets, instead of having to depend on imports. Evaluations of these programs have been carried out in numerous countries. The constraints found have included inadequate training of staff in case management, need for improved supervision, inadequate information, and excessive use of antidiarrheal drugs. By 1987, another pandemic of cholera had spread to 94 countries in all regions except Latin America. WHO has continued to advocate control of cholera through the general diarrheal control programs, properly managed. Efforts to produce an effective immunization against cholera also continue, with some promise for a possible oral vaccine.

SEXUALLY TRANSMITTED DISEASES

Special clinics for the diagnosis and treatment of syphilis and gonorrhea were established by public health authorities in Europe in the late nineteenth century. Under voluntary agencies (Society for Social and Moral Prophylaxis), such clinics were set up in the United States a little later. Attitudes were highly moralistic, and support often came on such grounds, rather than health protection. The early European clinics had functions connected with prostitution, which was legally permitted on condition that the prostitutes were found free or kept free of venereal disease.

Paul Ehrlich had discovered "salvarsan," an arsenic compound, for the treatment of syphilis in 1909. This provided a powerful tool for control and for rendering cases noninfectious, but the regimes of therapy were complex and long, usually several years. The tracing of contacts and follow-up of cases required much time from public health personnel. A further and greater breakthrough occurred in 1946, when penicillin was found to be a rapid and effective treatment of both syphilis and gonorrhea. New technology is often thought to increase expenses, so that cost–benefit analyses are required to justify the investments. Penicillin, however, clearly reduced costs, and achieved cures for the two commonest sexually transmitted diseases (STDs) far more efficiently than before.

In the 1930s, even before the effectiveness of penicillin was discovered, national campaigns were mounted against these diseases. In the United States, a special title to the Social Security Act gave grants to the state health departments for venereal disease (VD) control. In the World Health Organization, a unit was devoted to this field in 1948. Although most work was in the industrialized countries, VD control was also included in the normal functions of public health agencies in the developing countries.

As more has been learned about STDs, greater efforts have been directed to prevention, at least in the industrialized countries. This has meant education about sexuality in the public schools, as well as specifically about the hazards of STD. The value and use of condoms as barriers to disease transmission were taught. At the STD clinic, patients can participate in contact-tracing for the benefit of their partners and themselves. Screening for early detection of cases has been promoted in various population groups, such as industrial workforces or routinely on patients admitted to general hospitals. Laboratory services are required to examine serological specimens, and the follow-up of positive findings must be carefully done. In many industrialized countries, premarital examinations for syphilis are required by law, and prenatal tests of the pregnant woman are often done routinely in MCH clinics.

The treatment of syphilis and gonorrhea in a country naturally depends on the economic support mechanisms of the whole health system. In developing countries, hospital outpatient departments and health centers, financed mainly by a Ministry of Health, are intended to serve everyone; STD sessions are included in normal operations. In the United States, where national health insurance is lacking, but voluntary insurance is extensive, most patients seek care from private physicians. There are also STD clinics in state and local health departments, attended by low-income patients, without coverage by insurance or public aid to finance visits to a private doctor. These clinics are supported to general revenues of the federal, state, and local governments.

In Western Europe, the need for special STD clinics declined as national health insurance gave everyone access to doctors. Yet it is noteworthy that even so, these clinics in France and Germany have continued to serve many patients by their own choice; some people may not feel comfortable with a personal physician and they know that at the clinic they will receive expert care. In the British National Health Service, where generalists are paid by capitation, patients are encouraged to use the public clinics. In the 1950s there was a steady decline in syphilis and gonorrhea, and many public health authorities relaxed their control efforts. Then in the 1960s and early 1970s, there was a new rise in the worldwide incidence of gonorrhea and syphilis, as well as a "second generation" of STDs, caused mainly by viruses and parasites. New efforts were then put forward in popular health education, STD screening, diagnosis and treatment of cases, contact tracing, and training of health personnel.

By the end of the 1970s, the bacterial but not the viral STDs had been contained in the industrialized countries. In many developing countries, however, they remained a priority public health problem, especially because of the seriousness of their sequelae.

Then in 1981, the world was stunned by the discovery a new and extremely dangerous sexually transmitted disease—acquired immunodeficiency syndrome or AIDS. It was soon found to be caused by a virus, the human immunodeficiency virus (HIV), with a very long incubation period (several years) before development of a full-blown case of AIDS. Evidence suggested origins in Africa, but wide dissemination was occurring everywhere. Case fatality rates for full-blown AIDS were virtually 100%. The final causes of death have been mainly a parasitic form of pneumonia and Kaposi's sarcoma.

The transmission of the etiological agent, HIV, occurs mainly through sexual contact with an infected individual. It also occurs through exposure to contaminated blood, passage from an infected mother to her baby (before, during, or shortly after birth), or by means of transplanted body organs from an infected donor. By far the most common form of spread is through certain sexual contacts, which in Europe and North America involve mainly homosexual males. In Africa, where the HIV prevalence is extremely high, the transmission is mainly through heterosexual partners. The rate of heterosexual transmission is increasing also in the industrialized countries.

Since homosexual behavior has figured so prominently in HIV transmission in the United States and Europe, the problem has generated moralistic attitudes, seen with syphilis a century before. These have retarded control efforts, which must rely on disseminating clear information and influencing personal behavior through widespread health education.

In the industrialized countries, especially in large cities, a second important mode of HIV transmission has been connected with drug abuse. The drug-dependent person uses contaminated needles for injection of addictive compounds; needles are passed around without sterilization. The infected person may then transmit the disease to a heterosexual partner. Control efforts have included provision of clean needles to addicts, so long as the basic addiction has not been cured—a strategy that has naturally been controversial.

In western industrialized countries, health education efforts have been concentrated in high-risk groups—homosexuals and drug addicts. More general education is also conducted in public high schools. In Africa, all health education efforts are directed to the general population. New legislation on the control of AIDS has been enacted in more than 60 countries, as discussed in Chapter 11. Issues of confidentiality, discrimination, and human rights play a large part in policies laid down by these laws.

For persons who are HIV-positive or developing symptoms of AIDS, certain chemical therapies have been found. These drugs are very expensive, over and above the cost of hospital care of advanced cases. The search for a preventive vaccine is occupying hundreds of scientists, but for the present the best hope seems to be use of chemotherapy for HIV-infected persons.

Considering STD control as a whole, including AIDS, the movement requires the classic strategy of public health. Prevention calls for education on sexuality and human behavior. The focus may be targeted or generalized. Prostitution in industrialized countries can be controlled to limit its extent to small enclaves in the large cities. In developing countries, where rural poverty leads young women into prostitution, the dimensions are overwhelming, as in Thailand, the Philippines, or Brazil. The social rehabilitation of prostitutes (with job training), accomplished in China, shows what is possible with political will. When venereal disease has not been prevented, cases can be detected by testing—voluntary or mandatory for certain groups. Partner notification (contact tracing) is very important for all STD control, as in screening programs for several communicable diseases. Early controversies on syphilis detection are being replicated currently, regarding routine testing to detect HIV infection. The AIDS situation is more critical, however, because of the lack of a preventive vaccine or a cure.

When prevention has failed treatment must be given. This has been the major role of the STD clinic, which is now a standard component of local public health programs. The treatment of terminal cases of AIDS is very costly and its feasibility depends on the national health system. If economic support is universal, the costs are absorbed even though they may be high. In the United States, special legislation was required to finance medications for impoverished patients. In developing countries, the treatment of advanced cases of AIDS is tragically unaffordable for all but the richest persons. The only hope is prevention.

MENTAL DISORDERS

Every country is faced with problems of the mentally ill, for which special strategies are necessary. In contrast to the requirements for coping with somatic illness, the treatment and prevention of mental disorders must deal with patients who are not ordinarily seeking care. Society must take the initiative for both helping the individual and protecting other people. Historically the protection of the general population against harm from the mentally disordered was the primary objective.

The earliest actions of governments were to isolate the mentally disturbed in places where they had no contact with other people. It was many years later before ambulatory services were organized, in the hope that mental deterioration would be prevented. Eventually strategies developed that combined both types of care for different types of mental patients.

Mental Hospitals

Mental disorders were long believed to be caused by mysterious demonic influences. The early response of communities was to put these people away into asylums. As noted in Chapter 3, psychotic patients were even kept in prisons, to isolate them from the community. The French Revolution led to the first movement in defense of "the insane." Asylums were still places of isolation, rather than treatment, but they became more humane. In the United States around 1840, a Massachusetts school teacher led a similar movement. Restraints on patients were lightened, and various sorts of group activity were organized. Patients were encouraged to talk with the staff and with other patients, rather than sitting alone or staying in bed. With more advanced knowledge, there arose the concept of mental illness, rather than insanity, and the need for treatment rather than isolation.

In the late nineteenth century, asylums throughout Europe and America were gradually transformed into mental hospitals. With recognition of the vast proportions of mental illness and the high cost of prolonged hospital care, these were typically large hospitals built adjacent to urban centers. They were usually financed by central or provincial governments, rather than social security funds. Administratively, mental hospitals are typically public facilities under the control of the Ministry of Health or its geographic subdivisions. Because the operating costs depend on provincial and local general revenues—perhaps with some national level subsidy—and because the hospitalized psychotic has low political priority, the funding of mental hospitals is rarely adequate. They have typically been overcrowded and understaffed. In the language of a WHO report for Europe in 1975 (but repeated in 1981): "Impersonal custodial regimes, lack of privacy and of normal social and intellectual stimuli lead to apathy and the aggravation of symptoms, especially in patients with psychotic illness." These conditions have gradually improved, not so much because of greater funding, but because of reduced occupancy of the mental hospitals, improved internal organization, and policies favoring discharge of mental patients to general hospitals and other forms of community care.

In the large mental hospitals, the wards are generally organized, not according to diagnoses, but according to case severity. There are "open wards" for short-stay acute cases, and various other levels of wards for long-stay cases. On some wards patients receive active therapy, including rehabilitation attempted through group psychotherapy. On other wards, the care may be simply custodial. Influence from Germany has stressed therapy through disciplined work, and this modality is prominent also in Latin America and the former socialist countries of Eastern Europe. The variations in the internal organization of mental hospitals are very great.

Before World War II, commitment or admission to mental hospitals, which had usually been involuntary, was through a judicial procedure. As discussed in Chapter 11, the patient lost his freedom, and this required decision by a court of law. Then in the 1950s, a movement began to convert such admissions into voluntary medical procedures, with a psychiatric certification of the need for mental treatment. These medical admission procedures started in Europe, and spread to America and the rest of the world. In both the industrialized and the developing countries, that were formerly colonies, mental hospital commitment policy was influenced by the general movement for human rights.

After World War II and especially in the 1960s, the discovery of effective psychotherapeutic drugs infused mental hospital care with greater optimism. Many long-stay patients could be rehabilitated and discharged. On the wards the concept of the "therapeutic community" improved the atmosphere. Energetic medical care was shown in the use of procedures such as electric shock therapy.

The active therapeutic approach to mental illness in Europe and America was shown in the policy of the 1960s to admit mental patients to general hospitals. This was done mainly for short-stay cases likely to respond to active therapy. Such arrangements could shift the cost of mental illness from general tax funds to health insurance. Although special wards were usually set aside for these patients, the stigma of mental disease was far less in a general hospital, and resources for general medical care were much greater. In the Netherlands, for example, in 1975 some 13,000 mental patients were admitted to general hospitals, in comparison with 17,000 to mental hospitals.

In 1978, Italy passed legislation for a National Health Service (NHS)—an entitlement of everyone to comprehensive health services. As part of this law there was a provision that all mental hospitals must close down, and be replaced by services in general hospitals and in ambulatory care clinics. In reality, both the NHS and its mental hospital features are being only partially implemented. The northern Italian regions are making much greater progress than the southern. Many general hospital sections for mental patients are described as segregated and repressive. Nevertheless, a national movement, known as "Democratic Psychiatry," promotes the reforms in each locality.

In very affluent countries, there are often separate institutions for the mentally retarded. Sometimes these people are served in special sections of mental hospitals. As almost lifelong patients, the care of the mentally retarded is often under the administration of Ministries of Education. In this field, one purely preventive measure was the public health correction of iodine shortages (usually through iodized salt) to prevent cretinism, a form of retardation.

In developing countries, hospital care for the mentally disordered is much weaker than in the industrialized countries. In India, for example, beds in mental hospitals constituted 3.5 percent of all hospital beds in 1980. In Nigeria the equivalent figure was 2.7 percent. By contrast, even after discharge of mental patients to community resources, mental hospitals beds in France were 16.3 percent of the total in 1980, in Germany 15.2 percent, and in the United States 15.1 percent. The physical features of mental hospitals in most developing countries are generally extremely poor.

Some of the mentally ill in developing countries are admitted to general hospitals, but most are simply kept at home with the family. There are no organized follow-up programs to provide home care. In rural areas of African countries, traditional healers still try to exorcise evil spirits. Large general hospitals may sometimes operate psychiatric clinics, to which patients are referred for drug therapy.

In the developing countries of Latin America, at a transitional economic level, mental hospitals are stronger. In Mexico, for example, 9 percent of total beds are in mental hospitals, operated by the Ministry of Health and its subdivisions. This is associated with urbanization, which has grown rapidly. On the other hand, mental patients are being discharged, if they are covered by social security entitling them to obtain care in special polyclinics.

Community Mental Health Programs

Since about 1900 a mental health movement, quite separate from the mental hospitals, has grown in the industrialized countries. The provision of mental health service to the ambulatory person has been promoted in parallel with the efforts to improve the quality of mental hospitals. The origins of this approach are usually traced to the "mental hygiene" drive, initiated by voluntary groups in the United States.

With the notion of prevention, emphasis was given to clinics for children; if they were treated, it was believed, adult illness and hospitalization might be avoided. Although this theory has not been confirmed, the whole field of child psychiatry out-of-hospital has developed. Closely related is the field of child development under the discipline of psychology. Popular applications are seen in books on child rearing, such as those of Dr. Benjamin Spock, available in dozens of languages around the world.

The development of community mental health services in Europe was motivated less by preventive objectives than by provision of psychiatric help to patients discharged from mental hospitals. Services to patients at home were especially well planned in Great Britain. Most were elderly patients who were provided home visiting and nursing, meals-on-wheels, transport to hospitals and clinics, social clubs, and so on. Meanwhile, the patient gets primary care from a general practitioner and more specialized services at the outpatient departments of general hospitals. Elderly patients without acute mental symptoms can go to residential facilities.

In Austria, some special community psychiatric clinics have been developed, and in France and Germany, only a few of these. The

response to "deinstitutionalization" is generally more extensive in the countries with economic support for general medical care. In Canada, for example, between 1960 and 1976 the number of mental hospital beds was reduced from 48,000 to 15,000. The number of beds for mental patients in general hospitals increased from 840 to 5,840. The posthospital care of discharged patients is provided basically by physicians and hospital outpatient departments. Provisions are made for subsequent admission to a residential facility, if necessary, and home care is slowly developing to help mental patients get along in their own homes.

Japan is a highly industrialized country, where increasing numbers of elderly patients with senile dementia are being admitted to mental hospitals, and also to beds for mental patients in general hospitals. At the same time, this trend is being opposed by encouraging families to care for these patients at home. This has been the traditional form of care in Japan, and it is being strengthened with education and social clubs for the elderly. Even if there is no family, other living arrangements are made, so that the elderly person is not alone. Organized home care programs, stemming from general health centers (for preventive service) and public hospitals, are developing slowly.

The movement for decentralization and deinstitutionalization is, nevertheless, strong throughout Europe. The bold legislative action in Italy has been noted. A study of eight European countries by the World Health Organization showed the response to deinstitutionalization to be large increases in outpatient mental health service between 1972 and 1982. This trend was especially strong in France and Finland.

There are several unique projects in out-of-hospital care of the mentally ill in Europe. One involving foster care in family homes has been operating in Geel, Belgium for several hundred years. It was started with religious inspiration and was intended to avoid use of a custodial facility. Mentally ill patients from all over Belgium came to Geel for care, as though to a religious shrine. Eventually a mental hospital was built for 250 patients, but 1,500 patients were cared for in foster homes; these were long-term schizophrenics and some retarded. The Belgian health insurance program pays these guardian families, just as it supports care in mental hospitals.

In the United States—perhaps because national health care financing was absent—greater initiative was taken to develop organized clinic services for the mentally ill; this was not only for discharged hospital patients, but also for other people with mental and emotional problems. (Since high-income people saw private psychiatrists, these clinics served mainly middle- and low-income patients.) The first mental health clinics were mainly under voluntary auspices, but in 1963 the U.S. federal government launched a major public program. Federal grants were made to the states for establishing a national network of "community mental health centers." These were intended to provide all types of ambulatory care, as well as training, with an emphasis on follow-up of patients discharged from mental hospitals. (Such discharges had, of course, occurred earlier but without such systematic arrangements for community follow-up.) In the 1980s, federal support for these centers was greatly reduced, but many were kept open with purely state and local funding and even with some support through voluntary health insurance. Another adjustment to public policy trends in the United States has been for local government authorities to "contract out" to private medical resources for delivery of ambulatory mental health services.

From the movement that started in the United States as *mental hygiene,* there developed a whole spectrum of clinics for ambulatory care around the world. Aside from general mental health clinics, there were *crisis clinics,* suicide prevention clinics, *hot line* telephone services, and others. The theoretical foundations of this work were largely the doctrines of Sigmund Freud that spread from Europe to the rest of the world after World War I. Along with the clinics, there was a great deal of community education about mental disease and mental hygiene. Societies, advocating that mental hospitals be improved and community services be organized, have been established in many industrialized countries and in a few developing countries. The International Union of Societies for the Aid of Mental Health has representation in 25 countries that are mainly French speaking.

Very few developing countries can afford to develop community mental health centers, except occasionally in the capital city. The more widespread policy is to train physicians for psychiatric care in the all-purpose health centers. In Africa, where few physicians are found outside hospitals, medical assistants and even very briefly trained community health workers are taught to recognize patients with mental disorders. They refer them to a physician in a hospital or sometimes in a large urban health center. In several countries of South East Asia, family members, as well as medical assistants and community health workers, are educated to help mental patients. In India traditional Ayurvedic practitioners are asked to refer the patients that they have found difficult to treat to general hospitals and health centers.

The transitional developing countries, such as those in Latin America, have much greater resources, but they still have not been able to set up specialized mental health clinics. They operate mental hospitals, but other care is simply integrated with general health services. In Chile, for example, mental hospitals had 11 percent of the beds in 1980, but there has been increasing use of general hospitals for mental patients. Ambulatory care is given in the polyclinics and health centers by doctors who have had some psychiatric training. The World Health Organization, after a study of numerous developing countries in 1984, concluded that mental health service should simply be part of conventional polyclinic or health center functions.

Commentary

As a result of these developments in mental hospitals and in community mental health services, one can perceive the outlines of a contemporary strategy for coping with mental disorders in national health systems. Regarding hospitals, the movement is from large custodial facilities to smaller medically active ones. New drug therapies are prominent. Mental patients are increasingly being admitted to general hospitals. Mental hospitals are slowly evolving into places for treatment, rather than purely custodial care.

The basic strategy everywhere is to discharge patients from mental hospitals, and arrange for their follow-up care in a community clinic. This has been less successful in practice than in theory, and its deficiencies are evident in the United States. Follow-up is poor, and large numbers of discharged mental patients end up as "homeless." This may be compensated by more adequate public housing in European countries. The solution is seen, however, as strengthening of community health services.

Regarding extramural ambulatory care of mental patients, specialized mental health clinics and centers have been established extensively in Great Britain and the United States. They are only occasional in other European countries. The commonest site for ambulatory care is still the outpatient department of mental or general hospitals. Psychiatrists and other physicians with some psychiatric training see the patients. Voluntary agency clinics for special disorders, such as epilepsy or drug dependence, are sometimes subsidized by Ministries of Health.

In developing countries, ambulatory mental health services can seldom be offered in any specialized facility. The accepted strategy is to incorporate such services in the general programs for primary health care, provided usually by auxiliary personnel. Outpatient departments of large general hospitals in the capital city may occasionally have a psychiatrist to consult.

Mental hospitals and the promotion of community mental health programs are in most countries the responsibility of a mental or psychiatric subdivision of the Ministry of Health (MoH). Since the general population served by a mental hospital is ordinarily much larger than that served by general hospitals, the authority is usually exercised at higher administrative levels, even the national level. Special boards or commissions under the MoH may have a role. Community mental health programs are ordinarily supervised by lower echelons of the MoH.

In the states of the United States, where the historic background of public health agencies was quite different from that of public hospitals, authority over mental hospitals is usually vested in separate departments. Community mental health programs meanwhile come under the Department of Health. Sometimes a State Department of Mental Health is established, responsible for all aspects of treatment and prevention of mental illness, but separate from the State Department of Public Health.

A final element of ambulatory mental health care should be noted. Outside of government in the main cities of affluent countries, there is an expanding number of private psychiatric practitioners. Utilizing both Freudian concepts and psychopharmacology, they are seeing increasing volumes of patients. Their services are usually financed by insurance, voluntary in the United States and social in Europe. Private practice of psychotherapy in the United States and Canada is permitted also for psychiatric social workers and clinical psychologists. There is often some interchange between such private psychiatric care and services in organized clinics.

The fees of psychiatrists for private treatment are typically very high, so that they tend to serve high-income patients. Even if health insurance is available, there are often large co-payments and spending limits for private psychiatric care. Psychiatrists are numerous enough in North America and Western Europe, and the market for private services is large enough, to permit many to engage exclusively in private practice. In the rest of the world, where psychiatrists are scarce, the great majority serve in organized programs, with limited private practice to supplement their earnings.

Other Psychiatric Problems

Certain mental or emotional disorders have led to consumption of substances causing serious individual and social problems. Alcoholism and drug abuse are the most widely prevalent of these problems, leading to specially organized programs for their control throughout the world.

Alcoholism. Research on the cause of this addiction, in contrast to "normal social drinking," has been conducted for decades, but the exact determinants—as among biological and social factors—are still not clear. Strategies for both prevention and treatment, nevertheless, are applied in virtually all industrialized and many developing countries. Some controls are directed against traffic accidents caused by intoxicated drivers.

As the harmful effects of alcohol have become more evident, legal interventions have been possible. Certain hours of business may be imposed on public drinking places. Minors may be prohibited from purchasing liquor. Liquor stores may be entirely under government control, as in Norway and several Canadian provinces. In many European countries, there is random testing of motorists for blood alcohol level. Advertising of alcohol is subject to various constraints, and it may be completely prohibited on television; in France, advertising is barred almost entirely.

Psychotherapy of full-blown alcoholism has not been effective, nor has medication. The use of "antabuse" to make alcohol distasteful is of moderate value. Undoubtedly the most successful strategy of treatment has been organized self-help through a nongovernmental organization, such as Alcoholics Anonymous. There are chapters in more than 30 countries. Using a sort of spiritual self-analysis, Alcoholics Anonymous has a better record of long-term recoveries than any other method.

Drug Abuse. Addiction to narcotic drugs has led to control programs in all types of countries. The strong policies in China, after the 1949 revolution, included compulsory treatment of opium addicts and punitive measures against "drug pushers." Identification and punishment of drug sellers are the major strategies in Malaysia and other Asian countries.

In the United States and Western Europe, a major preventive approach has been the education of secondary school students. The adolescent age group is most susceptible to drug abuse, and the organization of job-training, sports clubs, and so on is promoted in response to problems of stress. Great Britain has been unique in legalizing the narcotic drugs, when dispensed or injected by a licensed physician. The net effect of this policy, which has yielded a higher consumption of narcotics but a reduced rate of crime and more successful rehabilitation, is debated.

In treatment, a major breakthrough occurred around 1970, with the discovery of methadone as a substitute for heroin. Public health clinics were organized to provide methadone maintenance therapy. In both Europe and America, these clinics were soon overcrowded with waiting lists. As a last resort drug addicts are hospitalized for rehabilitation, but there are not many beds for this.

In the United States, drug abuse has led to a great deal of crime—mostly petty theft. The addict steals to get money to support his habit. As a result, a high proportion of prison inmates, especially in large cities, are convicted addicts. Prisons have had to be enlarged, and this has naturally raised the issue of expanding treatment facilities rather than jails.

Much more fundamental is the international effort to stop the production of heroin, cocaine, marijuana, and other narcotics at the source in various countries. Colombia and Peru benefit economically, and international agreements are made. The "golden triangle" is an area of Burma, Thailand, and China where various tactics have been used to reduce opium output. The trafficking of cocaine from South America to Panama and the United States has entailed massive violence in the governmental attempts at intervention.

The problem of worldwide trafficking in narcotic drugs has so many economic and political aspects, that its international control is well beyond the reach of health agencies. Overall policy and enforcement of international legal conventions are managed by the United Nations Commission on Narcotic Drugs.

CHRONIC NONCOMMUNICABLE DISEASES

As the average length of life has increased throughout the world, more people live on to the ages when they succumb to chronic noncommunicable diseases. Disorders of the heart and cancer have been the major causes of death in the industrialized countries for many decades, and these are also coming to be leading disease problems in many developing countries, as the communicable diseases of childhood are reduced. Moreover, certain features of adult life, both environmental and personal, are leading to an increased incidence of these chronic diseases at specific age levels.

To combat the great social burdens of chronic disease, special control programs have been widely developed. They are more highly organized along several lines in the industrialized countries, but certain measures are also carried out in developing countries. The most extensive efforts have been applied to the control of cancer.

Cancer Control

Efforts to control cancer involve primary prevention, early detection, and prompt therapy. The earliest approaches of most countries have been oriented to treatment, which is usually given in general hospitals. Specialized cancer hospitals are relatively rare, insofar as general hospitals have the capabilities. Egypt has one cancer hospital out of a total of 1,470 facilities and Chile also has only one. On the other hand, India had 142 cancer hospitals in 1980 out of 8,500 hospitals in the country; perhaps this reflects dissatisfaction with the general hospitals. In the industrialized countries, where general hospitals are technologically advanced, there are usually only a few cancer hospitals in some major cities.

Much of the treatment of cancer entails very expensive radiological equipment and the use of numerous anticancer drugs. Surgical intervention by highly trained surgeons, however, is usually necessary, and such skills are scarce in the developing countries. In the industrialized countries, surgery of cancer or other disorders is highly remunerative, and the supply of competent surgeons is relatively large. Many countries have made hospitalized cases of cancer reportable, so that "cancer registries" can be used for epidemiological studies. Such registries, usually for certain regions or certain hospitals, are maintained in 75 countries.

The early detection of cancer through mass screenings is practiced throughout the world. In Europe, North America, and Japan it is done extensively in industrialized populations, in all patients admitted to hospitals, or even at festivals. Different techniques, of course, are used for various body organs—the breasts, the lungs, the uterus, the mouth, and so on. The breasts, for example, require physical examinations and mammogram X-rays. Detection of cancer in the cervix of the uterus requires a specimen, to be examined microscopically (Papanicoleau smear).

Conducting these screening tests on populations requires organization. Japan has carried out these tests at a large network of health centers, where equipment was available. In 1980, some 7 percent of the national population, considered to be at risk, was screened. In 1982, miniature chest X-rays were widely taken to detect lung cancer. In the Philippines, mobile clinic vans traveled through the country to offer various detection tests. In Indonesia, on the other hand, the policy has been to educate poeple about cancer and simply urge them to visit doctors for examinations. The same policy of attempted persuasion was followed in Singapore.

In many developing countries, cervical cancer screening is linked to family planning programs, which attract young women; but older women have higher cancer rates. The policy recommended by WHO is to have older women examined at the time of any visit to a health center. Cytological examinations of specimens by microscopy are quite impossible at most health centers, so that simple visual inspection of the cervix by nurses and assistant nurses must be done. Only a vaginal speculum and a light are necessary. Suspicious cases may then be referred to a hospital outpatient department.

In most European countries and in North America, special emphasis has also been put on screening for cervical cancer and for cancer of the breast. Such procedures have become routine features of the medical examination of adult women. They are routine also in preemployment examinations and on entry to prenatal clinics. As in developing countries, the greatest problem is to reach older women periodically.

Primary prevention is the most fundamental strategy for cancer control, and it is also the most complex. It has come latest in the control efforts. In industry and agriculture, workers may be exposed to carcinogenic chemicals, which can be identified and eliminated; human contact with these chemicals can, at least, be reduced. Such primary prevention has been feasible only in highly industrialized countries. General reduction of air pollution can also decrease susceptibility to lung cancer.

The most widely applied measure of cancer prevention is the reduction of exposure to tobacco through smoking cigarettes. As discussed in Chapter 11, the problem has been tackled first through legislation, designed to reduce both the supply of and demand for tobacco products. By 1990, such laws had been enacted in 91 countries. These laws are strongest in the industrialized countries, but they are slowly becoming more comprehensive in the developing countries. Complete bans on all cigarette advertising, for example, are imposed in 27 industrialized countries. In developing countries such laws apply only to certain media or they regulate only the content of advertising. Special cigarette taxes to raise their price, and health warnings on cigarette packages to discourage sales, are frequent strategies in affluent countries, but are exceptional in low-income countries.

A comprehensive cancer control program would include all three sets of strategies: for treatment, for early detection, and for prevention. Each of these efforts is part of the overall operation of a national health system, and depends on the resources and economic support of the whole system. In the health systems of very poor countries, control efforts are absent or ineffective, so that thousands of cases of terminal cancer occupy beds in hospitals or at home. For these unfortunate patients, nothing can be done beyond the relief of pain; the World Health Organization is, therefore, disseminating simple schemes for cancer pain management.

Cardiovascular Disease

Diseases of the heart and blood vessels are the chief cause of death in all industrialized countries and also are among the top few causes in the developing countries. Their characteristics, however, do not yield so readily to focused strategies as the control of cancer. The three basic approaches of primary prevention, early case detection, and proper treatment apply, but their implementation is inherently part of the overall health system.

Primary prevention depends substantially on diet, which can be influenced by national nutrition policy on animal and vegetable sources of food. The ingestion of fats is crucial, and the production of foods that result in low blood cholesterol call for national action. This extremely complex subject is being widely researched, but the crucial point is that nutritional prevention of heart disease requires far more than health education. It can be most effectively implemented by policies in agriculture and animal husbandry. (Prudent food preparation in families, of course, can also help.) Food preparation and table custom should favor low salt intake. Other aspects of primary prevention are the battle against smoking and the encouragement of exercise for persons in sedentary occupations. Health education plays a part but, as we have noted, antitobacco legislation has many other features.

Among strategies for early detection of heart disease, aside from routine medical examinations, blood pressure readings can be done on population groups. The prompt treatment of hypertension calls for diet and weight control, but many patients require antihypertensive drugs. The reduction of hypertension can contribute to the prevention of heart disease and cerebrovascular accidents.

Treatment of cardiovascular disease includes medication, diet, exercise, life-style changes, and attention to the many aspects of life that cause stress. There are numerous effective drugs for different cardiac disorders. Open-heart surgery to replace coronary blood vessels is done in a few affluent countries. Significant reductions of heart disease mortality were achieved in the United States and some Western European nations between 1950 and 1980. Epidemiologists studying these trends to determine their causes have not been able to separate the impact of prevention from that of treatment. They have concluded that both strategies have played a part.

Despite the great importance of cardiovascular disease as a cause of both morbidity and mortality, the many strategies developed have not been formulated as explicit "heart disease control" programs. This is probably reasonable, insofar as heart disease prevention and treatment permeate every aspect of a health system. Beyond the actions discussed, one must consider, for example, the content of medical education, the production or importation of anticancer drugs, the equipment of health centers and hospitals, and the amplitude of fund raising.

All the relevant strategies require national leadership, which may be expected from the Ministry of Health. But that leadership can be effective only by mobilizing the principal actors in agriculture, education, foreign trade, the universities, the health professions, and numerous bodies representing the general population. Insofar as legislation is necessary, lawmaking authorities must be reached or citizen campaigns mounted for a specific law. All these undertakings are more feasible, where the general literacy level is high and democratic participation is strong.

Heart disease control strategies have been the objective of applied research in many special demonstration projects. In the 1970s and 1980s a WHO-sponsored study of "multifactorial prevention" was conducted in five European countries, applying interventions to people at the workplace. Each program attempted to reduce dietary fat intake, to control hypertension, and to promote nonsmoking and vigorous exercise. After 6 years, heart disease mortality was reduced in all five places, most successfully in North Karelia, Finland. The extension of these strategies to larger populations has depended mainly on education of the people and training of the health professions.

All the policies discussed here are being implemented far more successfully in the most highly industrialized countries than in both middle-income and very poor developing countries. Although cigarette smoking is declining in the former, it is slowly increasing in the latter. (The international tobacco industry adjusts for losses in affluent countries by gains in poor countries.) Cardiovascular mortality is slowly rising in the poor countries, whereas it is declining in the rich and democratic ones.

The implications for policy in the developing countries would seem to be clear.

Severe Disabilities

In all industrialized countries with national social security programs, there are special provisions for helping the severely disabled. These are mainly oriented to vocational rehabilitation, so that the disabled person may work under protected conditions. Physical rehabilitation is provided in the facilities of the national health system. Sometimes very technologically advanced rehabilitation centers have been established by voluntary agencies.

Policies in Great Britain may be taken to illustrate industrialized countries with comprehensive or welfare-oriented health systems. Numerous laws help to ensure employment for the disabled. There are pensions for invalids and allowances for reduced mobility. Organized home care helps the disabled get along in a personal home. Training centers and sheltered workshops facilitate employment. Medical treatment and phsyical rehabilitation, however, are given in the hospitals of the National Health Service and in specially staffed rehabilitation centers. Some of these focus on paralytic disorders, some on patients with psychosomatic problems, and some on the visually impaired. Local governments and nongovernmental agencies have taken the initiative in establishing specialized facilities.

There are many issues in Great Britain and other affluent countries about the most appropriate arrangement for the education of handicapped children. For some years, special schools were provided, but in the 1970s policy shifted to enrollment of these children in regular schools, with physical adjustments in school design to accommodate to their needs. Equivalent issues are debated on the use of sheltered workshops for handicapped workers, as against special adjustments in job placement. Voluntary organizations have been active in arranging residential settings for young disabled adults, but this has not reduced local governmental initiatives; it has stimulated them.

In the United States, special federal grants to the states have provided for the rehabilitation of adults of working age, and of "crippled children" of low income. The vocational rehabilitation program for adults provides job training and guidance in finding employment, but its efforts affect only a small percentage of the disabled. Treatment and physical rehabilitation are provided in community hospitals or a few rehabilitation centers under private auspices. Low-income disabled children ("crippling" is defined by each state) are typically treated by private physicians, paid fees by the State Department of Health. Quality standards for medical care of crippled children are federally determined and applied by the states.

Egypt is an example of a developing country of transitional economic level with a welfare-oriented health system. In Egypt there are laws requiring employment of handicapped persons in large firms (over 500 employees), but these affect only a small percentage of the national workforce. Since 1975, the Ministry of Social Welfare has financed high-cost rehabilitation services, especially prosthetic appliances, for severely disabled adults and children of low income. Large hospitals have physical medicine departments, and there are two children's hospitals with such departments.

India is a very poor country with a welfare-oriented health system, where the problems of severely disabled children and adults are overwhelming. Because of its extreme poverty, nearly all efforts must go into the general organization of its national health system. Special concern for the disabled has focused almost entirely on blindness in children and adults. Campaigns are conducted on prevention, through treatment of eye infections, and on education of blind children (see below).

Zambia is an unusual African country in having established agricultural settlement centers, the main objective of which is to provide vocational employment to the disabled. In 1977 there were 11 such rural units, but there is no special program for medical or physical rehabilitation services.

Blindness is a major cause of disability throughout the world, and especially in developing countries. National voluntary organizations to advance the education and improve the whole quality of life of the blind are found in almost all countries. Even in the poorest countries, these organizations function to put pressure on government for special assistance, and in more affluent countries they operate schools to teach Braille reading, train "seeing eye" dogs, and provide appropriate residential living. Many Ministries of Education in industrialized countries maintain residential schools for blind and sometimes for deaf children.

The problem of blindness in India has been so great that special schools for blind children have been established, through voluntary initiative, since the late nineteenth century. In 1981, India had at least 9,000,000 economically and legally blind people, and still more suffering from visual handicaps. The state of West Bengal has 9 schools for the blind, each of which had been started and financed by some charitable group, mainly before national independence (1947). In 1964, the first planned effort at rehabilitation was started at one of the schools; a 9-month course was given in light engineering. The numbers of children and adolescents reached by these special educational programs are only a small fraction of the blind.

For prevention of blindness, other strategies are applied by Ministries of Health in many developing countries. Of an estimated 28 million blind persons in the world, some 90 percent live in low-income developing countries. The major causes of blindness in such countries are infections, including trachoma, onchocerciasis, and ophthalmitis. The first leadership has often come from voluntary agencies, working with the Ministry of Health. The World Health Organization has been promoting comprehensive "prevention of blindness programs," and these have been formally established in 50 countries. Case finding and limited treatment are supposed to be incorporated in primary health care. In some African countries, briefly trained medical assistants are taught to treat trachoma with eye medication.

A comprehensive prevention of blindness program must apply diverse interventions. Onchocerciasis requires combatting the insect vector, xerophthalmia requires food containing vitamin A, and cataracts require surgery. To be effective, therefore, various subdivisions of the Ministry of Health must be mobilized at provincial and local levels, with cooperation from other branches of government and voluntary agencies. Because of the large numbers of elderly in both developing and industrialized countries, cataracts are of increasing importance in causing very poor vision and even blindness. Surgical correction with artificial lens implants has become a simple and effective procedure, but it can be done only where proper resources are available.

There are so many national groups concerned with the problem of blindness that three separate international organizations are devoted to this field. The largest is the World Blind Union, including its merger with the World Council for the Welfare of the Blind, second is the International Agency for the Prevention of Blindness, and third is the International Council for the Education of the Visually Impaired. These bodies reflect the intensity of concern for helping the blind and preventing blindness throughout the world.

DENTAL DISEASES

The organized provision of dental care is another type of special service that has been developed in the health systems of countries. Unlike most other disease-specific health programs, it is not found in all countries, but in a minority that has attached a high priority to this component of health care, that is seldom life-threatening. These countries are essentially those with welfare-oriented or comprehensive health systems.

Under the national health insurance programs of many countries, such as Germany or Belgium, dental care from dentists is a regular benefit. Many such countries also operate preventive dental clinics for children, staffed by dental hygienists. In the British National Health Service, dental care is a basic benefit for everyone (paid by fee-for-service), and there are also school dental clinics, staffed by dentists and auxiliaries with limited functions. In general, countries with high priority for dental care have developed clinics for children with two types of staffing: fully trained dentists or specially trained dental auxiliary personnel.

The Scandinavian countries make use of fully qualified dentists who are trained in un-

usually large numbers. In Europe as a whole, dentists constitute about one-quarter of the number of physicians, but in Scandinavia it is one-half. With this large supply of dentists, public dental clinics for children are abundant. There are many chairside assistants, but only to help the dentist—not to work independently. In Sweden, adult dental care is financed by the National Health Service with 50 percent copayment, and in Norway adult care is entirely a private matter. In France, the school-based dental clinics are operated by the education authorities.

Mexico is a developing country with a welfare-oriented health system that has an exceptionally low supply of dentists. Yet the Ministry of Health organized dental clinics for the poor, staffed by dentists. Similar clinics were organized in Venezuela, staffed by new dental school graduates, as an obligation. Several chairside assistants are furnished by the public health authorities at the state or provincial level.

The second type of dental program for children, using broadly trained auxiliaries who work independently, has shown great promise for the extension of dental care. The pioneering of this pattern was done by New Zealand in 1921. High school graduates, young women, were given 2 years of training in complete dental care and designated by the innocent term *dental nurse*. They were stationed in the public schools, to examine all the children, and to give necessary treatment including fillings and extractions. Supervision by a dentist in the Ministry of Health was quite indirect.

This innovative pattern was found to give excellent results qualitatively and at a low cost. It was soon emulated by Australia, then by Malaysia, and up to about 20 countries mainly from the former British Commonwealth. In North America, however, the dental profession was generally resistant. Only in Saskatchewan, Canada, was the New Zealand school dental nurse adopted; there was some further development by providing her with a chairside assistant. Comparative cross-national studies have shown the status of oral health in children, served by the New Zealand pattern, to be generally superior to that in conventional populations of children.

Dental care programs, of course, require

much more than the operation of clinics. The World Health Organization has emphasized the need for outreach into communities, training of personnel, and program administration. With the promise of the dental nurse idea, training is all important and can be integrated with the training of other health personnel. Administration has been mainly in the Ministry of Health, but financing may also involve social security programs.

In the prevention of dental disease, a major development of the mid-twentieth century has been the discovery of the value of *fluorides.* Fluoridation of public water supplies has achieved about a 50 percent reduction in dental caries, and yet many communities have resisted this intervention. In the United States, the issue has been politicized, with popular referendums held—often with negative outcomes. Only about 60 percent of the U.S. population is served by fluoridated water. In Europe, water fluoridation has been achieved in nearly all countries, although Switzerland has adopted a policy of fluoridating salt. In certain jurisdictions fluoridation of water supplies has been made mandatory: Greece, Ireland, Bulgaria, and one republic of Yugoslavia in Europe, plus one Canadian province and five U.S. states. In other countries, legislation is typically "enabling"—that is, authorizing national authorities to act.

In Latin America, Brazil was one of the first countries to authorize fluoridation, and in the planning of all new public water supplies, the inclusion of fluoridation must be considered. Implementation, however, is not mandatory. On the other hand, in Ecuador, a law requires fluoridation in cities, so that 31 public water supplies were being fluoridated in the 1980s. In most developing countries, the fluoridation of urban water supplies presents many technical problems. After installation of fluoridation machinery, it frequently cannot be properly maintained.

In the absence of water fluoridation, other preventive approaches have been used, but these too are largely limited to the industrialized countries. Fluoride tablets are taken by children daily (similar to vitamins). Individual or "topical" application of fluorides is employed in the dental care clinics. Salt fluoridation is carried out in eight countries of Latin America. The fluoridation of toothpaste almost everywhere has had beneficial effects.

These programs of organized treatment or prevention of dental diseases operate in health systems where special priority has been assigned to dental needs. Unfortunately in most countries of the world, the priority for dental care is low. Dental disease is seldom life-threatening, like so much else confronted by health systems. The supply of dentists in the very poor countries is grossly deficient, and trained dental nurses are lacking. Personal dental care is not available, except to very affluent individuals. Oral health among the general population is conspicuously poor, with extractions leaving many elderly people edentulous or nearly so. Organized dental clinics for children have been the most widely applied policy for treatment in the industrialized countries, but these are far below the needs in developing countries. Prevention through fluoridation of water and personal dental hygiene are the most promising strategies everywhere.

REFERENCES

Communicable Diseases

Bulla, A., *Trends in Tuberculosis Hospital and Sanatorium Beds Throughout the World* (1960–1975). Geneva: World Health Statistics Report, 1977.

Ekunwe, Ebun O., "Expanding Immunization Coverage through Improved Clinic Procedures." *World Health Forum,* 5:361–363, 1984.

Fenner, F., D. A. Henderson, I. Arita, Z. Jezek, and I. D. Ladnyi, *Smallpox and Its Eradication.* Geneva: World Health Organization, 1988.

Henderson, Donald A., "How Smallpox Showed the Way." *World Health,* 19–21, December 1989.

Hinman, A. R., et al., "The Case for Global Eradication of Poliomyelitis." *Bulletin of the World Health Organization,* 65(6):835–840, 1987.

Holm, J., "Tuberculosis Control in the Developing World: It's Time for a Change." *World Health Forum,* 5:103–119, 1984.

International Union Against Tuberculosis, "Activity Report, September 1976–September 1977." *Bulletin of the International Union Against Tuberculosis.* 68–80, October 1977.

Keja, Ko, Carole Chan, Gregory Hayden, and Ralph H. Henderson, "Expanded Program on Immunization." In *World Health Statistics Quarterly,* Vol. 41. Geneva: World Health Organization, 1988, pp. 59–63.

LaForce, F. Marc, et al., "The Expanded Program on Immunization." *World Health Forum,* 8:208–215, 1987.

Lechat, M. F., M. Vanderveken, E. Declerq, and C. B. Misson, "Analysis of Trends in the Occurrence of Leprosy." *World Health Statistics Quarterly*, 39(2):129–137, 1986.

Martinez, C. Ann, Dhiman Barua, and Michael H. Merson, "Control of Diarrheal Diseases." *World Health Statistics Quarterly*, 41(2):74–81, 1988.

Maurice, John, "Leprosy: Light at the End of the Tunnel." *World Health*, 13–15, July 1988.

Mosley, W. Henry, Dean T. Jamison, and Donald A. Henderson, "The Health Sector in Developing Countries: Problems for the 1990s and Beyond." *Annual Review of Public Health*, 11:335–358, 1990.

Najera-Morrondo, J. A., "Malaria Control: History Shows It's Possible." *World Health*, 4–5, September–October 1991.

Noordeen, S. K., L. Lopez Bravo, and D. Daumerie, "Progress in Leprosy Control Through Multidrug Therapy." *World Health Statistics Quarterly*, 44(1):2–15, 1991.

Padmavati, S., "Rheumatic Fever and Rheumatic Heart Disease in Developing Countries." *Bulletin of the World Health Organization*, 56:543–550, 1978.

Pollitzer, R., *Cholera*. Geneva: World Health Organization (Monograph Series No. 43), 1959.

Salk, Jonas E., "Poliomyelitis Vaccine Preparation and Administration." *Journal of the American Medical Association*, 169(16):1829–1838, 18 April 1959.

Sidel, Victor W., and Ruth Sidel, *Serve the People: Observations on Medicine in the People's Republic of China*. New York: Josiah Macy Jr. Foundation, 1973.

Toman, K., *Tuberculosis Case-Finding and Chemotherapy*. Paris: Masson & Co., 1979.

Trigg, Peter, "Different Strategies (of Malaria Control) for Different Situations." *World Health*, 10–12, September–October 1991.

World Health Organization, "Malaria and Other Parasitic Diseases Vector Control." In *The Second Ten Years of WHO (1958–1967)*, Geneva: WHO, 1968, pp. 159–201.

World Health Organization, Expert Committee on Tuberculosis, *Ninth Report*. Geneva: WHO (Technical Report 552), 1974.

World Health Organization, *Tuberculosis Control*. (Report of a Joint IUAT/WHO Study Group). Geneva: WHO (Technical Report 671), 1982.

World Health Organization, Expert Committee. *The Control of Schistosomiasis*. Geneva: WHO (Technical Report No. 728), 1985.

World Health Organization, Parasitic Diseases Program, *Major Parasitic Infections: A Global Review*, in *World Health Statistics Quarterly*, 39(2):145–160, 1986.

World Health Organization, Division of Control of Tropical Diseases, "World Malaria Situation, 1988." *World Health Statistics Quarterly*, 43(2):68–79, 1990.

Sexually Transmitted Diseases

Anderson, Odin W., *Syphilis and Society—Problems of Control in the United States 1912–64*. Chicago: Center for Health Administration Studies, 1965.

Bayer, R., *Private Acts, Social Consequences: AIDS and the Politics of Public Health*. New York: The Free Press, 1989.

Cousse, Georges, and Andre Meheuse, "Control of Sexually Transmitted Diseases." *World Health Statistic Quarterly*, 41(2):100–102, 1988.

Creese, Andrew, and Anthony Battersby, "The Cost of Cold Chain Equipment." *World Health Forum*, 5:165–167, 1984.

Fee, Elizabeth, and Daniel M. Fox (Editors) *AIDS—The Burdens of History*. Berkeley, CA: University of California Press, 1989.

Hira, Subhash, K., "Sexually Transmitted Disease—A Menace to Mothers and Children." *World Health Forum*, 7:243–247, 1986.

Mann, Jonathan, "The Global AIDS Situation." *World Health Statistics Quarterly*, 40:185–192, 1987.

Mann, Jonathan, "Global AIDS in the 1990s." *World Health*, 6–7, October 1989.

Willcox, R. R., *The Management of Sexually Transmitted Diseases: A Guide for the General Practitioner*. Geneva: WHO, 1979.

World Health Organization, *Social and Health Aspects of Sexually Transmitted Disease: Principles of Control Measures*. Geneva: WHO (Public Health Papers No. 65), 1975.

World Health Organization, *Venereal Disease Control: A Survey of Recent Legislation*. Geneva: WHO, 1975.

World Health Organization, *Social and Health Aspects of Sexually Transmitted Disease: Principles of Control Measures*. Geneva: WHO (Public Health Papers No. 65), 1976.

World Health Organization, *AIDS—A Worldwide Effort Will Stop It*. *World Health* October 1989 (entire issue).

Mental Disorders

Abiodun, O. A., "Mental Health and Primary Care in Africa." *International Journal of Mental Health*, 18:48–56, 1990.

Beers, Clifford, *A Mind That Found Itself*. New York: Doubleday Doran, 1935.

Breemer Ter Stege, Chris, and Martin Gittelman (Editors), "Trends in Mental Health in Europe in the Past 25 Years." *International Journal of Mental Health*, 16:3–20, 1987.

Crepet, Paolo, and Giovanni De Plato, "Psychiatry without Asylums: Origins and Prospects in Italy." *International Journal of Health Services*, 13(1):119–127, 1983.

Curran, W. J., and T. W. Harding, *The Law and Mental Health: Harmonizing Objectives*. Geneva: World Health Organization, 1978.

Deutsch, Albert, *The Mentally Ill in America.* New York: Doubleday Doran, 1938.

Eisenberg, Leon, "Preventing Mental, Neurological and Psychosocial Disorders." *World Health Forum,* 8:245–253, 1987.

El-Guebaly, N., "Mental Health Services for the Elderly: European Models." *World Health Forum,* 4:63–68, 1983.

Goldberg, David, and Digby Tantam, "The Public Health Impact of Mental Disorders." In *Oxford Textbook of Public Health, 2nd ed.,* Volume III, Chapter 16. 1991, Oxford: Oxford University Press, pp. 267–280.

Goldman, Howard H. (Editor), "International Perspectives on Deinstitutionalization." *International Journal of Mental Health,* II(4), 1982–1983.

Hasegawa, Kazuo, "Aspects of Community Mental Health Care of the Elderly in Japan." *International Journal of Mental Health,* 8(3):36–49, 1979.

Hetzel, B., and J. Orley, "Correcting Iodine Deficiency—Avoiding Tragedy." *World Health Forum,* 4:260–264, 1985.

Hubbard, Robert L., and Don C. Desjarlais, "Alcohol and Drug Abuse." In *Oxford Textbook of Public Health, 2nd ed.,* Volume 3. Oxford: Oxford University Press, 1991, pp. 523–537.

Jones, Kathleen, *A History of Mental Health Services.* London: Routledge & Kegan Paul, 1974.

Kuwabara, Haruo, and Reiko H. True, "National Social Policy Toward the Mentally Ill in Japan and Its Consequences." *International Journal of Mental Health,* 5(3):95–108, 1976.

Leighton, A. H., and Jane H. Hughes, "Cultures as Causative of Mental Disorder." In *Causes of Mental Disorders.* New York: Milbank Memorial Fund, 1961, pp. 341–383.

Leon, Carlos A., "Perspectives on Mental Health Care for Latin America." *International Journal of Mental Health,* 11(4):84–97, 1983.

Mangen, S. P. (Editor), *Mental Health Care in the European Community.* London: Crown Helm, 1985.

Mechanic, D., "Correcting Misconceptions in Mental Health Policy: Strategies for Improved Care of the Seriously Mentally Ill." *Milbank Quarterly,* 65(2):203–227, 1987.

Mollica, Richard F. (Editor), "The Unfinished Revolution in Italian Psychiatry: An International Perspective." *International Journal of Mental Health,* 14(1–2), 1985 (entire issue).

Murthy, R. Srinivasa, "Treatment and Rehabilitation of the Severely Mentally Ill in Developing Countries of South-East Asia." *International Journal of Mental Health,* 12(3):16–29, 1984.

Ohashi, H., K. Nakayama, M. Saito, and B. Saletu, (Editors), *World Psychiatric Association, Regional Symposium: Proceedings.* Tokyo: Japanese Society of Psychiatry and Neurology, 1982.

Roth, Martin, and C. Q. Mountjoy, "Mental Health Services for the Elderly Living in the Community: A United Kingdom Perspective." *International Journal of Mental Health,* 8(3–4):6–35, 1979.

Rosen, George, *A History of Public Health.* New York: MD Publications, 1958.

Shen, Yu-cun, "Mental Health Care in China: A Time of Transition." *World Health Forum,* 8:379–382, 1987.

Straathof, L.T.A., "General Policies in the Development of Mental Health Services in the Netherlands." *International Journal of Mental Health,* 5(3):59–63.

R. O. Tegede, A. O. Odejide, and A. Sijuwola, "Rural Health Care in Nigeria." *International Journal of Mental Health,* 12:159–169, 1983.

Tims, F. M., *Effectiveness of Drug Abuse Treatment Programs.* Washington, D.C., National Institute on Drug Abuse, 1981.

U.S. Institute of Medicine, *Prevention and Treatment of Alcohol Problems.* Washington, D.C.: National Academy Press, 1989.

Volovik, V. M., and R. A. Achepitski, "Deinstitutionalization in Soviet Psychiatry." *International Journal of Mental Health,* 11(4):108–128, 1983.

Wig, N. N., "Indian Concepts of Mental Health and Their Impact on Care of the Mentally Ill." *International Journal of Mental Health,* 18:71–80, 1990.

World Health Organization, Regional Office for Europe, *Health Services in Europe,* 2nd ed. Copenhagen: WHO, 1975.

World Health Organization, *Mental Health Care in Developing Countries: A Critical Appraisal of Research Findings.* Geneva: WHO (Technical Report Series 698), 1984.

Chronic Noncommunicable Diseases

Albrecht, Gary L. (Editor), *Cross-National Rehabilitation Policies: A Sociological Perspective.* Beverly Hills, CA: Sage Publications, 1981.

Bikas, C. Sanyal, et al., *Education and Employment of the Blind—The Case of West Bengal.* Paris: UNESCO (South Asian Publishers), 1985.

Breslow, Lester, et al., "Cancer Control: Implications from Its History." *Journal of the National Cancer Institute,* 59(2):671–686, August 1977.

Cole, P., and A. S. Morrison, "Basic Issues in Population Screening for Cancer." *Journal of the National Cancer Institute,* 64:1263–1272, 1980.

Copeland, Lois S., "International Trends in Disability Program Growth." *Social Security Bulletin,* 44(10):25–36, 1981.

Doll, Richard, "Prospects for Prevention." *World Health Forum,* 4:219–227, 1983.

Farquhar, J. W., et al., "Community Education for Cardiovascular Health." *The Lancet,* 1:1192–1195, 1977.

Folsom, A. R., et al., "Improvement in Hypertension Detection and Control." *Journal of the*

American Medical Association, 250:916–921, 1983.

Gillum, R. F., et al., "Decline in Coronary Heart Disease Mortality." *American Journal of Medicine,* 76:1055–1065, 1984.

Havas, S., and B. Walker, "Massachusetts Approach to the Prevention of Heart Disease, Cancer, and Stroke." *Public Health Reports,* 101:29–38, 1986.

Hiroyama, T., *Cancer in Asia: Opportunities for Prevention, Detection, and Treatment.* Tokyo: University of Tokyo Press, 1976.

Kasili, Edward G., "Coping with Cancer in Sub-Sahara Africa." *World Health Forum,* 4:149–152, 1983.

Kornizer, M., and G. Rose, "WHO European Collaborative Trial of Multifactorial Prevention of Coronary Heart Disease." *Preventive Medicine,* 14:272–278, 1985.

Luthra, U., "Organization of Screening Programs in Developing Countries." In M. Hakama et al. (Editors), *Screening for Cancer of the Uterine Cervix.* Lyon, France: International Agency for Research on Cancer, 1986.

Miller, A. B., and R. D. Bulbrook, "Screening, Detection, and Diagnosis of Breast Cancer." *The Lancet,* 2:1109–1111, 1982.

Osuntokun, B. O., "The Changing Pattern of Disease in Developing Countries." *World Health Forum,* 6:310–313, 1985.

Puska, P., J. Tuomilehto, J. Salonen, L. Neittaanmäki, J. Maki, J. Virtamo, A. Nissinen, K. Koskela, and T. Takalo, "Changes in Coronary Risk Factors during Comprehensive Five-year Community Programs to Control Cardio-vascular Diseases." *British Medical Journal,* 2:1173–1178, 1979.

Rehabilitation International, *The Economics of Disability: International Perspectives.* New York, 1981.

Roemer, Ruth, *Legislative Action to Combat the World Smoking Epidemic.* Geneva: World Health Organization, 1982.

Roemer, Milton I., "The Value of Medical Care for Health Promotion." *American Journal of Public Health,* 74(3):243–248, 1984.

Rose, Geoffrey, et al., *Coronary Heart Disease Prevention: Plans for Action.* London: Pitman, 1984.

Stjernsward, J., K. Stanley, D. Eddy, M. Tschekovski, L. Sobin, I. Koza, & K. H. Notahey, "Cancer Control: Strategies and Priorities." *World Health Forum,* 6:160–164, 1985.

Swerdlow, Mark, and Jan Stjernsward, "Cancer Pain Relief—An Urgent Problem." *World Health Forum,* 3(3):325–330, 1982.

Thylefors, Bjorn, "Foresight Prevents Blindness." *World Health,* 3–5, May 1987.

Topliss, Eda, *Social Responses to Handicap.* London: Longman, 1982.

United Nations, Department of International Economic and Social Affairs (Decade of the Disabled Person, 1983–1992), *Diability: Situation, Strategies and Policies.* New York: United Nations, 1986.

United Nations (Economic and Social Council), *Recent Trends in Legislation Concerning Rehabilitation Services for Disabled Persons in Selected Countries.* New York: United Nations, 1977.

United Nations (Economic and Social Council), *Integration of Disabled Persons into Community Life.* New York: United Nations, 1981.

Watson, Frederick, *Civilization and the Cripple.* New York: Arno Press, 1980.

World Health Organization, *Community Prevention and Control of Cardiovascular Diseases.* (Report of WHO Expert Committee, Technical Report Series No. 732). Geneva: WHO, 1986.

Yamagata, S., et al., "Mass Screening for Cancer in Japan—Present and Future." In *Recent Advances in Cancer Control* (Proceedings of Asia-Pacific Cancer Conference, September 1983). Amsterdam: Excerpta Medica, 1983.

Dental Diseases

Ingle, John I., and Patricia Blair (Editors), *International Dental Care Delivery Systems.* Cambridge, MA.: Ballinger, 1978.

Murray, J. J., *Appropriate Use of Fluorides for Human Health.* Geneva: World Health Organization, 1986.

Roemer, Ruth, "Water Fluoridation: Public Health Responsibility and the Democratic Process." *American Journal of Public Health,* 55:1337–1348, September 1965.

Roemer, Ruth, *Legislation on Fluorides and Dental Health.* Reprinted from *International Digest of Health Legislation,* 34:1–34, 1983.

World Health Organization, *Planning Oral Health Service.* Geneva: WHO (Offset Pub. No. 53), 1980.

World Health Organization. *Oral Health Care Systems: An International Collaborative Study Coordinated by WHO.* London: Quintessence, 1985.

World Health Organization, *Alternative Systems of Oral Care Delivery.* Geneva: WHO Expert Committee, 1987.

CHAPTER SIXTEEN

Programs for Special Health Services

A third dimension by which special-purpose health programs may be defined is by their provision of special types of service. These programs are concerned with all types of persons and with any type of disorder, for which the service is provided. The list of such special services is long; it results from the many subdivisions of technology that have been developed to diagnose and treat disease or to prevent it.

The numerous specialties of medicine and the personnel engaged in them might be regarded as special types of service, but as a practical matter they contribute to general personal health service. The programs that have entailed special forms of organization are generally outside the domain of regular clinical medicine. We consider here environmental sanitation, emergency medical services, and programs applying other special techniques. Our perspective is the organized and not the clinical aspects of these health services.

ENVIRONMENTAL SANITATION

The tasks of controlling the environment so that it is not harmful to human beings and is conducive to health are tremendous. They include provision of safe water, disposal of human and solid waste, reduction of air pollution, insect vector control, protection against ionizing radiation, and many other interventions. Our main focus here will be on water supply and sewage disposal.

Industrialized Countries

After more than 200 years of economic development, basic environmental protection services in the industrialized countries have generally become well established. In the cities a local unit of government, such as a Department of Public Works, obtains and delivers the water supply. Sometimes, in entrepreneurial health systems, a private water company is granted exclusive responsibility as a "public utility" under contract with government.

The costs of original construction of water supplies are usually derived from local general revenues, but operating costs are usually recovered from charges to water consumers. Continual surveillance of the quality of water delivered is generally a responsibility of the Ministry of Health at local or higher levels. Since urban populations have been growing rapidly in the industrialized countries, there are continual needs for acquiring new sources of water. Chlorination or other forms of water treatment, to ensure its safety, is routinely implemented in urban water supplies.

Rural water supplies in industrialized countries may be through piped delivery in small towns, but for isolated dwellings individual wells are often necessary. Education and technical advice are the usual response of local public health agencies to the needs of individual families.

Sewage disposal in cities of industrialized countries is always a major challenge. The sewer effluent usually goes into some river or body of water, and the resulting contamination must be minimized. Accordingly, there are sewage treatment facilities that should be carefully maintained. These are operated by various units of local government, with public health agency surveillance.

Rural sewage disposal in small towns occasionally may be handled by the piped method. The effluent, however, is usually discharged in some distant waterway without treatment. For isolated dwellings, there may be sanitary latrines or indoor toilets, connected to septic tanks. In spite of all the accomplishments for both water supply and sewage disposal in the cities of industrialized countries, the rural populations of those countries still live with many deficiencies. When water-borne infectious diseases are reported in these countries, they come usually from rural areas.

In the industrialized countries, certain aspects of both water supply and sewage disposal involve special public agencies. Aside from drinking water, overall water resources may be governed by regional authorities concerned with water requirements for agriculture, industry, and even recreation. Planning agencies are involved and also, of course, finance departments. In some countries there is an overall Ministry of the Environment, with broad regulatory authority and a role in the coordination of all relevant programs.

Since the basic requirements for clean water and proper sewage disposal have been met for the great majority of people in the industrialized countries, attention has shifted largely to other environmental hazards. The prominent issues have become air pollution and the disposal of various types of toxic waste. In large cities, many forms of smoke from industry blacken the air. Automobile exhaust adds to air pollution. In London, England a massive inversion of polluted air caused scores of deaths. In the Soviet Union and countries of Eastern Europe, urban air pollution has been devastating. Large cities of the United States have major problems from the automobile, even when industrial pollution has been controlled.

The corrective strategies for attaining clean air have depended largely on regulation. The design of automobile motors has been modified to reduce harmful exhaust. Factory emissions have been reduced, at the expense of the firm. Sometimes a compound used in production is changed to one that yields less air pollution.

The disposal of toxic waste is another growing problem; in the United States, this is an obligation of each enterprise, but in some welfare-oriented health systems of Europe, governments take responsibility. The greatest hazard of toxic waste is that through the soil it can seep into the water supply. Industrialized countries even ship their toxic waste to developing countries for disposal—for which they pay. In Denmark the program has been considered a model. Authority for toxic waste disposal is assigned to the Ministry of the Environment; this agency supervises and subsidizes a National Association of Danish Municipalities to manage hazardous waste. Germany also puts the responsibility for hazardous waste disposal on government agencies at the provincial level.

The general problem of pollution—atmospheric, water, toxic waste—has become a political issue, especially in Europe. It has assumed a place in political debate and spawned "Green Parties" in several countries. It has led to local programs for recycling common household and industrial waste, and contributed to the whole ecology movement. The preservation of endangered animal species has led to conflicts with labor over employment, as in the timber industry.

As industrialization proceeds in all countries, an ultimate social and ethical issue emerges. Countries are uneven in their economic and technological development, and yet they must compete in international markets. The question then becomes how much can a country invest in acquiring a good environment, which may result in a weaker competitive position and loss of jobs. Large self-sufficient countries with strong domestic markets have advantages over small ones dependent on foreign trade. Large foreign debts, furthermore, impair the ability of developing countries to absorb the additional costs of environmental controls. There are countless subtleties to this issue, but they ultimately point to the need for uniform worldwide policies in countries on environmental protection.

Developing Countries

The tasks of water supply and sewage disposal in the developing countries are far greater than they are in the industrialized countries because of the enormous needs and the weaker resources. Understandably, much greater progress has been made in the cities than in the rural areas. Since urbanization is growing rapidly in most developing countries, this means the location of people in places where public water and sanitation (sewage disposal) programs are feasible.

The World Health Organization has compiled information on water and sanitation in the developing countries for 1983. For access to safe water, 74 percent of the urban population were covered—a rise from 68 percent in 1970. The quality of urban water supply also improved, as reflected by house connections between 1970 and 1983 increasing from 51 to 61 percent.

The rural population served by safe water was 41 percent of the total in 1983, which was a substantial increase from 12 percent in 1970. A safe water supply in rural areas, of course, does not necessarily mean a network of pipes leading to each house, but a single village source, as discussed below.

Sanitation facilities were less available in 1983. In developing country cities, about 51 percent of the population had proper excreta disposal. Of these people only about half were served by a sewer connection from their homes. In rural areas, sanitation has extreme deficiencies. In 1983, only 11 percent of the population had proper facilities—an increase from 7 percent in 1970.

In the cities of developing countries, the construction and management of water supplies are typically the responsibility of the Department of Public Works in city government. Sanitary engineers are often available to design and construct a piped network. Financial support may be contributed by the national government, and this is often the purpose of foreign aid (as in Egypt). Personal charges to water consumers may be too difficult to collect, so that funds are derived from local property taxes. With wealth concentrated in the cities, and an articulate middle-class population, urban improvements are continually being made in water and sanitation facilities. Yet they can hardly keep up with urban population growth. Both water supplies and sewage facilities are deteriorating and need replacement.

An even greater problem is in the periurban slums that have been growing up rapidly around the metropolitan centers in developing countries. These miserable living conditions call, first, for minimum adequate housing, to

which water supplies and sanitation could be connected. Financial support for construction must be expected from the central government, rather than solely from the municipality. Voluntary groups often wish to help on education and private fund raising. Ministries of Health may exercise some surveillance, and assist in small construction projects, such as drilling wells or building latrines.

The greatest problems of water supply and sanitation are in the rural areas of developing countries. Even though the percentages of national populations that are rural have declined, the absolute number of rural people has remained about the same. Responsibilities for promoting safe water supplies in rural areas are vested mainly in the Ministry of Health and its geographic subdivisions. (There are exceptions in Africa, where Ministries of Agriculture are most important.) Important for this work is the trained sanitarian or sanitary assistant of different levels.

The commonest method for providing safe water in rural villages is the drilling or digging of wells with hand pumps. Even this simple technology requires maintenance, for which someone has to be trained. Women transport the water in jugs to their homes for drinking, cooking, and washing. Cisterns, springs, and carefully chosen streams are alternative water sources. In a properly constructed well, the costs of maintenance must be assumed locally. Consumption charges may even be levied, as in Kenya. Water purification in a proper well needs only safe storage.

For human waste disposal in a rural community, the commonest method is by construction of pit latrines. There are many varieties, which reflect the socioeconomic and cultural diversity in developing countries. Ministries of Health often provide, for a subsidized price, the concrete slab that facilitates latrine construction. A problem everywhere is the continued use by families of latrines, because they may be poorly maintained. This calls for health education in the community and in the schools, as well as advice from sanitarians. The maintenance of wells and latrines furnishes a basis for local community participation for both women's and men's groups. This usually means involvement in planning and implementation through voluntary labor. Concentrated national "demonstration" efforts, combining central government support and strong local participation, have sometimes achieved remarkable results, such as those in Ayadaw township, Burma.

The general strategy of WHO is to link rural water supply and sanitation efforts to the movement for primary health care. All health personnel are urged to include education about safe water in their daily work. The sanitarians needed to provide technical guidance are unfortunately scarce in many developing countries, and medical leadership in Ministries of Health often gives low priority to training such personnel. An objective of WHO and UNICEF, therefore, has been to heighten this priority in the leadership of Ministries of Health.

International Drinking Water Supply and Sanitation Decade

The supply of safe water in the world was recognized as so important an objective that in the 1970s the Economic and Social Council of the United Nations decided to launch a global program for promoting progress. Each country, of course, would have to show its support through national initiatives. The decade 1980–1990 was chosen, and great efforts went into acquiring baseline data, so that subsequent changes could be determined. The principal findings on water and sanitation in developing countries, classified by urban and rural populations, have been reported above. The great disparities of conditions between these two populations were clear.

Many developing countries have set up *National Action Committees* to promote plans for water supply improvement. These committees usually represent the several ministries of government, as well as universities, professional associations, and engineering firms. Plans are worked out and strategies formulated. Results achieved over the decade of the 1980s are not yet available, but the gains in safe water access in the rural areas of developing countries from 1970 to 1983, reported earlier, forecast further progress.

Reports published outside the United

Nations or WHO give data on rural water supplies in individual countries. Analysis suggests a crude positive relationship in certain regions between rural water supply coverage and the percentage of national wealth (GNP) spent by government on health. In Latin America the relationship seems significant. Countries with higher rural water supply coverage spend three times the public money for health as those with lower water supply coverage. The data are given in Table 16.1. Similar analysis of data from the Middle East shows a weakly positive relationship, whereas in the South Asia and Africa regions, the relationship between the two variables seems to be random.

Economic support from central governments, which can mobilize national wealth, is undoubtedly basic for environmental health services in rural areas. At the local level in developing countries, appropriate technology and community education are required. Wells and latrines often become nonfunctional when there is no locally trained person to offer guidance. Sanitarians in the local units of the Ministry of Health are most suitable, but community health workers may have to play this role. All the strategies for access to safe water and

Table 16.1. Rural Water Supply Coverage in Relation to Government Expenditures on Health: Latin American Countries 1985

Country	Percent of Rural Population Covered	Government Health Expenditures as Percent of GNP
Trinidad and Tobago	95	3.00
Costa Rica	82	5.41
Brazil	71	1.30
Panama	63	5.37
Mexico	50.6	1.70
Venezuela	50	2.69
Honduras	45	2.60
Average	(65.23)	(3.15)
Guatemala	39	0.66
Ecuador	31	1.10
Haiti	30	0.87
Chile	29	2.05
Bolivia	27	0.40
Colombia	20	0.80
Argentina	17	1.50
Peru	17	1.00
Average	(26.25)	(1.05)

Source: Derived from *The International Drinking Water Supply and Sanitation Decade Directory.* 3rd ed. London: Thomas Telford, 1987.

sanitation in developing countries depend ultimately on the social values in the national health system.

On a larger scale in the developing countries, the growth of population is beginning to outstrip the global supply of safe water. (Desalination of seawater, for example, might solve the problem, except for its enormous cost.) In the judgment of a water expert, Peter Bourne, offered in 1984:

> There is little doubt that the world will increasingly face a global water crisis over the next 20 years. The ability to provide drinking water for people will clearly be tied to our ability to manage this crucial resource for all our needs, preventing worldwide industrial contamination, avoiding over exploitation for agricultural purposes, and preventing the diversion of scarce water resources to meet the needs of a powerful minority at the expense of the general population. On the other hand, growing concern about water in both the developed and developing world will demand that rough decisions be made, and large and important steps be taken to head off the impending crisis. The result may well be that the need to deal with the water issue as a whole may result in a continuing enhancement of interest in water for human consumption and a more vigorous effort to incorporate this concern into national and regional planning programs dealing with this resource.

EMERGENCY MEDICAL SERVICES

Emergency medical services (EMS) comprise a complex of activities to cope rapidly with urgent health needs. We consider briefly four aspects: medical services, ambulance transportation, disaster relief, and blood transfusions.

Medical Services

Medical help to an accident victim can, of course, be given anywhere, but the usual place for providing such services effectively is the outpatient department of a general hospital. In almost all countries, general hospitals have an EMS section where anyone can come day or night for urgent attention. Some industrialized countries have developed standards to show the level of case severity that a particular hospital can handle.

With an open door to everyone, the EMS sections of hospital outpatient departments are visited by patients with all sorts of illness, not necessarily emergencies. This practice is widespread in developing countries, where a physician may not be available to most people in any other way. EMS care becomes a back-up and substitute for primary health care. Also in industrialized countries, where a general physician provides primary care, the physician may not always be available, so that EMS care is used as a replacement. In the United States, most people do not have strong ties to a primary physician, so that they resort frequently to EMS care.

The medical staffing of EMS departments is done ordinarily by the hospital physicians providing inpatient care. In small hospitals, this work may be rotated. In large hospitals, there are usually young physicians in training who are assigned to this duty. In the open-staff hospitals of North America, outside physicians may be engaged specifically for EMS work. To elevate the quality of EMS care, a formal specialty of "emergency medicine" has been established in the United States.

When the volume of patients coming to a hospital outpatient department is very high, it may be possible to separate those requiring true EMS care from those requiring nonurgent care. This process of triage is often handled by well-trained nurses. The patient with a critical problem must then get further diagnosis and treatment on an inpatient ward or in one of the outpatient specialty clinics.

The financial support of EMS care varies with the general arrangements for economic support in the national health system. Where there is national health insurance or a national health service, as in Europe, EMS care is financed like any other hospital service. It may simply be part of a global budget or may warrant a fee payable to the hospital. There may be some personal copayment obligation, but most of the fee is paid by the insurance.

In developing countries, where national insurance is unavailable, EMS programs are financed mainly by the general revenues supporting the hospital; sometimes there are overall registration fees. In India emergency cases are seen along with all other cases in hospital outpatient departments, but there are no special arrangements for their treatment.

In the United States EMS financing is especially complex. A traditional notion that hospitals give emergency care free was slow to die. General hospitals, in fact, make charges for EMS service, like any other. For low-income people covered by Medicaid, and elderly people covered by Medicare, these programs pay the charges. Voluntary health insurance may pay, but many low-income people (even when employed in low-wage jobs) lack such insurance and are not protected by Medicaid nor Medicare. Voluntary hospitals, therefore, often refer such cases to public hospitals, a practice known as "patient dumping." This aggravates the solvency of public hospitals, which are typically underfinanced from local taxation.

In Great Britain, where the National Health Service finances all but a handful of private hospitals, emergency services are supported along with other outpatient care. Large hospitals usually have a *casualty department,* with a staff structure of hospital specialists and doctors in training (registrars). The exact method of staffing hospital EMS departments differs in the welfare-oriented and comprehensive health systems of Europe, but there is usually some mechanism for dealing with the clinical requirements of emergency cases.

The dramatic aspects of emergency services point everywhere to the leadership role of hospitals. Yet when one recognizes the great extent to which hospital outpatient departments are misused for primary health care, this role can lead to policies that are medically inappropriate and economically wasteful. The most effective and economical health system should have broad foundations in primary health care, with hospital emergency services as back-up to the extent necessary.

Ambulance Services

Ambulances are available in almost all countries to bring patients to EMS departments in hospitals. Ambulance transportation is used also for other purposes: for moving patients from home to hospital or vice versa and for transporting patients from isolated rural places to a city hospital. Ambulances in the nineteenth century were used by military forces in battle, and then they became attached to hospitals. As motorized vehicles became available, the Red Cross Society in many countries sponsored fleets of ambulances. In some countries, local public Fire Departments operate ambulance services, with carefully trained personnel.

In an entrepreneurial health system, like that in the United States, ambulance firms may be operated as private businesses. Where the population is small, funeral directors may use their hearses to transport patients.

The staffing and equipment of ambulances are the major determinants of their quality of service. Red Cross ambulance drivers and attendants are often trained in first aid, and in the industrialized countries the service may be quite sophisticated for trauma, heart attacks, and so on. When ambulances come to emergencies from hospitals, physicians may go along.

In the British National Health Service ambulance operations are a standard responsibility of all local health authorities. The Scandinavian countries assign repsonsibility to the county governments, which make use of ambulances attached to hospitals, fire brigades, and to some of the larger communes. In the former Soviet Union, a very impressive pattern of emergency services using ambulance transport was implemented in the major cities.

The program in Leningrad was regarded as a model. Anyone there could telephone a central exchange for help. Whether an emergency or not, an ambulance with trained staff was dispatched to take the patient to an appropriate polyclinic or hospital. No one was rejected, so that this was really a scheme for primary health care. Although this was an expensive way to provide back-up for primary care, it was extremely popular and was retained for political reasons.

A major resource for operating ambulances, especially in developing countries, is the Red Cross. Most of the costs are actually supported by the Ministries of Health and allocated to the

Red Cross for operating the program. Each country is typically divided into ambulance regions, corresponding to the MoH organization. The Red Cross in many countries also conducts courses on "first aid" for any group. It has made a special goal of disseminating cardiopulmonary resuscitation methods as widely as possible.

Even in Europe, the Red Cross is financed principally by government grants. Red Cross ambulances are used most often in the rural regions. In the main cities, local governments are more likely to be directly responsible for ambulance service. In recent years, however, private ambulance companies have been entering the field, creating problems of coordination. Sometimes a single telephone number is used to gain access to any ambulance, public or private, at the closest location.

Airplane ambulance transport is a special response to rural emergencies, discussed in Chapter 14. Essentially it is used for transporting patients (emergencies and others) from isolated rural locations to urban hospitals. This service usually comes under the Ministry of Health, often jointly with the Red Cross. It is organized in countries with large thinly settled territories, such as Canada, Australia, and the Russian Republic (Siberia).

Because of their consumption of fuel and their staffing, modern ambulance services are usually expensive. As long as they play a required role in the health system, therefore, it is reasonable that the costs be borne by social sources rather than individuals.

Disaster Relief

Closely related to EMS are the more intense demands coming from natural disasters (hurricanes, earthquakes, floods, etc.) or human disasters of war and revolution. The initial response is to tackle the basic disruption, such as water supply and electricity. Second is the need for immediate relief to families that are suddenly homeless and without food. Third is the need for management and coordination of the multiple agencies usually involved. For water and sanitation problems, Ministries of Health play the major role; for basic relief it is usually the Red Cross and diverse charitable agencies; and for general management it is often a coun-

cil chaired by a high general official of government.

Norway illustrates a country with an explicit scheme for coping with natural disasters. The police in each district are in charge, and they mobilize the services of hospitals, fire brigades, voluntary agencies, and even the military resources. Ministry of Health subdivisions allocate patients to different hospitals. Rescue of disaster victims requires transportation by railroads and airplanes. Problems arising are to be brought to the attention of police stations.

The World Health Organization has a headquarters unit on disasters, the function of which is to persuade countries to organize similar units—to be prepared. In the actual implementation of disaster relief, as well as in the basic planning, the Red Cross usually plays a key role. It is especially important in providing immediate food and shelter to disaster victims.

There are many examples of inappropriate responses to major disasters, due to lack of planning. After the Peruvian earthquake of 1970, portable hospitals were sent into the devastated area at high cost and with no significant benefit. A similar medicalized response came after the Nicaraguan earthquake of 1972, with little benefit. Relief goods were sent to these countries, without provision for their transportation to the needy areas.

A WHO official in charge of "emergency preparedness and disaster relief coordination" summarizes the practical response to most disasters, saying

> Most sudden impact disasters do not affect the entire country. Generally citizens from unaffected areas of the country donate an abundance of food, clothing, and other personal items which are well-suited to local needs. What is needed and what is not available locally: specialized skills, sophisticated technology and replacement of medical supplies used during the emergency.

Donated supplies and personnel from other countries often have greater symbolic meaning than practical value in response to disasters.

In the aftermath of disasters there is, of course, the long-term need to reconstruct community life or perhaps to undertake some basic changes. Sometimes the devastations of an urban area provide the opportunity for wholly new city planning, which improves future living conditions. This usually depends on mobilizing funds and resources from the entire nation.

Blood Transfusions

The transfusion of human blood is a special type of health service provided in various ways. Although it is strongly associated with emergencies, it is relevant to many other aspects of medical care. The need for blood in hospitals is so great that programs for its collection, storage, and distribution have been organized in many countries.

The earliest organized blood programs were developed in the 1920s in Great Britain, France, and the Soviet Union. Direct transfusions with human blood had been attempted even in the seventeenth century, but the four blood types were not discovered until 1900. Then anticoagulants were discovered, permitting the storage of blood in "blood banks."

Blood transfusion activities are, in principle, organized in four ways: (1) individual hospital blood banks, (2) governmental blood transfusion programs, (3) Red Cross blood programs, and (4) commercial blood enterprises. In most countries, there are combinations of these four types of sponsorship.

Governmental programs, usually under the Ministry of Health, operate in France, Great Britain, Ireland, New Zealand, and Hungary. These countries operate national networks of blood storage facilities that distribute blood to all hospitals. Most of the former socialist countries also operated centralized governmental schemes. Some developing countries have established a governmental network of blood services, such as Uruguay and Venezuela in Latin America, Kenya in Africa, Algeria, Egypt, and Iran in the Middle East, and Malaysia and Sri Lanka in Asia. Sometimes the Red Cross assists these countries in recruiting blood donors.

Blood programs, based simply on hospital blood banks, are predominant in the developing countries. Where no national network exists, blood collection and use are simply left up to each hospital. Only a few affluent countries, such as Sweden and Denmark, manage to get along this way.

Commercial blood enterprises play a large part in many developing countries, where the supply of blood from voluntary donors is far below the demands of hospitals. Mexico, for example, has 500 commercial blood banks that sell their blood to hospitals and pharmaceutical companies at home and abroad. A meeting of the Pan American Health Organization estimated that 60 percent of the blood used in Latin America came from paid donors.

Small commercial blood banks in countries of the Middle East and southern Asia take advantage of the many unemployed people who will sell their blood to survive. The company pays $3 for a pint, and sells it to hospitals for $60. In India, most of the blood is acquired this way. The United States has also had many commercial blood banks, but these have been decreasing. In France and Costa Rica, commercial blood companies were banned in the 1970s and replaced by public schemes.

The organized blood programs, in which the Red Cross provides the major leadership, operate in 23 countries. Among industrialized countries these include Canada, Australia, Japan, Finland, Switzerland, Netherlands, and Belgium. Among developing countries, they include Indonesia, Thailand, South Korea, Ecuador, and several smaller ones. In these countries, the Red Cross usually has large regional storage depots, equivalent to those in government programs. National networks of blood banks are also maintained. The Red Cross in these countries derives most of its funding from government grants.

In 39 other countries, the Red Cross operates some blood transfusion centers, along with others operated by government and some private companies. These include the United States, Germany, Italy, Spain, and Norway among industrialized countries, and some 30 developing countries; the latter include such large countries as India, China, Iran, Mexico, and Argentina.

In some 80 countries, the role of the Red Cross has been limited essentially to promoting the recruitment of voluntary blood donors. No blood facilities are operated by the Red Cross, but assistance is given to government and individual hospitals. This role is played in Brazil and in most of the countries of Africa.

The central policy of Red Cross is to promote voluntary blood donation as the exclusive method. When the blood is paid for, various commercial difficulties are encountered, which ultimately compromise the blood supply. In 1971 a British social scientist explored this issue, comparing Britain, where all blood donations were voluntary, with the United States, where about half were commercial. A great deal more hepatitis, a virus infection, was found to contaminate U.S. commercial blood. The crucial issue, however, is moral as well as pathological.

Whatever method by which blood is collected, its distribution is ultimately through hospitals. Blood banks must provide proper testing and storage. Distribution has other requirements. Large hospitals may sometimes carry out all the functions, including the distribution of blood to other facilities nearby. If hospitals are regionalized, the management of blood services is facilitated. National or regional networks of blood programs can be most efficient and effective under a Ministry of Health, with assistance from the Red Cross. In countries where the Ministry is slow to act, the Red Cross should be expected to provide the leadership.

In 1984, the International Society of Blood Transfusion issued a statement on "National Blood Policy." Among other things, this called for collection of blood only from voluntary donors. It called for management of the program by the national public health authority or else delegation to the national Red Cross Society or "to another non-profit organization of proven integrity." The national health authority, it states "should ensure that adequate funding is available to maintain the highest possible standards of transfusion practice and quality management throughout the country, commensurate with the state of development of the national health program."

OTHER SPECIAL TECHNIQUES

In most health systems, a number of special techniques, not part of conventional clinical medicine, contribute to comprehensive health services. Organized efforts have been widespread for many such services, of which we take note of health education, nutrition, and still others.

Health Education

The education of people about health and disease and actions to be taken for improving health are aspects of virtually all organized health programs. Health education has its largest role in the many strategies for disease prevention and health promotion, but it is also relevant for certain aspects of medical care. Two major settings for health education are in the schools and in the general community.

School health education is generally included in the instruction about personal hygiene and biology. Regular teachers are responsible. Sometimes special health problems will be discussed in the classroom by nurses or other personnel from the local public health agency. In large school networks of affluent countries, there may be special teachers devoted entirely to health instruction. At the secondary school level, this field may be linked to athletics or physical education. In recent years, health education of secondary school students has focused on problems of drug abuse and sexually transmitted diseases.

Health education of the general population is a feature of all the specialized programs reviewed in Chapters 14, 15, and this chapter. In maternal and child health services, occupational health services, mental health programs, and the others there is always a health education component. At the same time, health education is valuable to clarify for people the benefits of using general medical care and how to obtain it. The communication techniques must naturally be adjusted to the diverse settings of these programs.

With very general objectives, health education may be used to promote reasonable self-care. This is an aspect of primary health care that can be especially helpful in health systems where physicians are scarce. In developing countries, the task is often to replace superstitious or magical procedures with sound self-care techniques. The concept of self-care should not be abused to conceal the lack of proper health service where it is needed.

In the highly industrialized countries, mortality from cardiovascular disorders and cancer has stimulated many strategies of health promotion. Important among these is education on personal habits harmful to health, such as smoking cigarettes, lack of exercise, or consumption of high-fat foods. The etiology of disease, as between personal behavior and environmental pressures, is complex, but the educational goal is often epitomized as influencing "life-style." Many debates have arisen over "blaming the victim," but health education is still widespread, along with other strategies, such as banning tobacco advertising or influencing food production.

Health education applies a set of techniques employed by many types of health personnel. The specialized "health educator" is widely available throughout the health systems of the United States and Great Britain. In almost all U.S. county and city Health Departments, there are persons devoted exclusively to health education, although some may not be formally trained. Also in the federal Public Health Service and in most state Departments of Health, there are sections for health education.

In Great Britain a District Health Education Officer is appointed in each local administrative area to provide advice and guidance to the local public health authorities. This officer also gives health education consultation to local general practitioners and visiting nurses. In London there is a national Health Education Council, established as an independent body but funded by the central government. The Council has contracted with commercial advertising agencies for large campaigns against smoking, improper diets, venereal diseases, alcoholism, and drug abuse.

The health education policy in Germany is more typical of the other European countries. The regular medical and nursing staffs of the "lander" (provinces) and teachers in the schools conduct education on the main problems. Voluntary health agencies offer education on selected matters. There is a Federal Health Education Center at Cologne, which distributes educational materials, but there are no formally trained health educators. Several

thousand physicians work full-time in the German Ministry of Youth, Family Affairs, and Health, but their services are, by law, exclusively preventive. Hence, they normally include a good deal of health education.

In developing countries, specialized health educators are rare anywhere in the Ministry of Health structure. Instead an occasional physician may get special training in educational techniques. In the very poor developing countries, health education may be made a task of briefly trained community health workers. In Nigeria, for example, such workers were able to teach about the hazards of contaminated irrigation waters, with a resultant decline in infestation by the guinea worm.

Health education requirements in developing countries are particularly great, since the problems of heart disease and cancer are increasing, while the burdens of malnutrition and infectious disease are still heavy. Where health personnel as a whole are far below the needs, a health message can have wider impact than a purely personal health service. The emphasis on health education as an integral part of primary health care alerts all sorts of nurses, midwives, medical assistants, and sanitarians to learn the skills of education.

A literature review of health education interventions in developing countries, emphasizing evaluation, reflected the programs in which education played a part. All the activities were focused on such objectives as environmental sanitation, diarrhea, nutrition, breast-feeding, family planning, immunization, dental health, and leprosy. Judgment on the evaluations yielded only the modest conclusion that "health education can sometimes lead to changes in behavior and in health status, although there remains room for legitimate skepticism."

All countries make use of mass media to spread educational messages. Even when formally trained health educators are not available, Ministries of Health and many voluntary agencies produce posters, pamphlets, and films to influence people. The techniques applied in media have been defined as those of "social marketing," which orients messages to the personal values of the intended audience. Education on nutrition, for example, would not simply delineate food groups to be consumed, but rather would portray an attractive meal. Mass media are the least expensive form of health education, but they are most effective where combined with discussions with individuals or groups. For nonliterate populations, the pictures in mass media have obvious advantages.

There is an International Union of Health Education, with representatives from 70 countries. In addition to promoting the educational components of all health programs, the Union is devoted to multidisciplinary research on the most effective strategies for coping with the problems of both developing and industrialized countries. As educational strategies become more effectively used by health personnel, they may serve a larger purpose in health systems. Particularly in developing countries, education is a major tool for stimulating community participation in total health program design and operation.

Nutrition

The promotion of health and prevention of disease through proper nutrition are objectives of organized programs in many countries. In general, there are four broad strategies, each having several ramifications: (1) education, (2) supplemental feeding, (3) food modification, and (4) food production policy.

Nutritional education takes many forms. Much of it is disseminated through the general press, beamed at the population as a whole. Nutritional education may also be an aspect of more focused programs in maternal and child health services or communicable disease control. The "social marketing" approach is especially important in nutritional education. Recommended dietary practices are advocated with respect to the foods locally available and customarily consumed. Developing countries of Asia have learned to avoid the mere translation of texts from Europe into local languages.

Encouragement of breast-feeding of small infants is necessary in cities, where employment and liberation of women often lead them to abandon this sound practice. The commercial sale of infant formula milk in cities has had mixed and often deleterious effects.

Supplemental feeding programs also take many forms. A routine distribution of food (rice) to low-income families, as in Sri Lanka, is quite rare. School lunches at low prices are provided extensively in large urban schools. They are common in the affluent countries, and less in the developing countries in proportion to economic level. Another feeding strategy is the government distribution of *food stamps* to low-income individuals and families, enabling them to obtain certain foods at any local shop; this is done in the United States.

Food may also be given directly to malnourished preschool children brought to health centers. Sometimes there are national drives for this purpose, spearheaded by voluntary agencies but funded by the Ministry of Health. Ministries of Agriculture are expected to provide the supplemental food. Occasionally a supplemental feeding program is designed with identification of specific families to be served in each locality.

The strategy of food modification simply calls for the application of scientific knowledge to improve the value of food consumed. To assure consumption of essential vitamins, for example, milk is *fortified* with vitamins A and D, salt is iodized, and bread may be enriched with B vitamins. In many industrialized countries, the content of packaged food must be identified on labels. The general objective is to prevent nutritional deficiency diseases, and to enable consumers to select a prudent diet.

The fourth approach to improving nutrition, food production policy, is most basic and also most difficult. The modification of practices in agriculture and animal husbandry can have long-term benefits, such as the greatly increased grain output in India. Crop selection and irrigation are involved. Shifts of investments from animals to poultry in the industrialized countries have affected the consumption of fats. Government subsidies and taxation policies can obviously influence agricultural options.

All four of the nutrition strategies are inevitably intermingled in a country. Food production and consumption have many roles in society, beside their meaning for health. They are important features of the whole economy, affecting employment and trade. They influence political relationships between nations. In times of famine, the struggle for food can lead to violence and revolution.

Within national health systems, nutrition involves every component. Norway is one of the few countries that has articulated these actions in a legally defined "national nutrition and food policy." As a part of health service delivery, nutrition is a feature of primary health care. As a long-term policy, WHO favors this approach as more enduring than the intervention of a dramatic campaign. Financial support should be expected from the same sources as those that support other health services. In several developing countries, such as Guatemala and the Philippines, there are major research institutes on nutrition, externally funded, that conduct studies that help to formulate nutrition policies.

Although health personnel can have their greatest influence on nutrition within national health systems they must always be aware that the ultimate solutions lie in the production of food, the provision of employment, and the elimination of poverty.

Additional Techniques

Other special techniques are highly organized in certain countries, so that they are conceived as national programs. They may serve almost any type of person, with many different disorders requiring the technique. All of these activities have been noted in various contexts, so that here they will simply be identified.

Rehabilitation is a service associated medically with exercise and physical treatment. Numerous other functions involve employment (job training and placement), education of children, prosthetic appliances, community relationships, other forms of medical intervention, and so on. For providing these services with skill, there may be *rehabilitation centers* as public or private facilities. To some extent every large general hospital may serve as a rehabilitation unit. Administrative personnel may come from various regional offices, concerned with the many nonmedical aspects. The management of severe disabilities through rehabilitation programs for children and adults is discussed in Chapter 15.

Organized home care is another special type of health service to which nurses and several other types of personnel contribute. It is sponsored by various types of health agency: by visiting nurse associations, public health agencies, hospitals, and independent companies. As noted in Chapter 13, the general objective is to provide services that enable patients to stay in a personal home and avoid institutionalization. In Great Britain, for example, the home nursing services provided by the District Health Authority are backed up by homemaker services, "meals on wheels," friendly visitors, and various activities for the elderly. In the United States under Medicare, there is statutory support for organized home care, which has stimulated the organization of many local programs. Well-designed home care programs offer the services of physiotherapists, dieticians, and social workers, as well as nurses. In developing countries, on the other hand, families simply take care of disabled adults or children, without assistance from organized home care programs.

Laboratory services contribute to the operation of national health systems in many ways. Broadly speaking, they have developed along two pathways: laboratories for examination of specimens in public health programs and laboratories for services to individual patients receiving medical care. These are often defined as "public health laboratory services" and "clinical laboratory services." In the affluent industrialized countries, these two types of laboratory service can readily exist side-by-side; the clinical laboratories are in hospitals and the public health laboratories are attached to administrative offices at the provincial level. In developing countries, however, this dichotomy is wasteful, and WHO recommends that all laboratory services be integrated in a national network of central, provincial, and local laboratories. The usual setting for these multipurpose laboratories is in hospitals, where trained personnel and equipment are available.

Finally one may ask about the value of delineating all these special types of service as organized programs in a national health system. The same question may be raised about the value of health programs for certain populations (Chapter 14) and for certain disorders

(Chapter 15). Each categorical program implies a certain fragmentation of efforts to prevent or to treat disease, and yet the specialized strategies mobilize resources and funds. Health personnel are energized to reach goals. Skills are developed to solve the technical problems emerging from each program. The coordination and integration of the various activities are, of course, necessary. This must be a responsibility of subdivisions of the Ministries of Health at the local level or an intermediate level of provinces or districts.

REFERENCES

Environmental Sanitation

Bourne, Peter G. (Editor), *Water and Sanitation: Economic and Sociological Perspectives.* Orlando, FL: Academic Press, 1984.

Deck, F.L.O., "Community Water Supply and Sanitation in Developing Countries: An Evaluation of the Levels and Trends of Services." *World Health Statistics Quarterly,* 39(1):2–31, 1986.

Goldstein, Bernard D., and Michael Greenberg, "Environmental Applications and Interventions in Public Health." In *Oxford Textbook of Public Health,* 2nd ed., Volume 3, Chapter 2. Oxford: Oxford University Press, 1991, pp. 17–28.

Isely, Raymond B., "Water Supply and Sanitation in Africa." *World Health Forum,* 6:213–219, 1985.

Miller, Morris, *Debt and the Environment: Converging Issues.* Geneva: United Nations Publications, 1991.

Okun, Daniel A., "Water and Waste Disposal." In Last (Editor), Maxcy-Rosenau, *Public Health and Preventive Medicine,* 12th ed., Chapter 19. Norwalk, CT: Appleton-Century-Crofts, 1986, pp. 807–874.

Roemer, Ruth, J. E. Frink, and C. Kramer, "Environmental Health Services: Multiplicity of Jurisdictions and Comprehensive Environmental Management." *Milbank Memorial Fund Quarterly,* 49(4):419–507, 1971.

Schaefer, M., *The Administration of Environmental Health Programs.* Geneva: WHO (Public Health Papers No. 59), 1974.

Schiller, E. J., and R. L. Drote (Editors), *Water Supply and Sanitation in Developing Countries.* Ann Arbor: Ann Arbor Science Publishers, 1982.

Scotney, N., "Water and the Community" (Kenya). *World Health Forum,* 5:233–235, 1984.

The International Drinking Water Supply and Sanitation Decade Director, 3rd ed. London: Thomas Telford, 1987.

Tin U, et al., "We Want Water, Not Gold" (Burma). *World Health Forum,* 9:519–525, 1988.

Van Wijk-Sijbesma, Christine, "Drinking Water and Sanitation: Women Can Do Much." *World Health Forum,* 8:28–32, 1987.

Wolman, Abel, "Give Health a Chance—with Healthy Surroundings." *World Health Forum,* 7:107–130, 1986.

World Health Organization, Division of Strengthening of Health Services, *Improving Urban Health—A Program of Action.* Geneva: WHO, 1988.

Emergency Medical Services

American Hospital Association, *The Hospital's Role in Emergency Medical Services Systems* (United States). Chicago: AHA, 1984.

Cliff, Kenneth S., *Accidents: Causes Prevention and Services* (Great Britain). London: Croom Helm, 1984.

Cuny, Frederick C., *Disasters and Development.* New York: Oxford University Press, 1983.

de Ville de Goyet, Claude, and Patricia Bittner "Should Disaster Relief Strike, Be Prepared." *World Health Forum,* 12:10–12, January–February 1991.

Foege, William H., "Public Health Aspects of Disaster Management." In Last (Editor), Maxcy-Rosenau, *Public Health and Preventive Medicine,* 12th ed., Chapter 6. Norwalk CT: Appleton-Century-Crofts, 1986, pp. 1879–1886.

Frey, R., and P. Safar (Editors), *Types and Events of Disaster Organization in Various Disaster Situations.* Berlin: Springer-Verlag, 1980.

Hagen, Piet J., *Blood: Gift or Merchandise.* New York: Alan R. Liss, 1982.

International Society of Blood Transfusion, "Guidelines for Legislation on National Blood Policy." *International Digest of Health Legislation,* 36(4):1080–1082, 1985.

League of Red Cross and Red Crescent Societies, *Blood—A Vital Gift of Life.* Geneva: The League, 1984.

Leikola, J., "Blood Transfusion in Developing Countries: Problems and Progress." *Vox Sang,* 46 (Suppl. 1):49–63, 1984.

Pan American Health Organization, *Emergency Health Management After Natural Disaster.* Washington: PAHO (Scientific Pub. No. 407), 1981.

Portnoy, William M. (Editor), *Emergency Medical Care.* Lexington, MA: Lexington Books, 1977.

Shapiro, L. B., and I. A. Ostrovskii (Editors), *Organization of Emergency Medical Care* (Soviet Union). Baltimore, MD: Johns Hopkins University Press, 1975.

Singh, N. P. (Editor), *Emergency and Disaster Medicine* (India). New Delhi: National Association of Emergency and Disaster Medicine, 1982.

Surgenor, D. M., "Human Blood and the Renewal of Altruism: Titmuss in Retrospect." *International Journal of Health Services,* 2(3):443–453, 1972.

Titmuss, R. M. *The Gift Relationship—From Huamn Blood to Social Policy.* New York: Pantheon, 1971.

Zmijewski, Chester M., and Walter E. Haesler, *Textbook of Blood Banking Science.* New York: Appleton-Century-Crofts, 1982.

Other Special Techniques

Beaton, G. H., and J. M. Bengoa (Editors), *Nutrition in Preventive Medicine.* Geneva: World Health Organization (Monograph Series No. 62), 1976.

Berthet, Etienne, "The International Union for Health Education." *World Health Forum,* 5:76–78, 1984.

Biswas, Margaret, and Per Pinstrup-Andersen (Editors), *Nutrition and Development.* New York: Oxford University Press, 1985.

Brown, E. R., and G. E. Margo, "Health Education: Can the Reformers Be Reformed?" *International Journal of Health Services,* 8(1):3–26, 1978.

Cassels, Andrew, and Katja Janovsky, *Strengthening Health Management in Districts and Provinces.* Geneva: World Health Organization, 1991.

Crawford, Robert, "You Are Dangerous to Your Health: The Ideology and Politics of Victim Blaming." *International Journal of Health Services,* 7(4):663–680, 1977.

Ginzberg, Eli, W. Balinsky, and M. Ostow, *Home Health Care: Its Role in the Changing Health Services Market.* Totowa, NJ: Rowman & Allanheld, 1984.

Green, Lawrence W., "Prevention and Health Education." In Last (Editor), Maxcy-Rosenau, *Public Health and Preventive Medicine,* 12th ed. Norwalk, CT: Appleton-Century-Crofts, 1986, Chapter 29, pp. 1089–1108.

Green, L. W., and D. C. Iverson, "School Health Education." *Annual Review of Public Health,* 3:321–338, 1982.

Habicht, Jean-Pierre, "Nutrition: A Health Sector Responsibility." *World Health Forum,* 4:5–24, 1983.

Hoble, John H., "Rehabilitating the Severely Disabled: The Foreign Experience." *Journal of Health Politics, Policy and Law,* 4(2):221–249, 1979.

Holland, Walter W., and Ellie Breeze, "Good Life-Styles for Good Health." *World Health Forum.* 7:380–386, 1986.

Jalore, Bushra, "Innovative Approaches in Nutrition Education in the Pacific Region." *International Journal of Health Education,* 24(2):95–101, 1981.

Jelliffe, Derrick B., and E. F. Patrice Jelliffe, "The Infant Food Industry and International Child Health." *International Journal of Health Services,* 7(2):249–254, 1977.

Klepp, K.-I., and J. L. Forster, "The Norwegian Nutrition and Food Policy: An Integrated Policy Approach to a Public Health Problem." *Journal of Public Health Policy,* 6:447–463, 1985.

Levin, L. S., *Self-Care in Health: Annotated Bibliography.* New Haven, CT: Yale University Press, 1976.

Loevinsohn, Benjamin P., "Health Education Interventions in Developing Countries: A Methodological Review of Published Articles." *International Journal of Epidemiology,* 19(4):788–794, 1990.

Makhoul, Najwa, "Agricultural Research and Human Nutrition: A Comparative Analysis of Brazil, Cuba, Israel, and the United States." *International Journal of Health Services,* 13(1):15–31, 1983.

Pan American Health Organization, *Health Education: Addresses Presented at the IX International Conference on Health Education.* Washington: PAHO, 1978.

Scrimshaw, Nevin S., "Nutrition and Preventive Medicine." In Last (Editor), Maxcy-Rosenau, *Public Health and Preventive Medicine,* 12th ed. Norwalk, CT: Appleton-Century-Crofts, 1986, Chapter 49, pp. 1515–1542.

Ward, Graham W., "How to Sell Health." *World Health Forum,* 7:169–177, 1986.

World Health Organization, Expert Committee on Health Laboratory Services, *The Planning and Organization of a Health Laboratory Service.* Geneva: WHO (Technical Report Series No. 491), 1972.

PART FIVE

WORLD PERSPECTIVE

CHAPTER SEVENTEEN

International Health Activities

As communications and trade have increased among nations in all parts of the world, people have come to recognize the interdependence of each country's health with the disease problems of other countries. In its broadest sense, international health work concerns the many health activities that must be carried out across national boundaries.

COLONIALISM, RELIGIOUS MISSIONS, AND PHILANTHROPY

The beginnings of internationalism in medicine and public health or cross-national health work must be traced to colonial takeovers in Asia and Africa. In the sixteenth century, the Portuguese established settlements in China, India, and the Malay Peninsula in southeast Asia. Later the Dutch and then the British became the principal European colonists in both Asia and Africa. Great Britain was the dominant imperial power in the eighteenth and nineteenth centuries. As colonial governments grew stronger and their military and civilian personnel increased, small garrison hospitals or medical stations were established for their care. Sometimes special wards would be set up for the "natives."

A customary course of events is illustrated by the British colonization of East Africa around 1890. The initial settlement was by the Imperial British East Africa Company (IBEA), which soon engaged British doctors to take care of its employees. In 1894, the British government's Foreign Office took control of this work, including the medical services. A few years later these services became a medical department in the British protectorate of Kenya and Uganda, but its resources were very small. In a book published in 1905 on *The East Af-rican Protectorate,* the medical services were considered necessary only to protect Europeans against tropical health hazards. Some attention was also given to workers imported from British India, but the health of native Africans was not considered a British responsibility. Colonial government medical services for the control of tropical diseases and for general medical care were generally not extended to the African population until after World War I (1914–1918).

The strategy of colonial health services was to provide support for the general objectives of colonial agriculture. This put the greatest emphasis on growth and export of cash crops, through transfer of male workers to areas of commercialized agriculture, with consequent reduction of traditional food crops at home. This led to extensive malnutrition, even as the income from foreign trade increased. This was evident under the German and later the British colonial policies in what is now Tanzania.

Recent historical research on European imperialism, however, has recognized a complex mixture of motives and strategies in the role of western medicine in Asian and African colonies. In the early nineteenth century, the health protection of European military personnel and civilian settlers was clearly the main objective. Colonial medical services were largely confined to the main cities, where Europeans were concentrated. When quinine was used by Europeans in an African expedition of 1854, it was described as "the prime factor in allowing the white man's conquest of Black Africa." After the 1880s and the great breakthroughs in bacteriology, the discipline of "tropical medicine" took shape, but its principal objective was to make tropical environments more congenial to European colonists.

In the late nineteenth and early twentieth centuries, the rationale of colonial medical services gradually changed. It was increasingly appreciated that the health of soldiers and other Europeans depended largely on the health of "native populations" around them. As early as 1865 a British official in the Bengal region of India wrote: "Even if we look no further than the protection of the health of the European soldiers, it will be evidently insufficient if we endeavor to improve the condition of our cantonments alone, and ignore the existence of the masses of the native population by which our troops are surrounded." The Indian Medical Service, nevertheless, though started by the British in 1714, did not really begin to serve the Indian people until the twentieth century. In Africa, a Colonial Medical Service for the British colonies was started only in 1927.

In mining and agriculture, disease among indigenous workers was increasingly seen as an impediment to production. It was an obstacle, in later terminology, to economic development. Reduced output of commodities likewise meant decreased tax collections. Also, as the political consciousness of native populations rose, health services were recognized as useful in displaying benevolent and paternalistic intentions among the foreign masters. For all these reasons, by World War I and even before the "national liberations" after World War II, colonial health services had acquired a much broader meaning—that is, to apply scientific medicine as well as public health strategies to the needs of general colonial populations.

Medical services sponsored by religious missions were entirely separate from the colonial government, and these were often provided to the Africans. A 70-bed hospital was built in 1897, for example, by the Church Missionary Society in Uganda, principally to serve African natives. The administration of the colonial government looked upon these mission services as a useful supplementation to the official program.

In the nineteenth and early twentieth centuries, Christian missions from Europe and North America came to spread the doctrines of Christianity. They developed hospitals or clinics in many small towns and villages as vehicles for their evangelism associated with humanitarianism. These facilities often provided the first contact of rural people with Western medicine. In Latin America hospitals founded by religious groups (mostly Catholic) from Spain and Portugal became the most numerous facilities in several countries. In the later twentieth century, most of these "beneficencia" hospitals were subsidized and then taken over by governments.

In 1799, John Vanderkemp became the first medical missionary in Africa. He was a Dutch physician whose work was sponsored by the London Missionary Society. Later in the mid-nineteenth century a Scottish physician, David Livingstone (1813–1873), served as a medical missionary in South Africa (what is now Botswana), and after 1850 he became a general explorer in central Africa. In the late nineteenth and early twentieth centuries, Albert Schweitzer (1875–1965) established the hospital at Lambaréné in French Equatorial Africa, eventually attracting worldwide attention.

Missionary work by physicians started in China at Canton around 1840. These evangelical physicians brought to imperial, and later republican China, its first acquaintance with western medical education. They introduced concepts of bacteriology and organ pathology, and demonstrated the role of nurses in caring for patients in hospitals. Several western-type medical schools were founded, leading up to the Peking Union Medical College (PUMC) started with support from the Rockefeller Foundation in 1914. After 1949 under the Communist government, western religious missions were terminated in China, but the PUMC was continued as a high-level medical school.

International health work was carried out in many countries by the Rockefeller Foundation from the United States. The Rockefeller International Health Division (started in 1913) promoted health activities in Latin America and Asia involving (1) basic health research, (2) training health personnel through supporting graduate education, and (3) setting up demonstrations of model health programs. Among its more notable achievements, the Rockefeller Foundation developed an effective yellow fever vaccine, mounted a campaign against the mosquito vector, and trained health personnel to carry out this preventive work.

Specific enterprises for mining, agriculture, or other forms of production often established medical units for the care of their employees and their families. In the nineteenth and early twentieth centuries some colonial governments required business enterprises with more than a certain number of workers to establish units for medical care. This was the policy in India, for example, and in Egypt and Nigeria. After national independence was gained, such requirements usually became more rigorous.

In addition to direct colonial domination, overt military hostilities promoted by foreign governments have seriously impaired health services in certain newly independent countries. This was evident in the support of counterrevolutionary *contras* by the United States, which eroded the health gains of the Sandinista government of Nicaragua in the 1980s. It is seen also in the insurrections supported by the government of South Africa against the FRELIMO independence movement that gained control over Mozambique in 1975.

On a nonreligious and nongovernmental basis, another sort of international health work was done by heroic figures such as Norman Bethune (1890–1939) of Canada. In support of the republican (Loyalist) cause in Spain, he performed surgery behind the battle lines in 1936 and then went to China in 1938 to work with the Red Army before its final victory in 1949. There can be little doubt that inspiration from religion or political conviction or a spirit of international good will has figured prominently in the extension of international health work.

INTERNATIONAL SANITARY CONFERENCES

The first truly international collaborative work, involving 12 European countries (including Turkey), was a meeting in Paris in 1851. It was designated as an International Sanitary Conference. Although it lasted from July 1851 to January 1852, the discussion of different policies on quarantine regulations at national borders failed to lead to any agreement. There were unresolved disputes among the delegates about the contagiousness of the

plague, yellow fever, and cholera—whether these dreadful scourges were communicated from the sick to the well or whether they were caused by certain atmospheric, climatic, and soil conditions creating an *epidemic constitution.* A majority of the delegates voted that cholera should be subject to quarantine regulations, but none of the participating governments acted to ratify such regulations. The only accomplishment of this 6-month meeting was the basic experience of several countries in meeting together to discuss international health problems.

Eight years later a second International Sanitary Conference was held in Paris in 1859. In that 8-year interval an Italian microscopist, Filippo Pacini (1812–1883), clearly described the *Cholera vibrio* as the pathogenic agent of cholera—a discovery overlooked for 30 years until it was reaffirmed by Robert Koch (1843–1910). Also in 1854, John Snow (1813–1858) dramatically demonstrated the contagiousness of cholera through ingestion of fecally contaminated water in London from the River Thames. After 5 months, the Second Conference adjourned with no resolution of the dispute between the contagionists and the miasmatists, and no subsequent ratification of the *draft convention* on quarantine of cholera by any country.

The third International Sanitary Conference was held in Constantinople in 1866, followed by a Fourth Conference in Vienna in 1874. Still no effective agreements could be reached, despite a fifth conference in Washington in 1881 and a sixth conference in Rome in 1885. It was only at the seventh International Sanitary Conference in Venice, held in 1892, that agreement was finally reached. It had taken 41 years of discussion to reach agreement on a proposal of very limited scope, quarantine of westbound ships with a case of cholera on board. This first historic convention also provided that the Pan-Arab Quarantine Board of Health in Egypt should prepare compatible provisions regarding plague and yellow fever, although their etiology and epidemiology were still quite unknown.

An eighth Sanitary Conference was held at Dresden in 1893, followed soon by a ninth one at Paris in 1894. At the tenth conference held in Venice in 1897, agreement was reached on a second international convention on plague (the spread of which by fleas on rats was to be discovered some years later). This conference of 21 nations also decided that an international committee should be constituted to codify the sanitary conventions and conclusions of the conferences of 1892, 1893, 1894, and 1897.

International Sanitary Conferences continued to be held periodically until the fourteenth in 1938. This conference brought to an end the international work of the Health, Maritime, and Quarantine Board that had been functioning in Alexandria (although largely under the control of the Egyptian Ministry of Health) since 1881. Later the structure that housed this Alexandria agency became the site of the Eastern Mediterranean Regional Office of the World Health Organization. Another border quarantine agency, founded in 1838 at Constantinople (now Istanbul) with field offices throughout the Ottoman Empire, was completely terminated by the League of Nations (see below) in 1923.

In 1902, as a sequel to these international quarantine efforts, the republics of Latin America, along with the United States, established the Pan-American Sanitary Bureau (PASB), with offices in Washington, D.C. The strong voice of the United States in this body was reflected in its first several Directors, each of whom was a recently retired Surgeon-General of the U.S. Public Health Service. Other leading U.S. figures continued to occupy this post until 1958, when the first Latin American health leader was chosen—Dr. Abraham Horwitz (1910–) of Chile. Since then several other notable Latin American figures have served in this role; a United States physician has always occupied a second place as Deputy-Director. In 1949 the PASB became the Regional Office for the Americas of the World Health Organization.

In addition to this long series of international conferences to halt the spread of infectious diseases, the nineteenth century spawned international congresses on other medical and related subjects. In 1867 the first general medical congress, with representatives from many nations, was held in Paris—followed every 2 years by similar meetings in Florence, Vienna,

and other European cities (except for 1887 in Washington) up to 1913 in London. International congresses on specialized health-related subjects had, in fact, been held earlier in Brussels—on statistics in 1851, demography and hygiene in 1852, and ophthalmology in 1857. Other international meetings were held in various European cities on veterinary medicine (1863), pharmacy (1865), tuberculosis (1888), dermatology (1889), psychology (1890), gynecology and obstetrics (1892), alcoholism (1894), leprosy (1897), dentistry (1900), surgery (1902), school hygiene (1904), physiotherapy (1905), cancer (1906), sleeping sickness (1907), epilepsy (1909), comparative pathology (1912), and the history of medicine (1920). These are only a sampling of the subjects of such international meetings—most of which seemed to be based on topics of interest to selected medical specialists.

THE RED CROSS AND GENEVA CONVENTIONS

Almost parallel with the International Sanitary Conferences and their development was another international initiative launched by private citizens. This was the Red Cross, founded by five leading citizens of Geneva, Switzerland in 1863. A Swiss philanthropist, J. Henri Dunant (1828–1910) had witnessed the bloody battle of Solferino (northern Italy) in 1859, and he formed the International Committee of the Red Cross—devoted to helping the wounded soldiers of any country. The impartial humanitarian spirit of the "Committée Internationale de Croix Rouge" (CICR) was closely linked to traditional Swiss neutrality in international affairs; all members and employees of the CICR, therefore, had to be Swiss citizens.

Very soon several European nations formed their own national Red Cross societies, and they met in Geneva in 1864. This First Geneva Convention agreed that "sick and wounded soldiers will be collected and cared for *irrespective of nationality.*" This remarkable impartiality was confirmed and extended at subsequent Geneva Conventions held in 1906 and 1929. The Third Convention in 1929 extended the Red Cross purposes to include help for prisoners of war and also for civilian victims of hostilities.

The several national Red Cross (and later in Moslem countries the Red Crescent) societies grew and developed during periods of peace after wars. In peacetime, they devoted their voluntary efforts to helping their own citizens in the event of various natural disasters, such as floods, hurricanes, earthquakes and fires; they also helped to care for people injured in domestic civil wars or other types of mass violence.

By the end of World War I, the national Red Cross societies, although still nongovernmental, had attained sufficient stability and recognition to be noted in the Covenant of the League of Nations (Article 25) in 1918. Then in 1919, under the leadership of the American Red Cross, there was formed, for the first time, an international League of Red Cross Societies. Initially there were member-societies from 26 countries; this grew to 113 countries in 1970 and to 164 in 1987. The League of Red Cross Societies headquarters is located in Geneva, but it is separate from the CICR, though obviously in close working relationship. The CICR is financed mainly by voluntary donations from the national societies.

The national members of the League meet every 2 years in Geneva, as a Board of Governors, with one vote per member (regardless of national population). In the Geneva secretariat there are several sections, most important of which are the Relief Bureau and the Health and Social Service Bureau. The latter has activities relating to (1) first aid and accident prevention, (2) blood transfusion services, (3) standardization of medical equipment, and (4) medical information and documentation. The League of Red Cross Societies as a whole is devoted to (1) assisting national societies in their development of programs and (2) coordinating collaborative international efforts of national societies. The League also maintains relationships with WHO and UNICEF.

OIHP AND THE LEAGUE OF NATIONS

Another milestone in international health was an agreement reached in Rome in 1907 among 23 European countries on the establishment of a permanent public health office in Europe. This was the *Office International d'Hygiene Publique* (OIHP), to be located in Paris. The functions of the "Office" concerned the collection and dissemination of new knowledge on infectious diseases that should be embodied in international quarantine regulations. The principal focus initially was on cholera, plague, and yellow fever—three diseases that had occupied the attention of the International Sanitary Conferences. Eventually OIHP had nearly 60 countries in its membership, including Persia, India, Pakistan, and the United States. French was the only official language.

Soon the concerns of OIHP were broadened to other communicable diseases, such as malaria, tuberculosis, typhoid fever, meningitis, sleeping sickness, and the overall suppression of insect vectors of disease. Interest was shown also in other public health subjects, such as food hygiene, the management of hospitals, and the hygiene of schools and factories. Although OIHP did not do any field work on these matters, it provided an international forum for their discussion among public health leaders of different nations. With the outbreak of World War I in 1914, all OIHP activities were suspended, except the publication of its *Bulletin.* Recommendations had been made to governments on environmental sanitation, notification of cases of tuberculosis, inoculation against typhoid fever, and isolation of cases of leprosy. The dissemination and discussion of such ideas had some value, in spite of no national action being taken for their implementation.

After World War I, a worldwide desire for peace resulted in the organization of the League of Nations. To carry out the League's activities relating to the "prevention and control of disease," it established a subdivision, known as the Health Organization of the League of Nations. The United States was not a member of the League, and—being a member of OIHP—it vetoed a proposal to move the Paris-based body into the League. Therefore, in 1921 there were three international agencies with very similar functions: the OIHP, the Pan American Sanitary Bureau, and the League's Health Organization. Cooperative agreements among these were obviously necessary.

After 1919, an epidemic of typhus fever

spread through Russia and Poland. Some 1,600,000 cases were reported in Russia; soon after, the unprecedented world pandemic of influenza arose, estimated to have caused as many as 15,000,000 deaths by 1920. In this catastrophic situation, an International Health Conference met in London, but it was attended by only five countries—Great Britain, France, Italy, Japan, and the United States. Eventually the Health Organization of the League of Nations became a Health Committee of the League, and of its eight members four served also as members of the Permanent Committee of the OIHP.

In spite of the diplomatic complexities of these relationships between the League's Health Committee and OIHP, several new international health activities were initiated by the League. Broadly speaking, these fell into two general categories: (1) international health studies, expert committees on selected subjects, and proposed international standards on certain issues; and (2) field assistance to countries on special health problems.

With modest funding, most League health activities were of the first type. Studies were made and expert committees appointed on major diseases (malaria, syphilis, tuberculosis, leprosy, etc.), on aspects of health care (school health service, health centers, medical care administration, health insurance, medical education, etc.), and on other matters. International classification of the "Causes of Death and Disease," the standardization of biological substances and potent drugs, and the methods of control of narcotics were solid achievements. Especially important studies were made and conferences were held on nutrition, the health aspects of housing, physical education, and the general provision of public health services in rural areas. As part of its epidemiological intelligence work in 1925 the League Health Organization set up a field office in Singapore to collect and disseminate reports on infectious diseases in the Far East.

The second main type of League health activities, on field assistance to countries, was limited by insufficient funding. In 1928, Greece was assisted in reorganizing its public health services, followed by a similar service to Bolivia. In 1929, China was assisted in developing its public health service, particularly for epidemic control. Smaller missions were sent to a few other countries, and study tours were made by health administrative officials from many countries to observe public health practices in selected European nations.

WORLD WAR II

With the invasion of Poland by Nazi Germany in 1939, the League of Nations soon collapsed and, with it, the League's Health Committee. This gave a clear lesson to the group of public health leaders, who later set out to establish a *World Health Organization* (WHO). The fate of WHO should not depend to the survival of its parent body, the United Nations. An Interim Commission was organized at an International Health Conference held in New York in 1946. The WHO Constitution drawn up by the Commission was ratified and took effect on 7 April 1948 with the signature of 26 member-states of the United Nations, but independent of the U.N. By 24 June 1948, when the first World Health Assembly, held in Geneva, Switzerland, adjourned, the WHO Constitution had 55 national signatories.

In December 1946 the United Nations General Assembly established an International Children's Emergency Fund (UNICEF) to be supported by the voluntary contributions of governments. The Interim Commission to plan a "World Health Organization" had just been formed, and the directors of the Emergency Fund did not wish to encroach on its jurisdiction. From the outset, therefore, UNICEF worked in close cooperation with WHO, using its own money essentially for the provision of supplies (food and drugs) and equipment. UNICEF is governed by an Executive Board of members from 25 countries, and comes under the general supervision of the U.N. Economic and Social Council (ECO-SOC). Although "emergency" was soon deleted from the name of UNICEF, it was retained in the acronym, and the agency's robust performance has kept it alive to the present time.

In these World War II years, other international organizations, with substantial health functions, were launched. To provide general relief, including health services, to the war-torn countries of Europe as well as to China, 43 nations formed the United Nations Relief and Rehabilitation Administration (UNRRA) in 1943. This was an intentionally temporary agency, in which representatives from the United States played a major role. The Health Division of UNRRA was transferred to WHO by a vote of its Council in 1946.

Another specialized agency of the United Nations, intended also to be temporary, was the International Refugee Organization (IRO) established in 1948. The former director of the displaced persons program in the Health Division of UNRRA was taken on the IRO executive staff, based in Geneva. In January 1949, the United Nations Assembly terminated the IRO, but continued its important work through the UN High Commissioner for Refugees (UNHCR). The UNHCR had a relatively small staff and did no international health work directly, but looked to WHO for technical advice. Health services to refugees were left in the hands of the host countries. The UNHCR still operates, with headquarters in Geneva, and works closely with WHO.

After World War II a new type of international work was developed through the initiative of the United States and several European countries—namely foreign aid from single industrialized countries to single developing countries. These *bilateral assistance programs* were designed to assist in many fields, including health service. By 1980, expenditures by most industrialized countries (principally the 17 member states of the Organization for Economic Cooperation and Development—OECD) were larger through bilateral than through multilateral programs.

Of a total of about U.S. $30 billion for all types of foreign aid in general, about $3 billion or 10 percent was earmarked for health projects. Of this amount, about one third was spent through WHO and other United Nations affiliated agencies and two-thirds through bilateral aid programs. The United States, for example, provided development assistance to 88 countries in 1980, of which health assistance applied to 60 countries. In the first postwar decades most bilateral U.S. expenditures were focused on population control through family planning, but in the latter 1970s and the 1980s U.S. policy shifted toward the support of the WHO strategy of emphasizing primary health care.

THE WORLD HEALTH ORGANIZATION AND ITS WORK

In 1948, after its first World Health Assembly, the World Health Organization took action to form a Secretariat in Geneva. It was given space for its initial years in the Palais des Nations, which had been the last home of the League of Nations. As stated in Chapter I of its Constitution, WHO was "to act as the directing and coordinating authority on international health work." This was a much broader scope than that of any other international agency in the orbit of the United Nations.

WHO's structure and functions expanded rapidly. Its program initially included activities acquired from the International Sanitary Conferences, the OIHP, the Health Committee of the League of Nations, and the Health Division of UNRRA, plus many new activities affecting the overall development of health systems in countries.

Soon after the establishment of WHO headquarters in Geneva, steps were taken to set up regional offices. The first was the South-East Asia Regional Office (SEARO), located in New Delhi, India, in January 1949. In July 1949, a second office for the Eastern Mediterranean Region (EMRO) was set up in Alexandria, Egypt, at the seat of the original pan-Arab Health, Maritime, and Quarantine Board, established previously in Alexandria.

In the same month, July 1949, negotiations with the Pan American Sanitary Bureau in Washington resulted in integration of the PASB with WHO, as the Regional Office for the Americas. In 1951, two more WHO Regional Offices were established for the Western Pacific Region, based in Manila, Philippines, and the African Region, based in Brazzaville, French Equatorial Africa—later the Republic of Congo. The last Regional Office, to be formed by the vote of a majority of its member states, was for Europe; located temporarily in

Geneva in 1952, it was moved to its final location in Copenhagen (EURO) in 1957. The WHO Constitution provides for election of the Regional Office directors by a majority of the countries in each region.

Within WHO, the highest authority is the World Health Assembly, convened once each year for about 3 weeks in May. The Assembly includes representatives of all member states—some 166 countries in 1990—with one vote each, regardless of size or financial contribution. Large countries, nevertheless, naturally have substantial influence. The Regional Boards in each of the six regions have a great deal of autonomy, since they are chosen by the countries in each region and they elect the Regional Director. In reality, the Regions tend to follow policy decisions of the global headquarters, but they are free to implement these in their own way.

Between assemblies, there are two meetings per year of an Executive Board, composed of 12 to 18 persons "technically qualified in the field of health," but not representing their own countries. The Executive Board prepares the agenda for the World Health Assemblies, and makes recommendations to the Assembly on all matters of world health policy.

For advice on almost every technical question, considered by WHO, the headquarters Secretariat appoints Expert Panels, and from these are selected Expert Committees that recommend policies. In 1990, there were expert panels on 47 subjects—for example, malaria, maternal and child health, pharmaceuticals, environmental health, medical care organization, and health manpower development—containing 2,600 persons from virtually all countries. The experts chosen for committee meetings are intended to represent all types of country concerned with the special problem discussed.

In its first decade, WHO focused major attention on specific infectious diseases afflicting millions of people in the developing countries. These included malaria, yaws, tuberculosis, and venereal diseases. There was also a high priority for maternal and child health services, for environmental sanitation (especially safe water), and for standardization of drugs and vaccines. In these years WHO developed close working relationships with other UN agencies.

The second WHO decade (1958–1968) was much influenced by the national liberation in Africa of several former colonies, which became voting members of the Organization. In 1960, the departure from the newly independent Democratic Republic of the Congo of nearly all foreign doctors, created a massive emergency. Working with the international Red Cross, WHO recruited 200 physicians and other health workers, and established a new fellowship program to enable scores of Congolese *medical assistants* to become fully qualified doctors. In this period, fellowships for health manpower development became a major WHO strategy in almost all countries.

WHO stimulated and even collaborated with the world chemical industry in the 1960s to develop new insecticides for fighting onchocerciasis ("river blindness") and for treating schistosomiasis, spread by snails. Demonstration that tuberculosis could be effectively treated, without expensive sanatorium care, was a great breakthrough of the late 1950s. Even the mundane standardization of the nomenclature of diseases and causes of death was an important contribution to international health communications.

The third WHO decade (1968–1978) included the great victory of eradicating smallpox from the earth. In 1967, smallpox was still endemic in 31 countries, afflicting 10 to 15 million people. The work was done by teams of public health workers in all the countries affected, with WHO serving as leader, coordinator, and inspiration. Millions of dollars were saved in countries by this achievement, which eliminated the need for surveillance of vaccination scars at national borders.

The momentum of this great campaign added strength to another drive, to expand the immunization of the world's children against six once-ravaging diseases—diphtheria, tetanus, whooping cough, measles, poliomyelitis, and tuberculosis (with BCG vaccine). After long hesitation for political reasons, in this period WHO finally entered the field of family planning (contraception) by promoting worldwide research and development on human reproduction. New efforts were also put into the control of malaria and leprosy. In this period WHO promoted the training of auxiliary health personnel, such as China's *barefoot doctor* and India's traditional birth attendants. Such training was a sounder investment in most developing countries than preparing physicians for predominantly urban medical practice.

The fourth decade (1978–1988) was ushered in by a great world conference of WHO and UNICEF in Alma Ata, a city in the Asiatic part of the Soviet Union. Thirty years after the birth of WHO, 134 member states of WHO reaffirmed their commitment to equity—as embodied in the slogan "Health for All." In reaction against excessive attention to high technology, the Alma Ata Conference emphasized the great importance of *primary health care*, preventive and curative, as the best approach to national health policy. This approach, stressing community participation, appropriate technology, and intersectoral collaboration, became the central pillar of world policy (see below).

In this period, every country was encouraged to develop a list of "essential drugs" for use in all public facilities, instead of the thousands of brand-name products sold in world markets. WHO's condemnation of the promotion of artificial infant formula products in developing countries also attracted worldwide attention. The control of worldwide infantile diarrhea with simple oral rehydration therapy was another great advance, based on very simple principles.

Most of the estimated 500,000 maternal deaths each year are preventable through family planning—to avoid illegal abortions—and hygienic education of traditional birth attendants. WHO has also mounted increasing efforts against cancer, which now takes as many lives in the developing countries as in the affluent ones. The fight against tobacco—the largest single cause of preventable death in both men and women—is part of WHO effort in every country. Disseminating the simple rules of diet, exercise, not smoking, prudent use of alcohol, and hygienic working conditions is a major objective of health education in WHO everywhere. The worldwide epidemic of AIDS (acquired immune deficiency syndrome) has presented another challenge to WHO in mounting global efforts to stem the spread of this lethal sexually transmitted viral disease. Underlying all these efforts is WHO's constant advisory activity to strengthen the official public health organization for health protection in all countries.

Interpreting the strategies of WHO work during its first four decades reveals a broad trend from the specific to the general. In its early years, the objectives were defined by specific diseases and conventional categories—such as preventive MCH services and environmental sanitation—within the established domain of public health. A massive crisis in the Congo led to a broader approach in one ex-colony of Africa, but the principal efforts went to the eradication of smallpox and the expanded program of immunization. In its first two decades WHO was young, perhaps fragile, and dominated by a few western industrialized countries. It was only in the third decade that the organization felt stable enough to explore the sensitive field of family planning (contraception), and even this was only to promote research in human reproduction.

It was not until the fourth decade that WHO felt strong enough to embrace a far-reaching objective of promoting worldwide equity for health. "Health for all by the year 2000" was a slogan with the broadest possible political implications. The pathway to this goal was through *primary health care,* which included all principal strategies of prevention, as well as appropriate treatment of common diseases and injuries. The implications of this approach were not concealed, but called frankly for community participation and political commitment. No longer did WHO confine its interest to purely technical matters, but addressed openly the countless issues surrounding the organization of national health systems in every country.

In the fourth decade, after 1978, the great majority of WHO member-states were young developing countries. No longer were policies dictated by a handful of western powers. The

United Nations was firmly established and, even in the Security Council, veto power rested with the Soviet Union and the People's Republic of China, as well as with the United States, France, and the United Kingdom. Among the several U.N. specialized agencies, WHO was probably the most universally respected. Its performance had won plaudits from countries of every political persuasion. Its Director-General at the time was an unhesitant idealist, born in a small country (Denmark) from a missionary family. The Regional Committees had become an additional source of political expression, and five of the six were dominated by developing countries. To these countries, dramatic national health problems were more important than the ideologies of European or American medical associations.

Cooperation of WHO with other specialized agencies of the U.N. has been effective in avoiding jurisdictional disputes. Cooperation with the International Labour Office (located also in Geneva) has concerned activities in occupational health and in the health aspects of social security programs. Regarding nutrition and control of animal diseases (zoonoses), there is substantial cooperation with the Food and Agriculture Organization (FAO), headquartered in Rome. School health programs and the health education of teachers involve cooperative relations with the U.N. Educational, Scientific, and Cultural Organization (UNESCO), based in Paris. Collaborative arrangements were even made with the International Civil Aviation Organization (ICAO) on the disinfection of aircraft landing across national borders.

Official relationships were also established between WHO and various international nongovernmental organizations (NGOs). Important among these is the International Committee of the Red Cross and the League of Red Cross Societies, but there are hundreds of others in special fields. Under the sponsorship of WHO and UNESCO, an overall NGO was established for maintaining relationships with various scientific bodies. It is known as the Council for International Organizations of the Medical Sciences (CIOMS), and its headquarters office is in the WHO building in Geneva. The 62 international members of the CIOMS

are reviewed every 2 years by WHO officials. Members of CIOMS include such NGOs as the World Federation for Mental Health, the International Planned Parenthood Federation, the World Medical Association, and the International Council of Nurses.

ALMA ATA AND PRIMARY HEALTH CARE

The International Conference on Primary Health Care, held in Alma Ata, has been noted. Out of this conference was issued the Declaration of Alma Ata, which states, among other things, that

> A main social target of governments, international organizations and the whole world community in the coming decades should be the attainment by all peoples of the world by the year 2000 of a level of health that will permit them to lead a socially and economically productive life.

This *primary health care* approach called for attention to major health promotive, preventive, and elementary treatment aspects of common disorders. Several overall strategies were emphasized, such as appropriate technology, community participation, and coordination of health work with other social sectors (education, agriculture, housing, etc.) or intersectoral collaboration. The governments of nearly all countries soon affirmed their support of this primary health care approach in their national health systems.

The Alma Ata Declaration reaffirmed the high priority that countries should give to at least eight well-established programs of health promotion and protection. These were listed fully in Chapter 12. As this array of primary health care elements were discussed, an even broader range of health activities was encompassed. As back-up for PHC there had to be small general hospitals at the *first referral level*. Community health workers, with training of only a few months, had to be prepared in large numbers for work in rural districts. In district hospitals or health centers for ambulatory care, appropriate simple laboratory and even X-ray equipment should be understood by PHC workers, if only for appropriate referral to other resources.

GENERAL PRINCIPLES OF INTERNATIONAL HEALTH WORK

By the late 1980s, several basic principles for international health work had become widely accepted by the World Health Organization and other agencies in the United Nations family. Abiding by these principles helps to explain the high respect accorded to WHO and UNICEF throughout the world and especially in the developing countries:

1. International health work in any country is done only at the invitation of the country. Multinational agencies are established by member states and have no supranational authority.
2. All international civil servants must be devoted only to the agency in which they work, not to their country of origin.
3. An international health agency must respond to requests for help, without regard to the political ideology of the government in power. It must not pass judgment on the ethical values of that government. (An exception to this policy has been applied to South Africa, because of its extremely unjust racial policies embodied in *apartheid*.)
4. The development of national health systems has become generally recognized as contributing to overall social and economic development. Healthy people are able to contribute more effectively to national productivity than people handicapped by disease and disability.
5. The health of a population is influenced by all social sectors, not only by the health services. Health objectives, therefore, demand the greatest possible emphasis on intersectoral collaboration.
6. In determining priorities among the countless health problems observed in all countries, the highest priority should be assigned to problems affecting the largest number of people. This criterion calls for less emphasis on high technology tertiary hospitals and greater emphasis on primary health care in all countries.
7. International health policies should promote national health systems that ensure the most equitable distribution of health services—preventive and curative—to all people.
8. While motivated initially by the objective of stopping the spread of communicable diseases, international health work has become increasingly concerned with all aspects of health and health services in countries. The promotion of world health is recognized as being dependent on the prudent use of all types of health resources, the control of all types of disease and disability, and the provision of adequate economic support.

The heightened appreciation of international health work is matched, of course, by a greater recognition of the value of health services in virtually all countries. In the early decades of the twentieth century, health and medical activities, as reflected in national expenditures, absorbed only 1 to 5 percent of national wealth (measured by gross national product or GNP). The fraction was greater in the more industrialized countries and less in the less developed countries, where so much had to be spent on food and shelter. As the potentialities of the health sciences expanded after World War II (around 1945), the share of GNP devoted to health systems increased almost everywhere—to a level of 6 to 11 percent in the affluent countries and 2 to 5 percent in the developing countries.

These higher expenditures were both a cause and a result of collectivized methods of financing, through general taxation and earmarked social insurance funding. They also provoked greater political interest in cost containment through increasing the efficiency of health systems, deliberate planning of the supply of various health resources (personnel and facilities), and controlling the demand for services through different types of cost-sharing by patients. In all but a few industrialized countries, most health expenditures came from government, and therefore served to make health services economically accessible to nearly everyone. In many of the poorest developing countries, however, governmental programs were seriously inadequate, and most health expenditures came from the private sector, with great resultant inequities.

Toward the end of the twentieth century, these inequities became a major concern of international health work—a far cry from the original narrow focus on border quarantine. The World Health Organization, the World Bank, UNICEF, and other international agencies have become concerned about how each country organizes and operates its own national health system. The horizon of good health is continually expanding, so that national health systems must become broader and stronger to achieve their goal.

One may wonder how this mounting interest in the overall national health system of each country has affected the "global" role of WHO. Has this focus constituted a departure from the sense of national interdependence that generated, for example, the early conventions to halt the spread of infectious disease? Not at all. In the modern world, the claim that "disease knows no borders" has become a cliché that no mature health leader repeats. The goal today is how to ensure *within* all countries—rich or poor, large or small—the full health benefits of modern science and civilization. This is not to avert the transmission of cholera from Asia to Europe, but to enrich the lives of Asian people for their own sake. "One world" should mean endowing each country with the resources and strategies to achieve maximum health for all its people. At this stage in world history, national sovereignty is still respected. Within this reality, the goal of world health means that all the people of every country will have equal opportunity to attain "the highest possible level of health."

REFERENCES

Aitken, J. T., H.W.C. Fuller, and D. Johnson (Editors), *The Influence of Christians in Medicine.* London: Christian Medical Fellowship, 1984.

Allan, Ted, and Sydney Gordon, *The Scalpel the Sword: The Story of Norman Bethune.* Boston: Little, Brown, 1952.

Arnold, David (Editor), *Imperial Medicine and Indigenous Societies.* Manchester (England): Manchester University Press, 1988.

Beck, Ann, *A History of the British Medical Administration of East Africa, 1900–1950.* Cambridge, MA: Harvard University Press, 1970.

Black, Maggie, *The Children and the Nations: The Story of UNICEF.* New York: UNICEF, 1986.

Council for International Organization of the Medical Sciences, *Organization, Activities, Members.* Geneva: CIOMS, 1989.

Dayton, Edward R. *Medicine and Missions: A Survey of Medical Missions.* Wheaton, IL: Medical Assistance Program, 1969.

Garrison, Fielding H., *An Introduction to the History of Medicine,* Fourth Edition. Philadelphia: W.B. Saunders, 1966, p. 789.

Goodman, Neville M. *International Health Organizations and Their Work.* London: Churchill Livingstone, 1971.

Howard, Lee M., "International Sources of Financial Cooperation for Health in Developing Countries." *Bulletin of the Pan American Health Organization,* 17(2):142–156, 1983.

Howard-Jones, Norman, *The Scientific Background of the International Sanitary Conferences 1851–1938.* Geneva: World Health Organization, 1975.

Howard-Jones, Norman, *International Public Health between the Two World Wars—The Organizational Problems.* Geneva: World Health Organization, 1978.

Howard-Jones, Norman, *The Pan American Health Organization: Origins and Evolution.* Geneva: World Health Organization, 1981.

Hume, Edward H., *Doctors Courageous.* New York: Harper, 1950.

Kanagaratnam, Kandiah, "The Concern and Contribution of the World Bank in Population Planning." *International Journal of Health Services,* 3(4):708–718, 1973.

Kohn, R., and S. Radius, "International Comparison of Health Services Systems: An Annotated Bibliography." *International Journal of Health Services,* 3(2):295–309, 1973.

Linsenmeyer, William S., "Foreign Nations, International Organizations, and Their Impact on Health Conditions in Nicaragua since 1979." *International Journal of Health Services,* 19(3):509–529, 1989.

Macleod, R. M., and Milton Lewis (Editors), *Disease, Medicine and Empire: Perspectives on Western Medicine and the Experience of European Expansion.* London: Routledge, 1988.

Mahler, Halfdan, "Health for All by the Year 2000." *World Health,* 2:3–5, February–March 1981.

Morgan, M., *Doctors to the World.* New York: Viking Press, 1958.

Musgrove, Philip, "The Impact of the Economic Crisis on Health and Health Care in Latin America and the Caribbean." *WHO Chronicle,* 40(4):152–147, 1986.

Ravenholt, Reinert T., "United States Agency for International Development (USAID) Contributions to International Population Programs."

International Journal of Health Services, 3(4):641–660, 1973.

Roemer, Milton I. *The Organization of Medical Care under Social Security.* Geneva: International Labour Office, 1969.

Salas, Rafael M., "The United Nations Fund for Population Activities." *International Journal of Health Services,* 3(4):679–692, 1973.

Turshen, Meredeth, "The Impact of Colonialism on Health and Health Services in Tanzania." *International Journal of Health Services,* 7(1):7–35, 1977.

Williams, Glen, "WHO—The Days of the Mass Campaigns." *World Health Forum,* 9:7–23, 1988.

World Health Organization, *The First Ten Years of the World Health Organization.* Geneva: WHO, 1958.

World Health Organization, *The Second Ten Years of the World Health Organization 1958–1967.* Geneva: WHO, 1968.

CHAPTER EIGHTEEN

World Trends in Health Systems

There is abundant evidence that in spite of all the difficulties, the health systems of the world are contributing to improved health in the population. Exploration of the reasons for this is a large subject, and we shall consider them along different lines. Because of the great problems in acquiring data from recent years, the review of trends must generally apply up to about the mid-1980s.

First, we consider health improvements in the world from 1950 to 1980, and their association with government health activity. Then we explore the basic social trends responsible for these improvements, as well as comparative data on public spending for health in different types of systems. Next we review trends in each of the five major components of health systems. Finally, we explore progress toward the WHO goal of "Health for All."

GLOBAL HEALTH 1950–1980

The shocking differences in health status between the rich and poor countries of the world have been widely noted and analyzed. Here we want to examine health *trends* in recent decades in both types of country and consider the reasons for them.

Health Improvements

In the early 1980s life expectancy at birth in Africa was about 51 years, in Latin America it was 64 years, and in all economically developed countries of the world it was more than 72 years.

Infants born in Africa in the early 1980s died at the rate of 116 per 1,000 live births per year, in Latin America at the rate of 63 per 1,000 live births, and in the United States and Canada at the rate of 12 per 1,000 live births. Within each of these regions, of course, there are substantial differences in the mortality rates of various countries and different social classes. Very affluent families of Africa or India, for example, may have a better health record than the very poorest families of the United States, but the figures apply to averages calculated for total populations.

In spite of these differentials, the great progress made in health status by the vast majority of developing countries over the last 40 or 50 years may not be so widely recognized. Continuing gaps in health between the industrialized and developing countries should not obscure our recognition of the accomplishments in both types of setting. The struggles of health workers and countless others, often against great odds, have not been in vain.

Measurements of population health status in most countries, especially showing historical trends, are not plentiful. Except for a few highly industrialized countries, data are limited largely to infant death rates and life expectancies at birth. Although mortality figures are representative of only the tip of the iceberg in the vast structure of human health, they are still widely recognized as reflections of social well-being in a larger sense.

According to data gathered by official international agencies, in Africa—composed almost entirely of European colonies in 1950—over the 30-year period from 1950–1955 to 1980–1985, life expectancy at birth rose from 38.0 to 49.9 years. In South Asia (largely India and Pakistan), it increased over this 30-year period from 38.8 to 54.4 years. The equivalent trend in Latin America was 51.2 to 64.5 years.

Trends in infant mortality can also be reported for the 30-year span from 1950–1955 to 1980–1985. Over these three decades the rate declined in Africa from 187 to 116, in South Asia from 189 to 113, and in Latin America from 126 to 63 infant deaths per 1,000 live births. The great decline of Europe's infant mortality from 62 to 15 deaths per 1,000 live births over the same period should not downgrade the achievements of developing countries in saving even greater numbers of infant lives.

The worldwide economic difficulties of the 1980s and persistent high military expenditures have slowed down the development of organized health programs in many countries. One might expect that health status measurements would reflect these deficiencies. Yet, to the present, significant evidence of health declines in the developing countries is lacking. Thus between 1982 and 1987 in Africa's largest country, Nigeria, the infant mortality rate declined further from 120 to 106 deaths per 1,000 live births; in Latin America's largest country, Brazil, it declined from 70 to 64 deaths per 1,000 live births; and in India, with more than 800,000,000 mostly impoverished people, infant mortality declined from 120 to 100 deaths per 1,000 live births.

Such data are not intended to belittle the tragic discrepancies in the nutrition, well-being, and survival of infants, children, women, and men in the developing countries, compared with others. The application of current epidemiological knowledge in Africa, Asia, and Latin America could soon save millions of lives. But the overall trends are, nevertheless, real.

These trends are not easy to interpret in view of the enormous problems not only in health systems but also in the overall living conditions of people. One might only speculate that the improvements achieved over the previous few decades in quality of life, including the health services, have persisted in spite of economic setbacks. This surely does not apply to all countries and all people in a country, but evidently to enough people to affect regional and national averages. What then is the explanation for these remarkable improvements in the health of people in developing countries?

Determinants of Improved Health

Three major types of change have contributed to improved health status in developing countries since World War II: (1) social and economic development, (2) international and cross-national influences, and (3) the impacts of national health systems.

Social and Economic Development. A central fact of global society after World War II was the independence achieved by former European colonies. Nearly all of the dependent lands of Africa and Asia—usually after massive struggles—became sovereign nations, running their own affairs. The world's largest country, China, made a revolution from semicolonial and feudal status to a self-reliant form of socialism. After initial turmoil, these national liberations led to countless social changes. Transformation from colonial to independent status is reflected by changes in the work done by people. Between 1965 and 1986, the proportion of the labor force in developing countries engaged in agriculture declined, whereas the share in industry and services increased.

Economic productivity worldwide has been increasing. From 1965 to 1987 the gross domestic product (GDP) per capita in developing countries as a whole has been growing each year. Another reflection of economic development is the consumption of energy. Between 1965 and 1986, in the middle-income developing countries commercial energy consumption per capita has nearly doubled; in the low-income countries it has nearly tripled. These data on trends do not tell us about the distribution of economic benefits within countries or the differentials between developing countries, but they do document overall economic advancement that contributes to health status.

Social improvements have been even more dramatic. Virtually every developing country is becoming increasingly urbanized. Around the edge of the large cities, however, miserable periurban slums arise. In spite of early difficulties, in the long run urban life yields many advantages for employment, education, health, and other social benefits. In developing countries city populations have better health status than rural populations, especially with regard to infant death rates.

The effects of strengthened education in developing countries have been enormous. For all countries, classified by the United Nations as "least developed," the adult literacy rate rose from 19.4 percent in 1970 to 32.4 percent in 1980. Concerning the status of women—a crucial reflection of overall social development—the number of females per 100 males in primary schools has increased markedly. The mother's educational level, of course, is generally recognized as a major determinant of infant survival.

Cross-National Influences. The second major determinant of improved health in developing countries has been international exchange in the broadest sense. This exchange has occurred in three forms: (1) increased trade among countries, (2) the spread of useful technology, and (3) worldwide affirmation of human rights.

The growth of international trade has brought to developing countries machinery for industrial production, for construction, for environmental sanitation, for improved agricultural methods, and for modern transport and communication. Such industry, housing, sanitation, agricultural output, and so on obviously contribute to overall standards of living, which have substantial long-term impacts on health. Between 1970 and 1986, the developing countries with market economies had nearly a fivefold increase in their foreign trade. Not that all foreign trade has been beneficial for health. One cannot overlook the U.S. policy of forcing developing countries to buy its own products, including tobacco, as a condition for accepting (without trade barriers) products exported from those countries.

The *spread of technology* to the developing countries has been vast and pervasive. Malaria has not been eradicated, but in many countries it has been greatly reduced, as a result of DDT developed in Switzerland and other chemical pesticides. Although the eradication strategy of the 1960s has been replaced by the approach of primary health care, vector control by appropriate techniques remains an important component of malaria control.

Penicillin, first discovered in England and followed by generations of other antibiotics produced in America and Europe, has prevented countless deaths and disabilities. The worldwide eradication of smallpox, of course, required sophisticated planning, organization, and intercountry cooperation far more than an effective vaccine; yet the international availability of such a vaccine was essential. The elimination of crippling poliomyelitis is another goal now in sight because of innovative immunological research in the United States.

The term *technology* may bring to mind magnetic resonance imaging (MRI) and other forms of sophisticated diagnostic equipment that is seldom affordable in developing countries. But the misuse of some technology should not block our recognition of the benefits of appropriate technology that has benefitted millions of people. This would include improved and effective methods of contraception, of techniques for obtaining safe drinking water, of low-cost refrigeration, of efficient transport and communication, of fertilizers and pesticides used cautiously to enhance agriculture and nutrition, and of the new therapeutic agents that can effectively treat leprosy, schistosomiasis, trachoma, onchocerciasis (river blindness), and other scourges of the developing world, once regarded as hopeless.

The third form of international exchange, worldwide affirmation of *human rights*, may seem less concrete than trade and technology, but its influence has been profound. For several centuries there has been a certain competition in all countries between two concepts of health service. Health care has been regarded on the one hand as a commodity for buying and selling in the market, and on the other hand as an obligation of society—a human right. The differences between these two concepts are subtle but strong. In the late nineteenth and twentieth centuries, the conception of health services as a social entitlement and human right has gained ascendancy in most of the world.

After World War I, the Versailles Treaty gave birth to the International Labor Organization (ILO) in 1919, based on the principle: "peace through social justice" (see Chapter 17). The ILO became the principal world body to promote social security for the protection of people against various hazards, including sickness. After World War II, the United Nations went further. A major purpose of the U.N., defined in its Charter, is "to promote and encourage respect for human rights and for fundamental freedoms for all, without discrimination as to race, sex, language, or religion."

To implement this broad purpose, in 1948 the U.N. adopted its Universal Declaration of Human Rights, which provides that

> Everyone has the right to a standard of living adequate for the health and well-being of himself and of his family, including food, clothing, housing and medical care and necessary social services, and the right to security in the event of unemployment, sickness, disability, widowhood, old age or other lack of livelihood in circumstances beyond his control.

Many other international documents reaffirm the right to health protection. The Constitution of the World Health Organization (1948) sets the objective of the attainment by all peoples of the highest possible level of health and states that "Governments have a responsibility for the health of their people which can be fulfilled only by the provision of adequate health and social measures." In 1978, 30 years after its founding, the World Health Organization, UNICEF, and WHO member states reaffirmed at Alma Ata that "health . . . is a fundamental human right."

Impact of National Health Systems. The maturation of national health systems is the third major force contributing to the improved health of people, seen in developing countries since the end of World War II. In virtually all developing countries, human and physical resources for health have been expanding more rapidly than the growth of populations. Increased personnel has meant not only more professional doctors and nurses, but many new forms of medical assistants and community health workers. The WHO concept of *primary health care* has influenced national policy in most developing countries, even though large hospitals remain politically attractive. Primary health care is intended to implement principles of health equity and social justice.

Systematic organizational networks have helped to disseminate health service to the provinces, districts, and communities throughout the nations of Africa, Asia, and Latin America. Rational health planning and effective management may not be successfully achieved in many countries, but they are processes that almost all governments want to employ. Health services are being provided increasingly by teams of personnel working in health stations, health centers, polyclinics, and hospitals—usually interrelated in some type of regional framework.

To finance these health resources, programs, and services, developing countries are devoting larger shares of their national wealth to the health system. Around 1950 total health expenditures in developing countries were typically 1–3 percent of gross national product (GNP). In the 1980s, health expenditures in these countries were more often 3–5 percent of GNP. Much of this increase has come from private spending, even though greater amounts have also been collectively mobilized, usually through government. This varies with the political ideology of the national health system.

General evidence of the association of governmental health programs with health status may be inferred from the relationship of health expenditures by government to life expectancy at birth in countries throughout the world. The strong association of overall national wealth, as reflected in gross national product (GNP) per capita, with health status is widely recognized. My own research in 1986 showed that life expectancy in 142 countries correlated positively with the country's GNP per capita (Pearson $r = 0.658$). Correlation of total health expenditures by government—at all levels and by all public agencies—as a percent of GNP with life expectancy in the 134 countries on which 1986 data were available was virtually the same (Pearson $r = 0.635$). Private sector health spending does not contribute to this high correlation.

SOCIAL TRENDS

Several broad social trends affecting all national health systems were summarized in Volume I. They apply here as a background for examining world trends. In various countries they differ in degree, of course, but the directions are clear.

Urbanization and Industrialization

Countries at all stages of economic development have become increasingly urbanized. Between 1965 and 1985, the urban population increased in affluent industrialized and capitalist countries from 70 to 75 percent, in formerly socialist countries from 52 to 65 percent, in middle-income developing countries from 37 to 48 percent, and in low income (or "very poor") countries from 17 to 22 percent. The squalor and misery of large city slums are well known—the central-city slums in the megacities of affluent countries and the periurban slums around the metropolitan clusters in developing countries. Yet urban life eventually yields many advantages over life in miserable rural villages in terms of employment, education, transport, energy, health care, and other social services.

Parallel with urbanization, almost every country has to some degree increased the proportion of its labor force working in industry and services versus agriculture. Between 1965 and 1980, this was obvious in all the industrialized countries—both under free market and centrally planned economies. Even in the developing countries this was the trend. In middle-income developing countries the percentage of nonagricultural workers rose from 44 to 57 between 1965 and 1980. In the lowest income developing countries, this percentage rose from 23 to 28.

These trends are doubtless a reflection of the decolonization occurring after World War II in Asia, Africa, and elsewhere. They imply much more than a change in type of work. They have meant that many countries produced less raw material for export to industrial powers and produced more goods and services for their own people. This has contributed to a spirit of pride in national independence. It has led to trade unionism, social class consciousness, and many types of democratic demands for self-determination and social advancement.

With urbanization, the conditions for effective public schools are greatly improved. The effects of strengthened educational systems almost everywhere in the world have been enormous. The advances have been greatest in the primary school years, but even in the secondary school years and at the university level progress has been measurable. The achievements of certain countries—with strong political commitment to popular education—have been spectacular, and the levels of adult literacy have risen almost everywhere.

Governmental Structure

Since decolonization and the extension of self-government, the infrastructure of public authority has become strengthened. Even though governments in many developing countries fell under military dictatorships, this did not always obstruct (sometimes it even facilitated) the establishment of a framework of governance. Of 113 major developing countries in 1987, 59 (or 52 percent) were essentially under military control. This usually meant forceful repression of human rights, elimination of democratic voting procedures, and various sorts of corruption.

At the same time, in these countries and in the other 48 percent of developing nations, some framework of central as well as regional and local government was usually established. Whatever the principles of authority may have been in the health system—highly centralized, decentralized, or some combination of these—a viable governmental infrastructure can usually be helpful. Lines of authority in the health system, especially in the Ministry of Health, are ordinarily parallel with those in the general governmental structure. There may be different channels for policy decisions, however, on administrative matters and on technical questions.

International Trade

When countries engage in international trade, it can generally benefit their social and economic development, although interpretation of the exact consequences is always difficult. World Bank reports indicate that developing countries, on the whole, have engaged in foreign trade that seems to have contributed to their development. Thus, between 1965 and

1986, all middle-income developing countries reduced their imports of food from 15 to 10 percent of their total imports; meanwhile they increased their imports of machinery and transport equipment from 30 to 33 percent of the total. Data for China and India are unfortunately lacking, but in the other low-income developing countries, food imports declined from 19 to 14 percent of the total between 1965 and 1986, whereas machinery imports rose from 29 to 32 percent of the total. (Over these years, we know that China and India increased their food production immensely, and also imported machinery on a vast scale.) In the industrialized countries, the same differentials favoring the import of machinery were even more striking.

This sort of international trade has many implications for health systems. Machinery includes equipment for drilling wells and making pipes for environmental sanitation. Agricultural equipment can contribute to better nutrition, and construction equipment can multiply human dwelling units. Machinery may also include equipment for manufacturing and packaging pharmaceutical products. All sorts of basic diagnostic and therapeutic instruments in hospitals and health centers can be fabricated if the proper equipment is available. This should not imply excessive technology, but even the simplest primary health care requires certain basic instruments for clinics and laboratories. Proper maintenance, however, is always difficult.

Demographic Changes

The worldwide reduction in infant mortality and the crude birth rate, combined with the longer survival of elderly people, has contributed to *demographic transitions* in most countries. The health burden of the elderly is much greater than that of children, so that the problem perceived is usually described as the graying of the population.

If the number of people over 65 years of age is related to those 20 to 64 years, one derives a *dependency ratio*. On the basis of U.S. Census Bureau forecasts, this ratio in the United States was 20.5 percent in 1985 and will climb to 34.8 percent in the year 2025. In Great Britain over these years the ratio will change from 26.2 percent in 1985 to 32.8 in 2025. The same sort of increased ratio (or "burden" on the working population) applies to virtually all industrialized countries. More surprisingly it applies to most developing countries as well, though less consistently. If the smaller proportions of children are considered, as part of the dependent population, the change in dependency ratio everywhere is less marked.

All these basic social trends, quite prominent in the modern world, have significant implications for health systems, although some are indirect. In addition, several other major developments may be identified within the conventional boundaries of national health systems. The precise form and extent of these trends vary tremendously, of course, across systems. Yet, if we conceive of them very broadly, one finds numerous developments or tendencies that have shaped the characteristics of virtually all national health systems over the course of recent decades.

Demands for Privatization

Larger political events, maturing in the 1980s, stimulated a worldwide movement for privatization of health services. It was seen in welfare-oriented health systems, as a reaction against high taxes for social benefits. It was dramatically demonstrated in the wholesale rejection of socialism in Eastern Europe. Even in developing countries, it was seen in the main cities among middle-class people. The World Bank has promoted privatization. Although the vast bulk of any country's health expenditures is for medical care (not organized prevention), the World Bank has advocated that "most curative care, whether provided by the government or nongovernment sector, should be paid for by those who receive the care." The Bank contends that this policy will reduce government expenditures, limit inflation, and permit government funds to be used for the most needy.

The private sector in national health systems, however, has had largely antiegalitarian effects. The contention that private spending releases government health funds for the poor simply ignores the inequities of private claims on scarce social resources. As expressed in a WHO/UNICEF "Joint Health Policy" study of 1981:

> The private medical sector absorbs scarce health personnel trained mainly at the state's expense. It is predominantly curative in character, and its expensive practices lead . . . to inflated medical expenditure (and) . . . excessive foreign exchange cost for pharmaceuticals. . . . It has negative influence on medical education. . . . Private medicine undermines . . . attempts to rationalize . . . procedures on a cost-effective basis. . . . For these reasons the private medical sector now has negative effects on primary health care implementation.

In July 1989 the United Nations Economic Commission for Africa issued a scathing attack on the policies of the International Monetary Fund and the World Bank to increase the role of the private sector. Such programs, the U.N. Commission said, have often led to lower standards of living . . . to deindustrialization, poorer health, and falling educational standards.

It must be appreciated, furthermore, that the major health gains of developing countries in recent decades have come from actions by governments. Insofar as health services (both curative and preventive) have been more equitably distributed to rural and urban populations, to children, to the unemployed, and to the poor, it has depended on public action. This applies not only to functions inside health systems, but also to the broader sphere of socioeconomic development and international exchanges discussed earlier. The claim that private management of health services is more efficient than public management has been frequently asserted, but comparative studies in America have shown this to be false.

No one realistically expects to abolish the private sector from most national health systems in the modern world (although this has been attempted in certain African countries). But surely it could be kept to a minimal tolerable level, in the interests of health equity. Private resources may sometimes be used by public agencies and paid to provide public services. The solution to poor quality government health services, however, is not to privatize them, but rather to heighten the priority and enhance the support of governmental activities for advancement of health.

Public Expenditures and System Type

So much of the progress in health systems has come from the expanding role of government that this should be examined in more detail. To quantify the degree of government intervention in a private market of health services, embodied in the national health system, we can make use of data on total *governmental* health expenditures reported in a country. (It must be realized that the private market is a residual domain within the "organization" component of any national health system, but it is not shown here.) These figures on government health spending are drawn from the World Bank, the International Monetary Fund, the Organization for Economic Cooperation and Development (OECD) in Paris, and certain other official sources. Such government health expenditures include not only those of the Ministry of Health, but also of social security for health care, the health outlays

Economic Level of Countries	Health System Policies			
	Entrepreneurial	Welfare-oriented	Comprehensive	Socialist
Industrialized (high)	United States	France	Sweden	Soviet Union
Transitional (middle)	Philippines	Brazil	Costa Rica	Cuba
Very poor (low)	Ghana	Burma	Sri Lanka	China

Figure 18.1. Examples of national health systems: classified by economic levels and health policies, around 1986.

of other public agencies, health expenditures at provincial and local levels of government, and so on—all public expenditures for health but not those of the private sector. If we relate these public expenditures to the GNP—a measure of total national wealth, not simply the commonly used figure for total government spending—we derive a rough measure of the degree of government responsibility borne within the overall national health system.

We can explore the relationship between government health expenditures and the type of health system in a country by examining selected countries. This is done in Figure 18.1 according to the typology of national health systems developed in Volume I. The country in each cell is believed to be a fair example of the type conceptualized in that cell.

Then, in Figure 18.2 there is a graphic presentation of the total government health expenditures as a share of the country's GNP. These expenditures vary strikingly with the

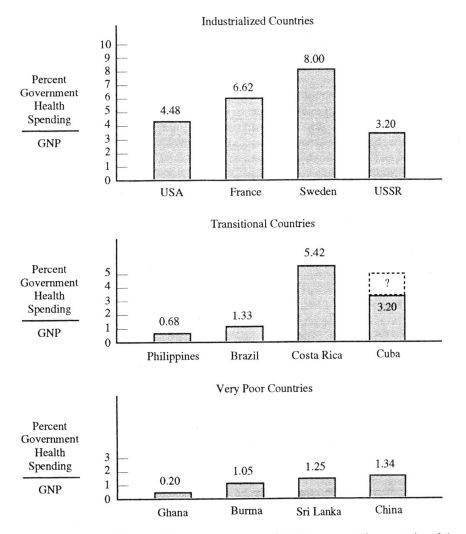

Figure 18.2. Government health expenditures as percentage of GNP: representative countries of three economic levels, 1986.

type of national health system. In industrialized countries, expenditures rise steadily from the entrepreneurial to the welfare oriented to the comprehensive system types, then decline in the socialist type. In the economically transitional countries, the same sequence is repeated. (For Cuba, the extended bar is intended to show the influence of indirect Soviet aid.) In the very poor countries, the gradient of health expenditures is slightly upward in all four system types, although the total health expenditures are relatively small.

The precise political and economic determinants of national health systems are, of course, much more complicated than this simplified analysis would suggest. Moreover, every health system is continually changing. Over the last 50 or 60 years there has been a verifiable movement of systems from the entrepreneurial toward the welfare oriented and then toward the comprehensive model of health system structure and function.

Since the upheavals in the socialist countries of Eastern Europe brought dramatically to the surface in 1989 and 1990, and also in the socialist economies of Asia and Africa, no further movement to the public side has occurred. Instead, in many formerly socialist countries, we are now seeing a movement in the other direction—that is, toward the comprehensive model of a health system. In this nonsocialist model, the entire population is entitled to comprehensive health service through various strategies other than socialist government control of all human and physical resources.

TRENDS IN HEALTH SYSTEM COMPONENTS

We may now take stock of the principal trends in each of the main components of health systems. As a result of basic social trends, public expenditures, and several other tendencies reviewed above, changes have been occurring in all national health systems. Taking a perspective going back to about 1900, one finds tremendous ferment in all system components. We analyze this under the five components formulated in Volume I: health resources, organization of programs, economic support, management, and delivery of health services.

Health Resources

All health services depend on resources of four types: personnel, facilities, commodities, and knowledge.

Personnel. The supply of doctors has been increasing throughout the world. Medical schools have been multiplying. The medical profession has become increasingly specialized. There is worldwide migration, with doctors moving from developing to industrialized countries (a brain drain). Continuing education is increasing to keep doctors informed about new advances. A dichotomy has taken shape between general practitioners in communities and specialists in hospitals. A reaction to specialization has occurred in recognizing *family practice* as a specialty.

Equitable geographic distribution of doctors within a country is a worldwide problem. It is most severe in developing countries, where large percentages of doctors (60 to 70 percent) settle in the national capital, with perhaps 10 to 20 percent of the population; the rest of the country is obviously medically starved. To a lesser extent this geographic imbalance occurs also in industrialized countries. Numerous strategies have been applied to reduce this problem. Now medical graduates are required to serve for a period with the Ministry of Health. Settlement in the capital city is barred for a certain number of years. Special amenities and financial rewards are offered for rural settlement. Immigrant physicians are granted entry to a country on condition that they settle in an area of great need. These and other strategies, however, have had only a limited impact on the problem.

The supply of nurses in the world is also rapidly expanding. Their functions are broadening from being the doctor's helper to independent caregiver in hospitals, clinics, and patient homes. In many countries their role as health leaders is being recognized.

The use of paramedical personnel or medical assistants, trained for 2 or 3 years, to replace doctors in both rural areas and urban health centers is increasing. They undergo a variety of training programs, and many specialize.

Community health workers are trained for very brief periods (3 to 6 months) to provide primary health care in developing countries, especially in rural areas. Proper supervision is sometimes lacking, but they have undoubtedly expanded coverage in very poor countries.

Traditional healers, not to be confused with conventionally trained personnel, are being recognized as a resource in Asia and Africa. Although mostly in private practice, in some countries certain healers are integrated into the government program.

Many other types of health personnel are expanding in health systems. Dental care involves not only dentists, but also school dental nurses, dental hygienists, and others. There are many types of laboratory, X-ray, and related technicians. The field of environmental sanitation has service from sanitarians and inspectors. Although this field is marked by serious shortages, the numbers are still expanding in developing countries.

The developing countries obviously have vast needs for innovative types of health manpower. The multiplication of conventional physicians and nurses is no longer appropriate. A WHO study on *International Development of Health Manpower Policy* (1982) showed that in the 32 years from 1948 to 1980, policy priorities evolved through eight steps with the following objectives:

1. Greater quantity of conventional personnel
2. Higher quality of medical and nursing education
3. Equality of credentials, cross-nationally
4. Greater geographic coverage in countries
5. Greater efficiency of health personnel
6. Planning of health manpower development
7. Relevance of health personnel to the needs
8. Integration of health manpower and health services

Implementation of these WHO policies was not in eight separate periods, but dovetailed across the 32 years, so that several policies are found at one time. The last four or five policies all prevailed during the most recent decade.

Facilities. Hospitals and the ratio to population of hospital beds are increasing almost everywhere, especially in developing countries.

In industrialized countries they are reaching a plateau, as other forms of facility are replacing the institution with beds. In all countries, general hospitals are assuming the roles formerly played by special hospitals.

The internal organization of hospitals is becoming increasingly structured. Pavilions with their own laboratory, pharmacy, X-ray, and so on are restructured into integrated facilities served by central technical services. Medical staff organization of hospitals has become dominated by full-time salaried staffs, rather than being open to every local doctor. Problems have developed between the elite hospital doctors and general practitioners in the community, although there are many approaches to break down this barrier.

Health centers, polyclinics, and other facilities for ambulatory care are the major new facilities of the twentieth century. In developing countries, they are the physical foundation of all organized ambulatory health services. Under Ministries of Health, thousands of health centers have been built to cover both rural areas and cities. Facilities of social security programs providing direct care, as in Latin America, have also increased. Ordinarily in rural areas there are hierarchies of main health centers, subcenters, and small health posts. The large health centers may have one or more physicians, but staffing is mainly by medical assistants and nurses. Much of the service is to expectant mothers and infants, but all types of patients are seen.

In the industrialized countries, health centers are generally a special innovation, but they are expanding. In the British NHS, about 35 percent of general practitioners are located in health centers, and in Sweden and Finland it is nearly 100 percent. The Italian NHS is established predominantly on the basis of health centers (local health units). In the United States, on the other hand, health centers of diverse types have expanded as a modality for the poor. In Australia and Canada also they are intended to help special groups of people.

The small health station in rural areas of developing countries, staffed by an auxiliary, in a sense attempts to replace the traditional healer. This is most striking in Africa, but true almost everywhere. In addition to first aid, these stations disseminate family planning materials and give immunizations. They cooperate in campaigns against vector-borne disease.

In addition to the many types of health center and hospital, other types of health facility must be noted. Pharmacies are generally stable in the industrialized countries, but are expanding in the developing ones. They are a source of medical care for self-prescribed drugs or drugs dispensed directly by the drug seller (rarely a pharmacist).

There is a whole spectrum of facilities for long-term care in the industrialized countries—nursing homes and custodial facilities. These are scarce in the developing countries but increasing rapidly in the industrialized ones. Many facilities provide simple but appropriate residential living for elderly persons without families.

Except for pharmacies, the majority of hospital and ambulatory care facilities in the world is sponsored by government. The situation in the United States, Canada, and Belgium—where most hospital beds are controlled by voluntary nonprofit agencies—is exceptional. Proprietary hospitals are rare, but expanding in a few entrepreneurial health systems. Nursing homes in North America are predominantly private and commercial. They have caused alarm about a "corporate takeover" of the entire health system, although only a small percentage of resources face such extreme profiteering. Regardless of ownership, the Ministry of Health generally has authority to oversee all facilities in relation to official quality standards.

Commodities. The production of drugs and equipment is a private enterprise in most of the world. Exceptions are in the formerly socialist countries: Soviet Union, China, and their former satellites. The output of the pharmaceutical industry has been expanding everywhere—much of it superfluous and requiring regulation. Major progress in economy and quality has come from the WHO program promoting the use of Essential Drugs. The widespread dissemination of penicillin, and other antibiotics, for example, has contributed importantly to the attacks on many infectious diseases.

Knowledge. Scientific knowledge may not be considered a resource, but it is obviously basic and cannot be taken for granted. Most knowledge is handed down from the past. New knowledge is produced by research, which is being conducted throughout the world. The output of health science research in scores of specialties is enlarging knowledge exponentially. The cost of research is underwritten predominantly by government in all countries, even though much of the work is done by nongovernmental entities. Using the device of special public grants, research can be directed along certain lines chosen by government.

Research results are disseminated by hundreds of health and medical journals, and by countless meetings. Special efforts are made to spread new findings to practitioners outside the main research centers. *Health systems research* is being conducted on methods of improving the operation of national health systems.

Organization of Programs

As more resources and money are being put into the operation of health systems, the programs in them are becoming increasingly organized. This is true for programs under either public or private auspices.

Ministries of Health. Every country has a principal national health agency, which may be called the Ministry of Health (MoH). Typically it operates at provincial and local levels, as well as at the national level. The world trend has been toward an increasing scope of responsibility in the MoH. Communicable disease control, maternal and child health services, health education, and environmental sanitation are basic functions everywhere. Although historically devoted mainly to disease prevention, the scope everywhere has broadened to medical care (hospitals and health centers) and to the planning and training of needed health personnel. Further strengthening of Ministries of Health has been a worldwide objective of WHO.

Other Public Agencies. In many countries, agencies other than the MoH play significant roles in health systems. Departments of labor conduct factory inspections, education authorities supervise the health of students, and various other agencies combat environmental hazards. Independent social security programs operate comprehensive health programs for their members. Other government agencies are responsible for health care of the military, military dependents, and veterans. These programs have a political strength of their own, and present problems of coordination with the MoH program.

Voluntary Health Agencies. Many new ideas are explored by voluntary health agencies, before government takes action. Campaigns on tuberculosis, sexually transmitted diseases, infant health care, community mental health, and other problems—started as voluntary efforts—developed into routine programs of the Ministries of Health. The early autonomous sickness insurance funds have become converted in many countries into branch offices of national health insurance programs. In these fields, voluntary agencies have become less important in health systems, as government's role has expanded.

Yet new challenges always appear, in which voluntary initiative has been crucial. In the 1980s, the struggle against the world AIDS epidemic and the fight against tobacco use have been spearheaded by voluntary agencies. Government, in fact, subsidized these agencies to do the work. The operation of many family planning programs is still largely through voluntary agencies, subsidized by government. The same applies to the widespread Red Cross ambulance services, linked to emergency medical service programs. Blood transfusion programs are often conducted by the Red Cross, in various sorts of collaboration with Ministries of Health.

The delegation of conventional child health programs to large voluntary agencies, as in Belgium and New Zealand, is exceptional in the world scene. The strength of voluntary health agencies is their undertaking of *new* tasks, for which government is not yet prepared.

Private Markets. In all countries, there is a residual private market for medical care. In the perspective of a century, it has undoubtedly been declining as organized public programs have grown. Still in the decades of the 1970s and 1980s, a reaction has occurred in many countries favoring return to privatization, as discussed earlier. The most dramatic demonstration of this has been in the several Eastern European countries that have rejected the entire concept of socialism. There is some evidence that these countries will retain much of their organized delivery patterns, but shift the financial support from general revenues to insurance, both social and private. The private market for medical care is in such turmoil that one cannot be sure of its future shape.

Economic Support

The clearest trend of all in health systems components has been the extension of organized methods of economic support, replacing individual expenditures. The early device of charity, although still growing, has been declining as a percentage of the total. Voluntary insurance emerged in Europe as an important collective mechanism in the early nineteenth century and remains so in the United States in the late twentieth century.

The commonest course of events has been for voluntary insurance to be converted to compulsory or social insurance. Some 70 countries now have such legislation, although about half of these cover much less than 90 percent of the population. With this control over costs, government naturally has substantial influence on the patterns by which services are delivered.

A further stage of economic support is through the use of general revenues of various types. This is the mechanism supporting MoH programs and the many specialized programs reviewed in previous chapters. General tax support, of course, is the most equitable, since theoretically it provides services according to need, rather than linking benefits to the source of contributions.

Within the accounts of a health system, hospital costs are generally the largest item. This has led everywhere to the search for alternative modes of care through home care, nursing homes, and other modalities. Modification of methods of paying hospitals is also being actively explored—shifting from flat per diem payments to various prospective payment methods for each type of care. Prospective *global budgeting* of hospitals is an ultimate strategy for cost-control, being used increasingly.

As noted earlier, in all countries—industrialized and developing—the percentage of GNP devoted to health has been rising since 1950. The increasingly collectivized methods of raising funds have made this possible. General taxation and social insurance are the commonest mechanisms.

Management

Management of health systems includes health planning, administration, regulation, and evaluation. In all four of these activities, progress has been clear. Almost all countries, at the national level, have been engaged in the *planning* of health resources to meet social needs. Activities have been greatest in developing countries. In industrialized countries, there is more microplanning of hospitals and health centers. Centralized planning theoretically draws on ideas from the periphery, but often this is more rhetoric than reality.

Administration. With hierarchies in the Ministry of Health, there is increasing delegation of responsibilities from the center to the periphery. In some places the movement is in the opposite direction—where independent local programs seek to achieve national uniformity. In former colonies, where central authority had been customary, decentralization in different forms is the principal strategy.

To enable local government to accept new responsibilities, health administrators must be trained. Both doctors and others are learning how to deal with large populations, money, supplies, logistics, and so on. Most leadership positions are held by physicians, even without public health training, since "medical chauvinism" still prevails almost everywhere. Schools of business administration have been organized, in which health administration is taught to nonphysicians. Schools of public health have also been increasing slowly, including curricula in health service administration.

Regulation and Legislation. The entire panorama of health systems has become increasingly subject to regulation and legislation, mainly in the interest of protecting quality. Laws have been enacted in six major fields, analyzed in Chapter 11.

First, for the protection of populations there are laws on communicable disease control, water and sanitation, food and drug control, and accident prevention. Second, for the regulation of health personnel, there are laws on professional licensure, medical ethics, traditional healing, and medical malpractice. Third, there are laws on the construction and operation of health facilities. Fourth, there is much legislation on personal health promotion, such as maternal and child health services, family planning, sound nutrition, drug abuse and alcoholism, the control of tobacco use, and other strategies for health promotion. Fifth is a large body of legislation on the financing of health systems. Sixth are the laws protecting the individual rights of patients.

Health legislation crystallizes policy so that it becomes explicit for everyone. If policy changes, the law should change. Legislative debate provides the opportunity for clarifying various viewpoints.

Evaluation. Statistical evidence on the operation of programs is a major basis for evaluation. This requires a scheme of information flow that yields data on both process and outcome. With computers, evaluation can be built into the daily operation of health programs. The strategies and interpretation of health program evaluation are being extensively studied in universities and government agencies.

Delivery of Health Services

The obvious world trend is toward the increasing organization of the delivery of all health services. The solo medical practitioner is declining everywhere and being replaced by teams of health personnel. The health center, staffed by allied health personnel, with or without a physician, is the major resource for primary medical care.

Primary health care, with strong preventive content, is a very broad component of health service delivery. It concerns environmental protection for water and disposal of human waste. It includes immunizations and education on healthy "life-style"—diet, exercise, avoidance of tobacco, and so on. Finally primary health care includes treatment of common ailments and availability of appropriate drugs. In each country the underlying national culture influences the principles of medical diagnosis and treatment, as shown by an insightful journalist in 1988.

Long-term care involves organized services of another type—increasingly prominent with the aging of the population. In addition to the range of facilities noted above, programs of home care, community activity for the elderly, and self-care are designed to avoid institutionalization. These services are mainly in the industrialized countries, but they are becoming organized in some developing countries.

In industrialized countries, where private medical practice is still viable, teamwork is shown in the growth of *group practice.* Although entirely private, the grouping of specialists and generalists achieves benefits in quality of care and in economies. Group practice clinics have a better record than solo practitioners in delivering preventive services and in using community resources, such as home nursing agencies, for their patients.

Among hospitals and health centers, regionalization has become the standard approach to planning and operating facilities and services in a region. The objective is to have each patient treated in the type of facility that is suited to his or her needs. Transportation is important. All of these strategies are special cases in the generally increased organization of health service delivery.

As a strategy for integrating all types of health service in communities, the World Health Organization has been promoting a policy of *district health systems.* An equivalent policy in the Pan American Health Organization refers to *local health systems.* The objective is not only to improve efficiency in the delivery of services, but also to encourage a spirit of community participation.

Adjustment of health service delivery to important new events must be rapid and appropriate. The appearance in 1985 of the autoimmune deficiency syndrome (AIDS) was a huge bombshell for world health. The identification of early infections, the treatment, the prevention, and the general struggle against this devastating, lethal disease mobilized resources in every country. Control required new strategies of health education everywhere.

All strategies for the improved delivery of health services are sometimes epitomized as *quality assurance.* The adequacy of resources, organization, management, and delivery of services determines the quality of the health system as a whole. The detailed attributes of each component should indicate plans for improvement. Some critics may allege that organization affects only the quantity of services, but careful analysis shows its value for quality assurance as well.

"HEALTH FOR ALL"

Since 1978, 30 years after its founding, the World Health Organization summarized its central policy goal as "Health for All by the year 2000." Endless debates on the meaning of this goal have followed, but one may regard it as basically a call for equity in society generally and health systems in particular.

It may be noted that the goal is not "health care," since so many other forces in the social and physical environment contribute to health. The operative word is *all,* which implies sweeping activities in social organization, both in health systems and in the society as a whole. The meaning of *all,* therefore, must be understood along three relevant dimensions: (1) coverage of all people, (2) provision of all the appropriate services, and (3) recognition of all other social sectors affecting health.

Coverage for All People

The history of health systems is one of piecemeal strategies to acquire health care coverage for selected population groups. The highest social classes had coverage in ancient times. Poor people were covered by religious and charitable sources. Later industrial workers were covered for general medical care by voluntary insurance, followed by social insurance. Gradually other types of working people were covered, including agricultural workers and farmers. In several industrialized countries, this gradual extension of coverage reached over 90 percent of the population by World War II.

Larger political events were necessary to extend the population coverage of *national health insurance* (NHI) to 100 percent in a *national health service* (NHS). The NHS strategy always meant a major shift of economic support from social insurance to general revenues. This was seen most dramatically in Great Britain and the Scandinavian countries; later NHS coverage extended to Italy and Greece. Another pathway to a NHS and universal coverage was through revolution, which occurred in the Soviet Union in 1918, and then in several other countries after World War II.

In developing countries, the effect of revolutions was varied. In Cuba, the revolution of 1959 led to universal coverage, as it did later in North Korea and Vietnam. In China, however, the socialist revolution of 1949 did not achieve universal coverage, although it greatly extended the population served; this huge country had too many economic problems to permit priority for health services.

The general trend of population coverage for health care in virtually all countries—industrialized and developing—has clearly been upward. The major strategy has been through social insurance. Next in importance is general revenue support, although—as we have seen in an earlier section—countries vary according to the political ideology of their health systems. In the face of declining government support, Ministries of Health have put major efforts into training medical assistants and community health workers to cover populations, especially in rural areas.

Provision of All Services

The meaning of "all services" obviously differs between an advanced industrialized country and a very poor developing country. In the former, such as Great Britain, it refers to medical and surgical specialists as well as primary care general practitioners. It involves laboratory and X-ray procedures and advanced endoscopic procedures. It refers to hospitals of different levels in a regional scheme, to polyclinics staffed by specialists, and to medically

staffed health centers. It also involves well-developed services in the home.

In very poor developing countries, services usually refer to those of medical assistants and auxiliary health personnel. Even more briefly trained community health workers are important. The emphasis is on preventive services for mothers and children, immunizations, health education, nutrition, communicable disease control, water supply, and sanitation. These are the elements of *primary health care* that WHO regards as the foundation for achieving Health for All.

Certain types of disorder demand specialized services in all health systems, although they are meagre outside the systems of industrialized countries. These include programs for the mentally ill, with special hospitals and mental health centers, emergency health services, with ambulances, and the complex field of long-term care with its spectrum of services in hospitals, nursing homes, custodial facilities, and varied home care services in the patient's home.

Other Social Sectors

Every public health professional realizes that the major determinants of health status lie outside the health system entirely. WHO speaks of *intersectoral coordination* as a feature of primary health care, but it is not realistic to expect health workers to influence all the other relevant social sectors. Instead, they must recognize and understand the large roles played by each of these, and cooperate with other sectors as much as possible.

Education is a major determinant of health. As reported in Volume I, the literacy level of women is the highest variable in a multiple regression of variables associated with life expectancy in some 140 countries. We know that educational level also implies many other features in a person's life situation.

Availability of safe water is another variable highly correlated with life expectancy. This feature is perhaps part of the health system, but also is determined by conditions in other sectors, such as city governments, land terrain, water sources, the availability of pipes and equipment, and so on. Sanitary housing is closely related to water supply and human waste disposal, as well as to questions of indoor space appropriate to family needs.

Even more basic than these social sectors is the economic sector of employment—in industry and agriculture. This depends, of course, on the whole economic system in the country, on the world economy, on international trade, and on the operations of capitalism.

By all three dimensions of Health for All, it should be clear that WHO and health leaders are speaking of goals. No one expects utopia to be reached by the year 2000. In 1981, Dr. Halfdan Mahler, Director-General of WHO, defined the goal in a way that is still valid, and should be quoted in full:

> "Health for all" means that health is to be brought within the reach of everyone in a given country. And by "health" is meant a personal state of wellbeing, not just the availability of health services—a state of health that enables a person to lead a socially and economically productive life. "Health for all" implies the removal of the obstacles to health—that is to say, the elimination of malnutrition, ignorance, contaminated drinking-water, and unhygienic housing—quite as much as it does the solution of purely medical problems such as lack of doctors, hospital beds, drugs and vaccines.

> "Health for all" means that health should be regarded as an objective of economic development and not merely as one of the means of attaining it.

> "Health for all" demands, ultimately, literacy for all. Until this becomes reality it demands at least the beginning of an understanding of what health means for every individual.

> "Health for all" depends on continued progress in medical care and public health. The health services must be accessible to all through primary health care, in which basic medical help is available in every village, backed up by referral services to more specialized care. Immunization must similarly achieve universal coverage.

> "Health for all" is thus a holistic concept calling for efforts in agriculture, industry, education, housing, and communications, just as much as in medicine and public health. Medical care alone cannot bring health to hungry people living in hovels. . . . The adoption of "health for all" by a government implies a commitment to promote the advancement of all citizens on a broad front of development, and a resolution to encourage the individual citizen to achieve a higher quality of life. . . . The rate of progress will depend on the political commitment.

The orientation of this statement is largely toward developing countries, which is reasonable in view of their enormous problems. Accepting this priority, there are certain other specific strategies to be emphasized.

Most important are the innovative health manpower strategies, reviewed above. Departure from the patterns of the past and formulation of new types of personnel, in proper response to the needs, are the top priorities in developing countries.

Another specific strategy, relevant also in health manpower development, is the establishment of an efficient managerial process. Many goals are not achieved simply because of poor management. This calls for training at many levels. Schools of public health in developing countries have been discussed. Such schools have increased over the years, but at a very slow rate.

Health systems research is another strategy to strengthen the operation of health systems. This should be directed to questions on population coverage, scope of services, quality, and costs. It can be done in Ministries of Health, schools of public health, and other departments of universities. Financial support must be sought from government and foundations. The important challenge in health systems research is to ask the right questions, so that the answers can contribute to the formulation of policy.

In summary of an assessment of health system progress made in 1988, a headquarters committee of WHO concluded:

> While there has beeen a progressive reorientation and strengthening of health sys-

tems based on primary health care, many issues still remain to be resolved. The district-health-systems approach appears to be providing a fresh opportunity to improve coordinated delivery of the elements of primary health care and to strengthen managerial capacity at local and intermediate levels, but a full understanding of this approach has still to be achieved among the different groups and partners involved in countries, if its implementation is to be accelerated.

Finally, it must be appreciated that the conversion of goals into action programs depends on political will. Health systems, like other social systems, are political issues. The potential achievement with one political party is bound to differ from that with another, and one cannot escape uncomfortable controversies. Civil servants are sworn to neutrality, but the objective facts on needs usually point to strategies required for improvement.

Political parties are concerned with many issues outside health. Questions of war and peace, of national employment, of foreign trade, and so on usually have top priority. Yet within the field of health, in the ideology of any political party, there is usually some flexibility. The worldwide acceptance of health service as a basic human right has taken centuries to evolve. This achievement favors some degree of political commitment in all countries to pursue policies that strengthen health systems.

FINAL COMMENT

As we conclude this account of issues in the national health systems of the world, the larger political scene abounds with problems. Considering only the 1980–1990 decade, the world has been aflame with violence and strife. Belligerence has led to open war in at least 20 places in the developing world. In the Middle East, there was the devastating war with Iraq provoked by its occupation of Kuwait, in addition to the embattlement of Iraq and Iran for several years before this. Afghanistan was the site of other warfare, as it strove to break away from the Soviet Union.

In Asia, wars have erupted in India over ethnic issues. In Burma (now Myanmar), battles have been continuous between the military government and the people. Indonesia has been violent in its invasion of East Timor. The Philippines and Cambodia are torn by internal political hostilities. The disruptive effect of all these hostilities on health services is obvious.

Warfare in certain sections of Latin America has been endemic. The small countries of Central America have been the scene of revolutionary movements to change the whole structure of society. In 1959, such a revolution had been successful in Cuba, and in the 1980s similar movements arose in Nicaragua and El Salvador—leading to domestic hostilities. Drug traffic issues led the United States to invade Panama in 1989, causing great disruption of the entire economy. In 1982, the pride of the British Empire was challenged by Argentina's occupation of the Falkland Islands, causing still another war between Her Majesty's navy and the military government of Argentina.

In Africa, wars have erupted due to a wide range of political issues. In Mozambique and Ethiopia, attempts to build socialist states have led to hostilities from both outside and inside the country. Sudan has had enormous internal strife between ethnic groups. Uganda's troubles under a military dictator, and the struggle to oust him, have been enormous. South Africa is the continent's most highly developed country, but—until its recent action to end *apartheid* policies—was a source of violent opposition to social change in all of Southern Africa. Health systems have been all but ruined by these hostilities.

In Europe, the enormous social changes of the 1980s did not take the form of open war, but rather of political cataclysm. The structure of Soviet-style socialism in all Eastern European countries collapsed. The origins of this peaceful revolution in the Soviet concepts of *perestroika* and *glasnost* have been explored in Volume I. The ultimate outcomes of these enormous changes are still not entirely clear, but they point generally to the adoption of the economic principles of capitalism. This would replace central planning with open markets, in which the flow of products and services is governed by supply and demand, quality, price, and competition. Application of these principles to health systems has not been easy.

One exception to this peaceful process of social change in Europe has occurred in Yugoslavia, in which the constituent republics of differing ideology have engaged in battle. Attempts of the United Nations European Region to mediate this warfare have not been successful. Yugoslavian health services have been almost destroyed.

The larger problems in the United States and Canada are economic and social. Throughout most of the 1980–1990 decade, the U.S. economy was in a period of decline. Productivity fell and unemployment rose. A huge national debt accumulated. Some of this was due to competition from Japan, but deficiencies in technology were more important. Scandalous non-regulation resulted in a loss of more than $600 billion in "savings and loan" agencies. The stock market showed extreme instability. Foreign trade declined and the United States changed from being a creditor to a debtor nation. Most people were deeply discouraged about the future. In the health systems, these failures of capitalism led to major cutbacks in the support of programs.

The social consequence of economic recession were visible everywhere. Thousands of homeless men and women lived on the streets of American cities. Neighborhoods in the center of cities were grim and unsanitary. Crime, much of it related to drug abuse, was steadily increasing. Rates of murder exceeded those in all other countries. In response to countless inequities, riots of African Americans against the ruling white social classes erupted in major cities, causing deaths and great destruction of property. Health facilities were not spared.

On a world scale, the social consequences of economic and political problems, aside from warfare, have been devastating. Refugees from a country of origin to a place of asylum in 1987 exceeded 13,290,000 people. Mortality rates in this population are always high. In Africa there were 3,577,000 refugees, the largest numbers being in Sudan and Somalia. In the Middle East there were 8,802,000 refugees, the largest number being in Pakistan and Iran. In East Asia, there were 560,000 refugees, in Latin America there were 290,000 refugees, and Europe has 69,000 refugees. Refugees come also to the United States and Canada, but their numbers are uncertain. They are not kept in camps, as is done in other countries. Camp settings, on the other hand, facilitate health services.

Beyond these man-made tragedies were natural disasters that aggravated economic and social affairs. The social structure cannot cope with earthquakes, hurricanes, floods, fires, and explosions, and the poorest sections of cities are usually hit hardest by them. Hospitals and clinics are not spared.

Thus, the world scene politically and economically has not been bright, as we ponder the realities of the 1980s. Confidence about the future of health systems, however, is derived from the perspective of more than one decade. Examining health issues and their trends over the last century gives grounds for optimism about the ultimate contribution of national health systems to the health of all people. To some degree, adversity is a challenge, which motivates people to work harder for worthy goals such as Health for All. Resolution of the health issues that this volume has explored will lead to the emergence of other issues in health systems. Successive responses move society ahead to cope better with future health problems.

REFERENCES

Abel-Smith, Brian, "Financing Health for All." *World Health Forum,* 12:191–200, 1991.

Altenstetter, Christa, and S. C. Haywood (Editors), *Comparative Health Policy and the New Right.* New York: St. Martin's Press, 1991.

American Public Health Association, *The Role of National Voluntary Health Organizations in Support of National Health Objectives.* Washington, D.C.: APHA, 1974.

Anderson, Odin, *The Health Services Continuum in Democratic States.* Ann Arbor, MI: Health Administration Press, 1989.

Basch, Paul F., *Textbook of International Health.* New York: Oxford University Press, 1990.

Bryant, John H., "Health for All: The Dream and the Reality." *World Health Forum,* 9:291–314, 1988.

Cassels, Andrew, and Katja Janovsky, *Strengthening Health Management in Districts and Provinces.* Geneva: World Health Organization, 1991.

Center for Human Rights, *Human Rights, A Com-*

pilation of International Instruments. New York: United Nations, 1988.

Cumper, George E. *The Evaluation of National Health Systems.* Oxford: Oxford University Press, 1991.

Dick, B., *Diseases of Refugees—Causes, Effects, and Control.* London: Transactions of the Royal Society of Tropical Medicine and Hygiene, 1984, pp. 734–741.

de Brun, Suzanne, and Ray H. Elding, "Cuba and the Philippines: Contrasting Cases in World-System Analysis." *International Journal of Health Services,* 17(4):681–701, 1987.

Elling, Ray H., "The Capitalist World-System and International Health." *International Journal of Health Services,* 11(1):21–51, 1981.

Fendall, N.R.E., *Auxiliaries in Health Care: Programs in Developing Countries.* Baltimore, MD: Johns Hopkins University Press, 1972.

Flahault, D., and M. I. Roemer, *Leadership for Primary Health Care—Levels, Functions, and Requirements Based on Twelve Case Studies.* Geneva: WHO (Public Health Papers 82), 1986.

Fries, James F., "The Compression of Morbidity." *World Health Forum,* 6:47–51, 1985.

Fulop, Tamas, and Milton I. Roemer, *International Development of Health Manpower Policy.* Geneva: World Health Organization (WHO Offset Publications No. 61), 1982.

Glaser, William A. *Health Insurance in Practice.* San Francisco: Jossey Bass, 1991.

Godber, George, "Striking the Balance: Therapy, Prevention, and Social Support." *World Health Forum,* 3(3):258–275, 1982.

Goodrich, L. M., et al., *Charter of the United Nations: Commentary and Documents,* 3rd ed. New York: U.N., 1969.

Gray, Alastair McIntosh, "Inequalities in Health. The Black Report: A Summary and Comment." *International Journal of Health Services,* 12(3):349–380, 1982.

Gray, Bradford H. (Editor), *For-Profit Enterprise in Health Care.* Washington, D.C.: Institute of Medicine, 1986.

Gunn, Selskar M., and Philip S. Platt, *Voluntary Health Agencies: An Interpretive Study.* New York: Ronald Press, 1945.

Halstead, S. B., Julia A. Walsh, and Kenneth S. Warren (Editors), *Good Health at Low Cost.* New York: Rockefeller Foundation, 1985.

Hofoss, Dag, and Peter F. Hjort, "Health Systems Research—Health Services: Finding Out What Is Wrong and Trying to Put It Right." *World Health Forum,* 9:315–321, 1988.

Institute of Medicine, *Homelessness, Health, & Human Needs.* Washington: National Academy Press, 1988.

International Planned Parenthood Federation, "Privatization 'Backfiring' in the Third World." *IPPF Open file.* London: IPPF, 21 July 1989.

Jamison, Dean T., and W. Henry Mosley, "Disease Control Priorities in Developing Countries: Health Policy Responses to Epidemiological Change." *American Journal of Public Health,* 81(1):15–22, January 1991.

Kleczkowski, B. M., M. I. Roemer, and A. Van der Werff, *National Health Systems and Their Reorientation towards Health for All.* Geneva: WHO (Public Health Papers No. 77), 1984.

Kovner, Anthony R., and Duncan Neuhauser (Editors), *Health Services Management.* Ann Arbor, MI: Health Administration Press, 1978.

Levey, Samuel, and N. Paul Loomba (Editors), *Health Care Administration: A Managerial Perspective.* Philadelphia: Lippincott, 1973.

Mahler, Halfdan, "The Meaning of 'Health for All by the year 2000'." *World Health Forum,* 9:291–314, 1988.

Maxwell, Robert J., *Health and Wealth: An International Study of Health Care Spending.* Lexington, MA: Lexington Books, 1981.

McKeown, Thomas, *The Role of Medicine: Dream, Mirage, or Nemesis.* Oxford: Blackwell, 1979.

McLachlen, Gordon, and Alan Maynard (Editors), *The Public/Private Mix for Health: The Relevance and Effects of Change.* London: Nuffield Provincial Hospitals Trust, 1982.

Pan American Health Organization, *Development and Strengthening of Local Health Systems in the Transformation of National Health Systems.* Washington, D.C.: PAHO, 1989.

Payer, Lynn, *Medicine and Culture.* New York: Holt, 1988.

Raffel, Marshall W. (Editor), *Comparative Health Systems: Descriptive Analyses of Fourteen National Health Systems* (emphasizing hospitals). University Park, PA: Pennsylvania State University Press, 1984.

Rayner, Geoffrey, "Lessons from America? Commercialization and Growth of Private Medicine in Britain." *International Journal of Health Services,* 17(2):197–216, 1987.

Roemer, Milton I., *The Organization of Medical Care under Social Security: A Study Based on the Experience of Eight Countries.* Geneva: International Labour Office, 1969.

Roemer, Milton I., "More Schools of Public Health: A Worldwide Need." *International Journal of Health Services,* 14(3):491–503, 1984.

Roemer, Milton I., "National Health Systems as Market Interventions." *Journal of Public Health Policy,* 10(1):62–77, Spring 1989.

Roemer, Milton I., and Ruth J. Roemer, *Health Care Systems and Comparative Manpower Policies.* New York: Marcel Dekker, 1981.

Roemer, Milton I., and Ruth Roemer, "Global Health, National Development, and the Role of Government." *American Journal of Public Health,* 80(10):1188–1192, October 1990.

Roemer, Milton I., and C. Montoya-Aguilar, *Qual-*

ity Assessment and Assurance in Primary Health Care. Geneva: World Health Organization (Offset Pubh. No. 105), 1988.

Rosen, George, *From Medical Police to Social Medicine.* New York: Science History Publications, 1974.

Ruderman, A. Peter, "Economic Adjustment and the Future of Health Services in the Third World." *Journal of Public Health Policy,* II:481–490, Winter 1990.

Saltman, Richard B. (Editor), *International Handbook of Health-Care Systems.* Westport, CT: Greenwood Press, 1988.

Scarpaci, Joseph L. (Editor), *Health Services Privatization in Industrial Societies.* New Brunswick, NJ: Rutgers University Press, 1989.

Seaman, J., *Medical Care in Refugee Camps.* London: Foxcombe Publications, 1981.

Sigerist, Henry E., in M. I. Roemer (Editor), *On the Sociology of Medicine.* New York: MD Publications, 1960.

Sivard, Ruth Leger, *World Military and Social Expenditures 1987–88,* 13th ed. Washington, D.C.: World Priorities, 1989.

Steffen, Monika, "Privatization in French Health Politics: Few Projects and Little Outcomes." *International Journal of Health Services,* 19(4):651–661, 1989.

Torrey, Barbara B., K. Kinsella, and C. M. Taeuber, *An Aging World* (International Population Reports Series P-95, No. 78). Washington, D.C.: U.S. Bureau of the Census, September 1987.

United Nations Children's Fund (UNICEF), *The State of the World's Children.* New York: Oxford University Press, 1985 and 1989.

State of the World's Children. New York: Oxford University Press, 1985 and 1989.

World Bank, *Financing Health Services in Developing Countries: An Agenda for Reform.* Washington, D.C.: the Bank, 1987.

World Bank, *World Development Report 1988.* New York: Oxford University Press, 1988.

World Health Organization, "Partners in Health." *Canada.* Ottawa: Royal Commission in Health Services, 1966.

World Health Organization, *Financing of Health Services.* Geneva: WHO (Technical Report Series No. 625), 1978.

World Health Organization and UNICEF, *Primary Health Care.* (Report of the International Conference on Primary Health Care). Geneva: WHO, 1978.

World Health Organization, *World Health Statistics Annual.* Geneva: WHO, 1982 and 1983.

World Health Organization, *Malaria Control as Part of Primary Health Care.* Geneva: WHO (Technical Report Series 712), 1984.

World Health Organization, *Intersectoral Action for Health: The Role of Intersectoral Cooperation in National Strategies for Health for All.* Geneva: WHO, 1986.

World Health Organization, *Strengthening Ministries of Health for Primary Health Care.* Geneva: WHO (Expert Committee, Technical Report Series 766), 1988.

World Health Organization, "Global Strategy for Health for All by the Year 2000: Development of Health Systems." *World Health Statistics Quarterly,* 42(4):201–227, 1989.

Index